Saunders' Pocket Essentials of

Clinical
MEDICINE

KT-567-371

Saunders' Pocket Essentials

Series Editors

Parveen Kumar and Michael Clark
St Bartholomew's and the Royal London School of
Medicine and Dentistry; Queen Mary and Westfield
College, London

For W. B. Saunders:

Commissioning Editor: Ellen Green
Project Development Manager: Janice Urquhart
Project Manager: Nancy Arnott
Design direction: Judith Wright
Illustrated by: Hardlines, Oxford

Saunders' Pocket Essentials of

Clinical
MEDICINE

Anne Ballinger
MD MRCP
Senior Lecturer, Digestive Diseases Research Centre,
St Bartholomew's and Royal London School of Medicine
and Dentistry

Stephen Patchett
MD FRCPI
Consultant Physician/Gastroenterologist,
Beaumont Hospital, Dublin

Series editors
Parveen Kumar and **Michael Clark**

SECOND EDITION

 W. B. SAUNDERS

Edinburgh • London • New York • Philadelphia • St Louis •
Sydney • Toronto • 2000

SAUNDERS
An imprint of Elsevier Science Limited

First published 1995
Second edition 2000
    Reprinted 2000 (twice), 2001 (twice), 2002 (twice)

ISBN 0-7020-2289-6
International edition ISBN 0-7020-2621-2

British Library Cataloguing in Publication Data
A catalogue record for this book is available from the British Library

Library of Congress Cataloging in Publication Data
A catalog record for this book is available from the Library of Congress

Medical knowledge is constantly changing. As new information becomes available, changes in treatment, procedures, equipment and the use of drugs become necessary. The authors and the publishers have, as far as it is possible, taken care to ensure that the information given in this text is accurate and up to date. However, readers are strongly advised to confirm that the information, especially with regard to drug usage, complies with current legislation and standards of practice.

ELSEVIER SCIENCE   your source for books, journals and multimedia in the health sciences

www.elsevierhealth.com

The publisher's policy is to use paper manufactured from sustainable forests

Printed in China by RDC Group Limited
B/06

Series Preface

Medical students and doctors in training are expected to travel to different hospitals and community health centres as part of their education. Many books are too large to carry on a regular basis but are still necessary for the basic understanding of disease processes. This series of books is designed to provide portable, pocket-sized companions to larger texts such as *Clinical Medicine*. They all contain core material for quick revision, easy reference and practical management. The modern format makes them easy to read providing an indispensable 'pocket essential'.

Parveen Kumar and **Michael Clark**
Series Editors

Preface

Medical students are confronted with the daunting task of assimilating a vast quantity of information during their training. After qualification the house officer will be expected to retain this knowledge and also learn new skills and practical procedures.

This compact textbook of clinical medicine aims to facilitate the learning process by providing a concise yet comprehensive account of general medical topics. Certain restrictions become necessary in a compact textbook, with topics such as childhood diseases, psychiatry, and most basic physiology being deliberately omitted. The section on tropical medicine includes only those conditions that a medical student is likely to encounter in Europe.

The inclusion of sample examination questions at the end of the book will not only allow the student to test his knowledge of the subject, but also to focus his attention on areas most commonly addressed in the final medical examination.

In this second edition, each chapter has been extensively revised and updated particularly in the area of new approaches to diagnosis and management. A dictionary of terms, which also includes a brief description of some rarer conditions, has now been included as a separate section at the end of the book to facilitate reference. We have also included a series of emergency boxes, which cover most of the commonly encountered medical emergencies. The inclusion of a new chapter dealing with practical procedures, along with the inclusion of important drug doses should increase the value of this book not only to final year medical students but also to pre-registration house officers.

We would again like to thank Mike Clark and Parveen Kumar for their support and assistance in the preparation of this second edition of *Pocket Essentials*. We are also indebted to all the contributors of the parent text *Clinical Medicine* on which this book is based.

Anne Ballinger and Stephen Patchett   1999

Contents

Abbreviations

ACE   angiotensin converting enzyme
ACTH   adrenocorticotrophic hormone
ADH   antidiuretic hormone
AF   atrial fibrillation
AIDS   acquired immunodeficiency syndrome
ANA   antinuclear antibodies
ANCA   antineutrophil cytoplasmic antibodies
ANF   antinuclear factor
ARDS   adult respiratory distress syndrome
AST   aspartate aminotransferase
AV   atrioventricular
AXR   abdominal X-ray
BCG   bacille Calmette-Guérin
BNF   *British National Formulary*
BP   blood pressure
CAL   chronic airflow limitation
CAPD   continuous ambulatory peritoneal dialysis
CCF   congestive cardiac failure
CCU   coronary care unit
CLL   chronic lymphatic leukaemia
CM   *Clinical Medicine* (Saunders 1998)
CML   chronic myeloid leukaemia
CNS   central nervous system
CRP   C-reactive protein
CSF   cerebrospinal fluid
CT   computerized tomography
CVP   central venous pressure
CXR   chest X-ray
DIC   disseminated intravascular coagulation
DNA   deoxyribonucleic acid
DVT   deep venous thrombosis
ECG   electrocardiogram
EEG   electroencephalogram

ERCP	endoscopic retrograde cholangiopancreatography
ESR	erythrocyte sedimentation rate
FBC	full blood count
GABA	γ-aminobutyric acid
γGT	γ-glutamyltranspeptidase
GFR	glomerular filtration rate
Hb	haemoglobin
5HIAA	5-hydroxyindoleacetic acid
HIV	human immunodeficiency virus
HLA	human leucocyte antigen
Ig	immunoglobulin (e.g. IgM = immunoglobulin the M class)
INR	international normalized ratio
iu/IU	international unit
iv	intravenous
IVP	intravenous pyelogram
JVP	jugular venous pressure
LP	lumbar puncture
LVF	left ventricular failure
MCV	mean corpuscular volume
ME	myalgic encephalomyelitis
MRI	magnetic resonance imaging
MRSA	methicillin-resistant *Staphylococcus aureus*
MSU	mid-stream urine
NSAIDs	non-steroidal anti-inflammatory drugs
P_aco_2	partial pressure of carbon dioxide in arterial blood
P_ao_2	partial pressure of oxygen in arterial blood
PCV	packed cell volume
PR	per rectum (rectal instillation)
PT	prothrombin time
PTC	percutaneous transhepatic cholangiography
PTCA	percutaneous transluminal coronary angioplast
PTTK	partial thromboplastin time with kaolin
RCC	red cell count
RNA	ribonucleic acid
SLE	systemic lupus erythematosis
STD	sexually transmitted disease
SVC	superior vena cava
SVT	supraventricular tachycardia
TIA	transient ischaemic attack

Normal Values

....

Haematology

Haemoglobin

Male	14.0–17.7 g dL^{-1}
Female	12.0–16.0 g dL^{-1}

Mean corpuscular volume (MCV) 80–96 fl

White cell count $4–11 \times 10^9$/litre

Platelet count $150–400 \times 10^9$/litre

Serum B$_{12}$ 160–925 ng L^{-1}
(150–675 pmol L^{-1})

Serum folate 4–18 μg L^{-1}
(5–63 nmol L^{-1})

Erythrocyte sedimentation rate
(ESR) <20 mm in 1 hour

Coagulation

Partial thromboplastin time (PTTK) 24–31 s

Prothrombin time 12–16 s

Serum biochemistry

Alanine aminotransferase (ALT) 5–40 U L^{-1}

Albumin 36–53 g L^{-1}

Alkaline phosphatase 25–115 U L^{-1}

Amylase <220 U L^{-1}

Aspartate aminotransferase (AST) 7–40 U L^{-1}

Bicarbonate 22–30 mmol L^{-1}

Bilirubin <17 μmol L^{-1}
(0.3–1.5 mg dL^{-1}

Calcium	2.20–2.67 mmol L^{-1} (8.5–10.5 mg dL^{-1}
Chloride	95–106 mmol L^{-1}
Creatinine	0.06–0.12 mmol L^{-1} (0.6–1.5 mg dL^{-1})

Ferritin
  Female
  Male
  Postmenopausal
	
	6–110 μg L^{-1}
	20–260 μg L^{-1}
	12–230 μg L^{-1}

Glucose	4.5–5.6 mmol L^{-1} (70–110 mg dL^{-1})
Potassium	3.5–5.0 mmol L^{-1}
Sodium	135–146 mmol L^{-1}
Urea	2.5–6.7 mmol L^{-1} (8–25 mg dL^{-1})

Medical Emergencies

Infectious diseases and tropical medicine

Infectious diseases are the most common diseases of humans and a major source of morbidity and mortality in both developed and developing countries. Upper respiratory tract infections and gastroenteritis are commonly seen in the community and do not often need admission to hospital. With increasing travel abroad more tropical diseases are now seen in the UK and, with the emergence of AIDS, opportunistic infections are seen more commonly. In the UK some infectious diseases must be notified to the local Medical Officer for Environmental Health; these are indicated by the abbreviation ND where appropriate.

Fever of unknown origin

Fever of unknown origin (FUO) is defined as a documented fever (>38°C) lasting more than 3 weeks in which a clinical history, repeated thorough physical examination and routine investigations have failed to reveal a cause. Occult infection remains the most common cause in adults. Connective tissue diseases, drug hypersensitivity and malignancy are other causes (Table 1.1).

Investigations

First-line investigations should be repeated as the results may have changed since the tests were first performed:

- Full blood count, including a differential white cell count (WCC) and blood film
- Erythrocyte sedimentation rate (ESR)
- Serum urea and electrolytes, liver biochemistry and blood glucose
- Blood cultures: several sets from different sites at different times
- Microscopy and culture of urine, sputum and faeces
- Baseline serum for virology

Table 1.1 Some causes of fever of unknown origin

Infection (40%)
Pyogenic abscess: e.g. liver, pelvic, subphrenic
Biliary infection
Urinary infection
Tuberculosis
Subacute infective endocarditis
Viruses, e.g. Epstein–Barr, cytomegalovirus, HIV-related
Brucellosis
Malaria
Acute HIV infection

Cancer (30%)
Lymphoma
Leukaemia
Solid tumours, e.g. renal carcinoma, hepatocellular carcinoma, pancreatic cancer

Immunogenic (20%)
Drugs (including drugs used to treat fever, e.g. aspirin, isoniazid)
Connective tissue diseases
Rheumatoid arthritis
Sarcoidosis
Polymyalgia rheumatica/giant cell arteritis

Factitious (1–5%)
Switching thermometers
Injection of pyogenic material
Remains unknown (5–9%)

- Chest radiograph
- Serum rheumatoid factor and antinuclear antibody.

Second-line investigations are performed in patients who remain undiagnosed and when repeat physical examination is unhelpful.

- Abdominal imaging with ultrasound, CT or MRI to detect occult abscesses and malignancy
- Echocardiography for infective endocarditis
- Needle biopsy of the liver
- Bone marrow examination
- Determination of HIV status
- Radio nuclide scanning: gallium–59 or ciprofloxacin-labelled polymorphs, or indium–111 or technetium-labelled leucocytes, can localize an abscess and may be useful when other imaging is unhelpful
- Exploratory laparotomy in patients who remain undiagnosed (very rarely needed).

Management

The treatment is of the underlying cause.

Septicaemia

The term bacteraemia refers to the transient presence of organisms in the blood (generally without causing symptoms) as a result of local infection or penetrating injury. The term septicaemia, on the other hand, is usually reserved for bacteria or fungi when they are actually multiplying in the blood, usually with the production of severe systemic symptoms such as fever and hypotension. Septicaemia has a high mortality without treatment, and demands immediate attention. The pathogenesis and management of septic shock is discussed on pages 439 and 447.

Aetiology

Overall, about 40% of cases are the result of Gram-positive organisms and 60% of Gram-negative ones. Fungi are much less common but should be considered, particularly in the immunocompromised. In the previously healthy adult septicaemia may occur from a source of infection in the chest (e.g. with pneumonia), urinary tract (often Gram-negative rods) or biliary tree (commonly *Enterococcus faecalis*, *Escherichia coli*). Intravenous drug abusers frequently get septicaemia caused by *Staphylococcus aureus* and *Pseudomonas* sp. Hospitalized patients are susceptible to infection from wounds, indwelling urinary catheters and intravenous cannulae.

Clinical features

Fever, rigors and hypotension are the cardinal features of severe septicaemia. Lethargy, headache and a minor change in conscious level may be preceding features. In elderly and immunocompromised patients the clinical features may be quite subtle and a high index of suspicion is needed.

Certain bacteria are associated with a particularly fulminating course:

- Staphylococci that produce an exotoxin called toxic shock syndrome toxin-1. The toxic shock syndrome is characterized by an abrupt onset of fever, rash, diarrhoea and shock. It is associated with the use of infected tampons in women but may occur in anyone, including children.

- Meningococci that produce the Waterhouse–Friderichsen syndrome. This is a rapidly fatal illness (without treatment), with a purpuric skin rash and shock. Adrenal haemorrhage (and hypoadrenalism) may or may not be present.

Investigations

In addition to blood count, serum electrolytes and liver biochemistry:

- Blood cultures
- Cultures from possible source: urine, abscess aspirate, sputum
- In some cases: chest radiography, abdominal ultrasonography and CT scan.

Management

Antibiotic therapy should be started immediately the diagnosis is suspected and after appropriate culture samples have been sent to the laboratory. The probable site of origin of sepsis will often be apparent, and knowledge of the likely microbial flora can be used to choose appropriate treatment. In cases where 'blind' antibiotic treatment is started, a reasonable combination would be intravenous gentamicin (3–5 mg/kg daily in divided doses) and piperacillin (200–300 mg/kg daily), with flucloxacillin if staphylococcal infection is a possibility. Therapy may subsequently be altered on the basis of culture and sensitivity results.

COMMON VIRAL INFECTIONS
Measles ND

Measles is caused by infection with an RNA paramyxovirus which is spread by droplets. With the introduction of immunization policies using a live attenuated vaccine in the west the incidence has fallen, but it remains common in developing countries, where it is associated with a high morbidity and mortality. One attack confers lifelong immunity.

Clinical features

The incubation period is 8–14 days. Two distinct phases of the disease can be recognized.

The infectious pre-eruptive and catarrhal stage There is fever, cough, rhinorrhoea, conjunctivitis and Koplik's spots in the mouth (small grey irregular lesions on an erythematous base, commonly on the inside of the cheek).

The non-infectious eruptive or exanthematous stage Characterized by the presence of a maculopapular rash which starts on the face and spreads to involve the whole body. The rash becomes confluent and blotchy.

Complications (uncommon in the healthy child)

Gastroenteritis, pneumonia, otitis media, encephalitis, myocarditis, subacute sclerosing panencephalitis (rare).

Management

The diagnosis is usually clinical and treatment is symptomatic. Measles vaccine is given to children between 12 and 18 months of age, in combination with mumps and rubella vaccine (MMR) to prevent infection.

Mumps ND

Mumps is also caused by infection with a paramyxovirus, spread by droplets. The incubation period averages 18 days.

Clinical features

Mumps is predominantly an infection of school-aged children and young adults. There is fever, headache and malaise, followed by the development of parotid gland swelling. Less common features are orchitis, meningitis, pancreatitis, oophoritis, myocarditis and hepatitis.

Management

Diagnosis is usually clinical. In doubtful cases demonstration of a rise in serum antibody titres is necessary for diagnosis. Treatment is symptomatic. The disease is prevented by administration of a live attenuated mumps virus vaccine.

Rubella ND

Rubella is caused by an RNA virus and has a peak age of incidence of 15 years. The incubation period is 14–21 days.

During the prodrome the patient complains of malaise, fever and lymphadenopathy (suboccipital, postauricular, posterior cervical nodes). A pinkish macular rash appears on the face and trunk after about 7 days and lasts for up to 3 days.

Diagnosis

Diagnosis is made by demonstrating a rising serum antibody titre in paired samples taken 2 weeks apart, or by the detection of rubella-specific IgM.

Management

Treatment is symptomatic. Complications are uncommon but include arthralgia, encephalitis and thrombocytopenia.

Congenital rubella syndrome

Maternal infection during pregnancy may affect the fetus, particularly if infection is acquired in the first trimester. Congenital rubella syndrome is characterized by the presence of congenital cardiac defects, eye lesions (particularly cataracts), microcephaly, mental handicap and deafness. There may also be persistent viral infection of the liver, lungs and heart, with hepatomegaly, pneumonitis and myocarditis. The teratogenic effects of rubella underlie the importance of preventing maternal infection with immunization.

Herpes viruses

Herpes simplex virus (HSV) infection
HSV-1 causes:

- Herpetic stomatitis with buccal ulceration, fever and local lymphadenopathy
- Herpetic whitlow: damage to the skin over a finger allows access of the virus, with the development of irritating vesicles
- Keratoconjunctivitis
- Encephalitis
- Systemic infection in immunocompromised patients.

HSV-2 is transmitted sexually and causes genital herpes, with painful genital ulceration, fever and lymphadenopathy. There may be systemic infection in the immunocompromised host. These divisions are not rigid, because HSV-1 can also give rise to genital herpes.

Recurrent HSV infection occurs when the virus lies dormant in ganglion cells and is reactivated by trauma, febrile illnesses and ultraviolet irradiation. This leads to recurrent labialis ('cold sores') or recurrent genital herpes.

Investigations

The diagnosis is often clinical but the virus may be cultured from lesions. Herpes simplex encephalitis is discussed on page 601.

Management

Aciclovir is used topically and systemically for both primary and recurrent infection of the skin and mucous membranes. Penciclovir is used topically as a cream for herpes labialis

Herpes zoster

Varicella (chickenpox) Primary infection with this virus causes chickenpox, which may produce a mild childhood illness, although this can be severe in adults and immunocompromised patients.

Clinical features

After an incubation period of 14–21 days there is a brief prodromal period of fever, headache and malaise. The rash, predominantly on the face, scalp and trunk, begins as macules and develops into papules and vesicles, which heal with crusting. Complications include pneumonia and central nervous system involvement.

Investigations

The diagnosis is usually clinical. Electron microscopy of vesicle fluid may reveal the virus.

Management

Healthy children require no treatment. Immunocompromised patients are treated with intravenous aciclovir and zoster-immune immunoglobulin (ZIG). Anyone over the age of 16 should be considered for antiviral therapy with aciclovir. Because of the risk to both mother and fetus during pregnancy, pregnant women exposed to varicella zoster virus should receive prophylaxis with ZIG and treatment with aciclovir if they develop chickenpox.

Herpes zoster (shingles). After the primary infection herpes zoster remains dormant in dorsal root ganglia and reactivation causes shingles.

Clinical features

Pain and tingling in a dermatomal distribution precede the rash by a few days. The rash consists of papules and vesicles in the same dermatome. The most common sites are the lower thoracic dermatomes and the ophthalmic division of the trigeminal nerve (pages 566 and 567).

Management

Treatment is with oral famciclovir given as early as possible. The main complication is postherpetic neuralgia, which can be severe and last for years. Treatment is with carbamazepine or phenytoin.

Infectious mononucleosis

Infectious mononucleosis is caused by the Epstein–Barr virus (EBV) and predominantly affects young adults. EBV is probably transmitted in saliva and by aerosol.

Clinical features

Many infections are asymptomatic. In symptomatic patients the main features are fever, headache, sore throat and a transient macular rash. There may be palatal petechiae, cervical lymphadenopathy, splenomegaly and mild hepatitis. Rare complications include splenic rupture, myocarditis and meningitis.

Investigations

Atypical lymphocytes on a peripheral blood film strongly suggest infection. The diagnosis is confirmed by a positive Paul–Bunnell reaction (agglutination of sheep red cells by heterophile antibodies) and IgM antibodies to EBV.

Management

Most cases require no treatment. Corticosteroids are given if there are systemic complications. Infection with *Toxoplasma gondii* or cytomegalovirus may produce a similar clinical picture in immunocompetent adults.

OTHER INFECTIONS

Lyme borreliosis (Lyme disease)

Lyme borreliosis is a zoonosis caused by the spirochaete *Borrelia burgdorferi*. The disease is transmitted by *Ixodes dammini* or related ixodid ticks (*Ixodes ricinus* in Europe).

Clinical features

The first stage of the illness consists of a characteristic skin rash – erythema chronicum migrans – which may be accompanied by fever malaise, headache or myalgia. The second stage, which follows weeks or months later, consists of neurological (*meningoencephalitis or polyneuropathy*) or cardiac (*myocarditis or conduction defects*) problems. The third stage consists of arthritis, which can occur in attacks for several years. Not all stages need appear and, conversely, clinical stages may overlap.

Investigations

Serology will show IgM antibodies in the first month and IgG antibodies late in the disease.

Management

Amoxycillin, doxycycline or cephalosporins are the treatments of choice in the early stages of disease. Intravenous benzylpenicillin should be given for later stages of disease.

Leptospirosis

This zoonosis is caused by a Gram-negative organism, *Leptospira interrogans*, which is excreted in animal urine and enters the host through a skin abrasion or intact mucous membranes. Individuals who work with animals or take part in winter sports are most at risk.

Clinical features

Following an incubation period of about 10 days, the initial leptospiraemic phase is characterized by fevers, headache, malaise and myalgia, followed by an immune phase, which is most commonly manifest by meningism. Most recover uneventfully at this stage. A small proportion go on to develop tender hepatosplenomegaly, jaundice, haemolytic anaemia, myocardial involvement and oliguric renal failure with microscopic haematuria (Weil's disease).

Investigations

Blood or CSF culture can identify the organisms in the first week of the disease. The organism may be detected in the urine during the second week.

Serology will show specific IgM antibodies by the end of the first week.

Management

Penicillin or erythromycin are most commonly used. The complications of the disease are treated appropriately.

··

TROPICAL MEDICINE

Fever in the returned traveller

Fever is a common problem in travellers returning from tropical countries. Malaria is the single most common cause of fever in recent travellers from the tropics. Falciparum malaria has the potential to be rapidly fatal, and so evaluation of fever in this group of patients is often regarded as a medical emergency. Table 1.2 lists the causes of fever in travellers from the tropics; in about 25% of cases no specific cause is found. The most common causes are discussed in greater detail below.

Table 1.2 Causes of fever after travel to the tropics

Malaria
Viral hepatitis
*Febrile illness unrelated to foreign travel
Dengue fever
Enteric fever
Diarrhoeal illness
Rickettsia
Amoebic liver abscess
Tuberculosis
Acute HIV infection
Others

* Includes respiratory tract infection and urinary tract infection. Accounts for 80% of specific infections.

Approach to diagnosis

An accurate history and physical examination will help formulate an appropriate differential diagnosis and guide initial investigations. In addition to a full medical history an accurate travel history must be obtained:

- Countries visited, arrival and departure dates (for assessment of incubation period; Table 1.3)
- Exposure to vectors: mosquitoes, ticks, flies and fresh water infested with snails containing schistosomes
- Vaccination and prophylaxis: recent vaccination against yellow fever and hepatitis A and B is extremely effective; subsequent infection with these agents is very unlikely.

Table 1.3 Typical incubation periods for tropical infections

Incubation period	Infection
Short (<10 days)	Arboviral infections (including dengue fever), enteric bacterial infections, paratyphoid, plague, typhus, haemorrhagic fevers
Medium (10–21 days)	Malaria (but may be much longer), typhoid fever (rarely 3–60 days) scrub typhus, African trypanosomiasis, brucellosis, leptospirosis
Long (>21 days)	Viral hepatitis, tuberculosis, HIV, schistosomiasis, amoebic liver abscess, visceral leishmaniasis, filariasis

Vaccination against typhoid or immunoglobulin for the prevention of hepatitis A is only partially effective, therefore infection is still a possibility. Malaria is always a possibility, even in those who have taken chemoprophylaxis

- History of unprotected sexual intercourse may suggest an acute HIV or hepatitis B seroconversion illness (page 103).

Investigations

- Full blood count with differential white cell count, and thick and thin blood malaria films. Repeat after 12–24 hours if initial films negative and malaria suspected

- Liver biochemistry – abnormal results found in many tropical infections
- Cultures of blood and stool
- Microscopy and culture of urine
- 'Acute' serum for storage and subsequent antibody detection with paired convalescent serum at a later date.

Malaria ND

Malaria is a protozoan parasite widespread in the tropics and subtropics (Figure 1.1). Each year 270 million people are affected, with a mortality rate of 1%.

Aetiology

Travellers abroad are infected following the bite of an infected female mosquito of the genus *Anopheles*. Rarely the parasite is transmitted by importation of infected mosquitoes by air (airport malaria).

Four malaria parasites may infect humans; by far the most hazardous is *Plasmodium falciparum*, the symptoms of which can rapidly progress from an acute fever with rigors to severe multiorgan failure, coma and death. Once successfully treated this form does not relapse. The other malaria parasites, *P. vivax*, *P. ovale* and *P. malariae*, cause a more benign illness which may relapse.

Pathogenesis

The infective form of the parasite (sporozoites) pass through the skin and via the bloodstream to the liver. After a variable number of days they invade red blood cells and pass through further stages of development, which terminate with the rupture of the red cell. Rupture of red blood cells contributes to anaemia and releases pyrogens, causing fever. Red blood cells infected with *P. falciparum* adhere to the endothelium of small vessels and the consequent vascular occlusion causes severe organ damage, chiefly in the kidney, liver and brain. All the different forms, except *P. falciparum*, may remain latent in the liver, and this is believed to be responsible for the relapses that may occur.

Clinical features

The incubation period varies:

- 10–14 days in *P. vivax*, *P. ovale* and *P. falciparum* infection
- 18 days to 6 weeks in *P. malariae* infection.

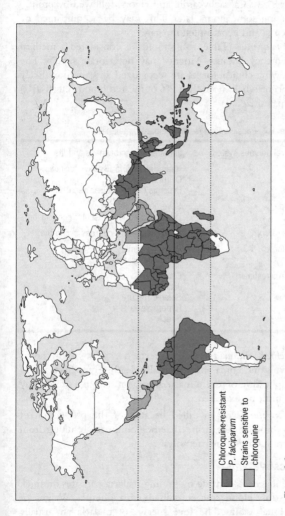

Figure 1.1
Malaria – geographical distribution.

Chloroquine-resistant
P. falciparum

Strains sensitive to
chloroquine

The onset of symptoms may be delayed in the partially immune or after prophylaxis. There is an abrupt onset of fever (>40°C), tachycardia and rigors, followed by profuse sweating some hours later. This may be accompanied by anaemia and hepatosplenomegaly.

P. falciparum (Table 1.4) should be considered a medical emergency because patients may deteriorate rapidly. The following clinical forms are recognized and are more likely to occur when more than 2% of the red blood cells (RBC) are parasitized.

Table 1.4 Possible features of falciparum malaria

Central nervous system	Impaired consciousness and fits
Renal	Haemoglobinuria (Blackwater fever)
	Oliguria
	Uraemia (acute tubular necrosis)
Blood	Severe anaemia
	Disseminated intravascular coagulation
Respiratory	Adult respiratory distress syndrome
Metabolic	Hypoglycaemia
	Metabolic acidosis
Gastrointestinal	Diarrhoea
	Jaundice
	Splenic rupture
Other	Hyperpyrexia
	Shock

Cerebral malaria is characterized by a high fever, convulsions, coma and eventually death. Hypoglycaemia, a complication of severe malaria, may present in a similar way and must be excluded.

Blackwater fever, so called because of the production of dark brown–black urine (haemoglobinuria) resulting from severe intravascular haemolysis.

Investigations

The diagnosis is made by finding malaria parasites on thick and thin blood smears stained with Giemsa, Wright or Leishman stains. The four species of malaria are usually distinguishable from each other on examination of peripheral smears. Other investigations include full blood count, serum urea and electrolytes, and blood glucose.

Management

The acute treatment and eradication therapy of malaria is summarized in Table 1.5 Antipyretics such as aspirin and paracetamol are given as necessary, and intravenous fluids may be required to combat dehydration and shock.

Severe malaria (more than 1% of RBCs infected), or any of the pernicious forms of falciparum malaria, constitutes a medical emergency. Ill patients may require intensive care.

Chloroquine is not used in treatment if it has been used as prophylaxis.

Table 1.5 Treatment of an acute attack of malaria

Treatment

Uncomplicated malaria in a chloroquine-sensitive area	Oral chloroquine 600 mg of base, 300 mg 6 h later, then 300 mg/24 h for 3 days*
Uncomplicated malaria in a chloroquine-resistant area	Oral quinine sulphate 600 mg three times daily for 7 days followed by a single dose of pyrimethamine 75 mg and sulfadoxine 1.5 mg (i.e. 3 tablets of fansidar). Other treatments: mefloquine halofantrine
Severe *P. falciparum* malaria	Rehydrate, maintaining CVP at approx 5 cm H_2O Intravenous quinine 20 mg/kg over 4 h followed by 10 mg/kg over 4 h at 8-hourly intervals until tablets tolerated Check BM stix frequently Treat seizures with i.v. benzodiazepine Transfuse if haematocrit <20% Artemisinin is an alternative agent which can be given orally or by i.m. injection

Eradication

For *P. vivax*, *P. malariae*, *P. ovale*	Oral primaquine 7.5 mg daily for 14 days

* The active component of many drugs, whether acid or base, is relatively insoluble and this presents a problem in formulation. This is overcome by using a soluble salt, e.g. adding a base to an acid, and vice versa. Hence, the base chloroquine is available as chloroquine sulphate or chloroquine phosphate. Chloroquine base 150 mg = chloroquine sulphate 200 mg = chloroquine phosphate 250 mg. The amount of drug prescribed is given as the active component, i.e. the base, to avoid confusion as to how much chloroquine is actually to be given.

Prevention and control

Effective prevention of malaria includes the following elements:

- Awareness of risk
- Use of mechanical barriers such as insecticide-impregnated nets and mosquito repellents
- Chemoprophylaxis.

As a result of changing patterns of resistance, advice about chemoprophylaxis should be sought before leaving for a malaria-endemic area. Prophylaxis does not afford full protection. Drug regimens should be started at least 1 week before departure and continued without interruption for 6 weeks after return. The rationale for this advice is to ensure therapeutic drug levels before travelling and to enable unwanted effects to be dealt with before departure. The continued use of drugs after returning home will deal with infection contracted on the last day of exposure.

Chloroquine In low-risk areas chloroquine 300 mg weekly is recommended. In areas of limited chloroquine resistance this is combined with proguanil 200 mg daily. This regimen has few side effects and is safe in pregnancy.

Mefloquine Mefloquine 250 mg weekly is used in areas where falciparum malaria is highly resistant to chloroquine (east and central Africa, South America and S. E. Asia).

Maloprim + chloroquine Maloprim + chloroquine is administered weekly to travellers to the Pacific Islands.

Dengue fever

Dengue fever is caused by a flavivirus. It is found mainly in Asia, Africa, Central and South America where it is a common cause of fever and may be fatal. The virus is transmitted by the mosquito *Aedes aegypti*. After an incubation period of 5–6 days there is an abrupt onset of fever, headache, retro-orbital pain and severe myalgia, often with a skin rash. Rare complications include shock and haemorrhagic manifestations, including purpura, epistaxis and melaena. Diagnosis is clinical and confirmed by acute and convalescent serum samples. Treatment is supportive.

Enteric fever

Typhoid fever and paratyphoid fever are caused by *Salmonella typhi* and *Salmonella paratyphi* (types A, B and C), respectively.

Typhoid fever ND

Humans are the only known reservoir of infection, and the spread is faecal–oral.

Clinical features

After an incubation period of 10–14 days there is an insidious onset of headache, dry cough and constipation, and a rising fever with relative bradycardia. In the second week of the illness an erythematous maculopapular rash that blanches on pressure and is referred to as 'rose spots' appears, chiefly on the upper abdomen and thorax, lasting for only 2–3 days. There is splenomegaly (75%), cervical lymphadenopathy and hepatomegaly (30%). Diarrhoea may develop. Complications, usually occurring in the third week, are pneumonia, meningitis, acute cholecystitis, osteomyelitis, intestinal perforation and haemorrhage. Recovery occurs in the fourth week.

Investigations

Culture of the organism from:

- Blood in the first 2 weeks
- Urine in the second week
- Stool cultures in weeks 2–4.

Blood count shows leukopenia.
Serology (Widal test) may show a sequential rise in antibody titre.

Management

Quinolone antibiotics e.g. ciprofloxacin are now the treatment of choice. Alternatives are chloramphenicol, co-trimoxazole and ampicillin.

Infection is cleared when consecutive cultures of urine and faeces are negative. Some patients become chronic carriers, with the focus of infection in the gallbladder. Treatment is with amoxycillin and probenecid for 6 weeks, but cholecystectomy may be needed. A live oral vaccine and a parenteral vaccine are available which both give protection for about 3 years respectively.

Paratyphoid ND

Paratyphoid results in a milder illness that is otherwise clinically indistinguishable from typhoid fever. Treatment is with co-trimoxazole for 2 weeks.

Entercolitis ND

Other *Salmonella* species (*S. choleraesuis* and *S. enteritidis*) cause a self-limiting infection presenting with diarrhoea and vomiting (Table 1.6).

Amoebiasis ND

Amoebiasis is caused by infection of the human gastrointestinal tract with the protozoal organism *Entamoeba histolytica*. Infection occurs worldwide, although much higher incidence rates are found in the tropics and subtropics. The modes of transmission are:

- Ingestion of cysts in contaminated food and water
- Person-to-person spread
- Sexual transmission among homosexual men.

Clinical features

Intestinal Amoebiasis (Amoebic Dysentery) Invasion of the colonic epithelium by *E. histolytica* leads to tissue necrosis and ulceration. Ulceration may deepen and progress under the mucosa to form typical flask-like ulcers. The presentation varies from mild bloody diarrhoea to fulminating colitis, with the risk of toxic dilatation, perforation and peritonitis. In 10% of cases an amoeboma (inflammatory fibrotic mass) develops, commonly in the caecum or rectosigmoid region, which may bleed, cause obstruction or intussusception, or be mistaken for a carcinoma.

Amoebic liver abscess An amoebic liver abscess develops when organisms invade through the bowel serosa, enter the portal vein and pass into the liver. The abscess is usually single and in the right lobe of the liver. There is tender hepatomegaly, a high swinging fever and profound malaise. There may not be a history of colitis.

Table 1.6 Bacterial causes and clinical features of food poisoning ND

Organism	Source	Incubation period (h)	Symptoms	Diagnosis	Recovery
Bacteria which colonize the gut					
Salmonella sp.	Eggs, poultry	12–48	Abrupt diarrhoea, blood, abdominal pain, fever, vomiting	Culture organism in faeces	Usually 2–5 days may be up to 14.
Campylobacter jejuni	Milk, poultry	48–96	As above: pain, diarrhoea	As above	7–21 days
V. parahaemolyticus (rare in UK)	Seafood	2–48	As above (blood less common)	As above	3 days
Y. enterocolitica	Milk, pork	2–144	Diarrhoea, fever, pain	As above	1–3 days
Clostridium perfringens	Spores in food, especially meat	8–22	Diarrhoea, pain	Culture of faeces and food	1–3 days
Preformed enterotoxins					
Staphylococcus aureus	Contaminated food, usually by humans	2–6	Vomiting, pain, (diarrhoea)	Culture organism in remaining food	Few hours
Bacillus cereus	Spores in food, reheated rice	1–6	As above	Culture of organism in food or faeces	Few hours
Clostridium botulinum	Spores in home-bottled or home-canned food	18–36	Transient diarrhoea, paralysis caused by neuromuscular blockade	Demonstrate toxin in food or faeces	10–14 days

Main clinical features are underlined.

Investigations

Serology Amoebic fluorescent antibody test (FAT) is positive in 90% of patients with liver abscess and in 75% of patients with active colitis.

Colonic disease The most important diagnostic investigation in suspected amoebic dysentery is sigmoidoscopy and immediate microscopic examination of a rectal smear. This shows the motile trophozoites which contain red blood cells. A fresh stool sample shows the same features but is less sensitive.

Liver disease Liver abscesses should be considered when the serum alkaline phosphatase is elevated. Liver ultrasonography or CT scan will confirm the presence of an abscess.

Differential diagnosis

Amoebic colitis must be differentiated from the other causes of bloody diarrhoea: inflammatory bowel disease, bacillary dysentery, *E. coli*, *Campylobacter* sp., salmonellae and, rarely, pseudomembranous colitis. Amoebic liver abscess must be differentiated from a pyogenic abscess and/or a hydatid cyst.

Management

Metronidazole is given for 5 days in amoebic colitis and a more prolonged course (10–14 days) in liver abscess. A large tense abscess may require percutaneous drainage under ultrasound guidance.

Control and prevention

Improved standards of personal hygiene and water supply are important. Travellers are advised to drink bottled water. Individual chemoprophylaxis is not advised because the risk of acquiring infection is low. There is no effective vaccine.

Shigellosis (bacillary dysentery) ND

Shigellosis is an acute self-limiting intestinal infection which occurs worldwide but is more common in tropical countries and in areas of poor hygiene. Transmission is by the faecal–oral route. The four *Shigella* species (*S. dysenteriae*, *S. flexneri*, *S. boydii* and *S. sonnei*) produce colonic inflammation, with liberation of a cytotoxin (predominantly *S. dysenteriae*) which results in diarrhoea.

Clinical features

After an incubation period of about 2 days there is an abrupt onset of fever, malaise, abdominal pain and watery diarrhoea, which may progress to bloody diarrhoea with mucus and tenesmus.

Investigations

The diagnosis is made on the basis of the stool culture.

Differential diagnosis

This is from other causes of bloody diarrhoea (see above). Sigmoidoscopic appearances may be the same as those in inflammatory bowel disease.

Management

Treatment is symptomatic with antidiarrhoeals, e.g. loperamide, and rehydration. In severe cases treatment is with trimethoprim 200 mg twice daily or ciprofloxacin 500 mg twice daily.

Cholera ND

Cholera is caused by the Gram-negative bacillus *Vibrio cholerae*. Infection is common in tropical and subtropical countries in areas of poor hygiene. Infection is by the faecal–oral route, and spread is predominantly by ingestion of water contaminated with the faeces of infected humans. There is no identified animal reservoir.

Infection is confined to the small bowel, where a powerful enterotoxin is formed. The B subunit of the toxin attaches to receptors on the enterocyte; this allows migration of the A subunit into the cell to stimulate adenylate cyclase activity and increase cAMP levels. This produces massive secretion of isotonic fluid into the intestinal lumen.

Clinical features

The incubation period varies from a few hours to 6 days. The illness varies from mild diarrhoea to profuse watery diarrhoea ('rice-water stools') resulting in dehydration, hypotension and death.

Investigations

The diagnosis is largely clinical. Fresh stool microscopy may show the motile vibrios.

Management

Management is aimed at effective rehydration, which is mainly oral but in severe cases intravenous fluids are given. Oral rehydration solutions (ORS) depend on the fact that there is a glucose-dependent sodium absorption mechanism not related to cAMP and thus unaffected by cholera toxin. The traditional World Health Organization ORS contains sodium (90 mmol/l) and glucose (111 mmol/l), along with potassium, chloride and citrate. New ORS solutions based on rice water may be more effective and are being evaluated.

Tetracycline for 3 days helps to eradicate the infection, decrease stool output and shorten the duration of the illness.

Prevention and control

Good hygiene and sanitation are the most effective measures for the reduction of infection. Oral cholera vaccines are under development.

Giardiasis

Giardia intestinalis (*lamblia*) is a flagellated protozoan that is found worldwide but is more common in tropical areas. It is a cause of traveller's diarrhoea (see later).

Clinical features

The clinical features are the result of damage to the small intestine, with subtotal villous atrophy in severe cases. There is diarrhoea, nausea, abdominal pain and distension, with malabsorption and steatorrhoea in some cases. Chronic giardiasis can result in growth retardation in children.

Investigations

The diagnosis is made by finding cysts on stool examination or parasites in duodenal aspirates.

Management

Metronidazole 2 g daily for 3 days will cure most infections; some patients need two or three courses.

ACUTE INTESTINAL INFECTIONS

Infections of the gastrointestinal tract are the most common intestinal disorders. Infection is acquired through the ingestion of faecally contaminated food or beverages. Individuals at increased risk of infection include infants and young children, the elderly, travellers (principally to developing countries), the immunocompromised and those with reduced gastric acid secretion.

After entry and attachment to the intestinal epithelium, organisms cause intestinal disease by two mechanisms: the production of secretory enterotoxins and cytotoxins, and/or invasion of the epithelium.

Three clinical syndromes are recognized:

- Acute food poisoning ND
- Watery diarrhoea
- Bloody diarrhoea (dysentery).

Gastroenteritis and food poisoning

Most cases of food poisoning in adults are caused by either *Salmonella* or *Campylobacter* spp. The clinical features associated with the causative organisms are summarized in Table 1.6. Listeriosis (infection with *Listeria monocytogenes*) is associated with contaminated coleslaw, non-pasteurized soft cheeses and other packaged chilled foods. The main feature of listeria infection is meningitis, occurring perinatally and in immunocompromised adults (see page 597).

Watery diarrhoea

Watery diarrhoea is produced by decreased absorption and/or increased secretion of water and electrolytes in the small bowel or colon.

Serotypes of *E. coli* produce diarrhoea by one of several mechanisms:

- Enterotoxigenic *E. coli* (ETEC) produces two enterotoxins, one of which is structurally similar and has a similar mode of action to cholera toxin (see below).
- Enteroaggregative *E. coli* also produces a secretory enterotoxin.
- Enteropathogenic *E. coli* (EPEC) attaches to and damages the small intestine and produces diarrhoea in children.

- Enteroinvasive *E. coli* induces a massive influx of polymorphonuclear leucocytes into the mucosa and submucosa, with an acute inflammatory colitis.
- Enterohaemorrhagic *E. coli* produces principally a bloody diarrhoea (see below). Serotype O157 may be associated with serious complications, particularly haemolytic uraemic syndrome in 5–10%.

Other infectious causes of watery diarrhoea are *V. cholerae*, *Salmonella* sp., *Giardia intestinalis*, *Cryptosporidium parvum* and viruses (rotavirus, adenovirus and Norwalk family of viruses). A number of other organisms cause watery diarrhoea in the immunocompromised.

Bloody diarrhoea

Dysentery is caused by organisms that produce invasive inflammatory disease, usually in the distal ileum and colon: *Salmonella* sp., *Shigella* sp., *Campylobacter jejuni*, enterohaemorhagic *E. coli*, *Yersinia enterocolitica* and *Entamoeba histolytica*. These organisms may also cause watery diarrhoea without blood. Cytomegalovirus causes bloody diarrhoea in the immunocompromised.

Traveller's diarrhoea

Acute gastrointestinal infection affects 30–50% of travellers from western countries to the developing world. Typically abdominal cramps and diarrhoea begin 4–6 days after arrival and last 1–3 days. Less commonly diarrhoea persists and may last for weeks. Infection is most commonly due to enterotoxigenic *E. coli* (Table 1.7). Investigation, with

Table 1.7 Common causes of traveller's diarrhoea

Pathogen
Enterotoxigenic *Escherichia coli*
Shigella sp.
Salmonella sp.
Rotavirus
Norwalk virus family
Aeromonas and *Plesimonas* spp.
Campylobacter jejuni
Entamoeba histolytica
Giardia intestinalis
Others

Shaded areas indicate invasive organisms

microscopy and culture of three serial stool specimens, is usually only necessary for individuals with dysentery when invasive organisms are involved, or when diarrhoea persists in the returning traveller. Colonoscopy and biopsy is occasionally necessary, particularly if an alternative diagnosis is considered, such as inflammatory bowel disease.

HELMINTHS

The helminths or worms that may infect man are of three classes (Table 1.8). In the UK only three species are commonly encountered: *Enterobiasis vermicularis*, *Ascaris lumbricoides* and *Taenia saginata*. Occasionally other species are imported from abroad, where they occur mainly in tropical and subtropical countries. A raised blood eosinophil count (eosinophilia) occurs at some stage in nearly all helminth infections.

SEXUALLY TRANSMITTED DISEASES

Sexually transmitted diseases (STDs) remain endemic in all societies and the range of diseases spread by sexual activity continues to increase. The three common presenting symptoms are:

- Urethral discharge (see below)
- Genital ulcers (see below)
- Vaginal discharge caused by *Candida albicans*, *Trichomonas vaginalis*, *Neisseria gonorrhoeae*, *Chlamydia trachomatis*, *Herpes simplex*, cervical polyps, neoplasia, retained tampon, chemical irritants. Bacterial vaginosis is also characterized by a vaginal discharge but it is not clear to what extent this is a sexually transmitted disease. It occurs when the normal lactobacilli of the vagina are replaced by a mixed flora *of Gardnerella vaginalis* and anaerobes, resulting in an offensive discharge.

STDs predominantly seen in the tropics are chancroid, granuloma inguinale and lymphogranuloma venereum. They may present with genital ulceration and inguinal lymphadenopathy.

Table 1.8 Summary of intestinal diseases caused by helminths (parasitic worms)

Organism	Site	Clinical manifestations	Diagnosis	Treatment
Nematodes (roundworms)				
Strongyloides stercoralis	SI	Malabsorption, disseminated disease	Serology: detection of specific antibodies in serum. Detection of larvae in fresh stool/duodenal aspirate	Thiabendazole
Hookworm: Ancylostoma duodenale & Necator americanus	SI	Iron deficiency anaemia	Detection of ova in faeces	Mebendazole
Capillaria philippinesis	SI	Malabsorption		
Ascaris lumbricoides (roundworm)	SI, lung	Malnutrition, intestinal obstruction, pulmonary eosinophilia	Detection of eggs in faeces	Levamisole
Trichuris trichuria (whipworm)	LI	Often asymptomatic, bloody diarrhoea	Detection of eggs in faeces	Mebendazole
Trichinella spiralis	SI	infection, from undercooked infected pork, causes pain, diarrhoea. Worms penetrate gut wall, migrate to striated muscle causing pain/tenderness	Detection of specific antibodies in serum. Encysted larvae demonstrated in muscle biopsy	Thiabendazole
Enterobius vermicularis (threadworm)	LI	Often asymptomatic, pruritis ani	Apply adhesive tape to perineum and identify eggs microscopically	Mebendazole
Toxocara canis or T. cati		Worm passed in dog/cat faeces, penetrates gut to lungs (bronchial asthma), liver (hepatomegaly) and eye (chorioretinitis)	Detection of specific antibodies in serum	Albendazole.
Cestodes (tapeworms)				
Taenia saginata		Beef tapeworm acquired by eating insufficiently cooked beef. Causes abdominal pain and malabsorption		Niclosamide

T. solium	Pork tapeworm from undercooked pork. SI infection and disseminated disease (cysticercosis) involving CNS (fits, dementia), eye, skin, muscle	
Echinococcus granulosus	Hydatid disease acquired by eating meat (sheep, cattle) contaminated with ova excreted by dogs. Large cysts develop in liver, lung, brain. Anaphylactic reactions if cyst contents escape	Plain X-ray, ultrasound and CT show the cysts — Diagnosis by serology — Surgical excision, albendazole
Trematodes (flukes)		
Schistosoma mansoni Schistosoma japonicum Schistosoma haematobium	Snail vectors release cercariae which penetrate human skin (causing 'swimmer's itch') during swimming, paddling. Worms migrate to pelvic veins and bladder (haematobium), or mesenteric veins and bowel (mansoni/japonicum), causing urinary frequency, dysuria, hydronephrosis or bloody diarrhoea, intestinal strictures, hepatic fibrosis and portal hypertension	Detection of eggs in stool, urine or on rectal biopsy — Detection of specific serum antibodies — Praziquantel
Fasciola hepatica	Spread by ingestion of organisms (via freshwater snails) in faeces of sheep, goats, cattle. Causes hepatomegaly, cholangitis	Serology, stool microscopy — Triclabendazole
Clonorchis sinensis	Life-cycle similar to above but fish form the intermediate host. Cholangitis, liver abscess and cholangiocarcinoma	

SI, small intestine; LI, large intestine.

The important aspects of management of all the STDs are:

- Accurate diagnosis and effective treatment
- Screening for other STDs (multiple STDs may coexist)
- Patient education
- Contact tracing: the patient's sexual partners must be traced so that they can be treated, thereby preventing the disease from spreading further
- Follow-up to ensure that infection is adequately treated.

Urethritis

Urethritis in men presents with urethral discharge and dysuria. It is often asymptomatic in women.

Gonorrhoea

The causative organism, *Neisseria gonorrhoeae* (gonococcus), is a Gram-negative intracellular diplococcus which infects epithelium, particularly of the urogenital tract, rectum, pharynx and conjunctivae.

Clinical features

The incubation period ranges from 2 to 14 days. In men the symptoms are purulent urethral discharge and dysuria. In homosexual men proctitis may produce anal pain, discharge and itch. Women are often asymptomatic but may complain of vaginal discharge, dysuria and intermenstrual bleeding. Complications include salpingitis and Bartholin's abscess in women, epididymitis and prostatitis in men, and systemic spread with a rash and arthritis (page 217). Infants born to infected mothers may develop ocular infections (ophthalmia neonatorum).

Diagnosis

Gram stain and culture of a swab taken from the urethra in men and the endocervix in women.

Management

- A single oral dose of amoxycillin (3 g) plus probenecid (1 g)
- Spectinomycin or ciprofloxacin patients allergic to penicillin

- A longer course of treatment is required in complicated infection.

Non-gonococcal urethritis (NGU)

The most common cause is infection with *Chlamydia trachomatis*, which in men presents with urethral discharge and dysuria. In women infection may be asymptomatic and only found during investigations for infertility (secondary to salpingitis and fallopian tube blockage). The organism is intracellular and diagnosis is made by direct detection of chlamydial antigens by ELISA in material obtained from swabs, or cell culture of swabs taken from the urethra or endocervix. Treatment is with oxytetracycline or erythromycin (in pregnancy). Other causes of NGU are *Ureaplasma urealyticum, Bacteroides* sp and *Mycoplasma* sp.

Genital ulcers

The infective causes of genital ulceration in the UK include syphilis, herpes simplex and herpes zoster. Non-infective causes are Behcet's syndrome, Stevens–Johnson syndrome (page 633), carcinoma and trauma.

Syphilis

The causative organism, *Treponema pallidum*, is a motile spirochaete which enters via a skin abrasion during close sexual contact. The organism may also pass transplacentally from mother to fetus.

Primary infection

After an incubation period of 10–90 days a papule develops at the site of infection. This ulcerates to become a painless, firm chancre which heals spontaneously within 2–3 weeks.

Secondary infection

This occurs 4–10 weeks after the appearance of the primary lesion. There may be one or more of the following features: fever, sore throat, arthralgia, generalized lymphadenopathy, widespread skin rash (except the face), superficial ulcers in the mouth (snail-track ulcers) and condylomata lata (warty perianal lesions). In most patients symptoms subside within 1 year.

Tertiary syphilis

Occurs after a latent period of 2 years or more. The characteristic lesion is a gumma (granulomatous lesion) occurring in the skin, bones, liver and testes. Cardiovascular syphilis is mentioned on pages 370 and 389 and neurosyphilis is described on page 602.

Congenital syphilis

This usually becomes apparent between the second and sixth weeks after birth, early signs being nasal discharge, skin and mucous membrane lesions, and failure to thrive. Signs of late syphilis appear after 2 years of age, when there are also characteristic bone and teeth abnormalities as a result of earlier damage.

Diagnosis

- *Dark ground microscopy of fluid* taken from lesions shows organisms in primary and secondary disease. Serological tests may be negative in primary disease.
- *Serology*. The VDRL (Venereal Disease Research Laboratory) test is detectable within 3–4 weeks of infection; it becomes negative in treated patients and in some untreated patients with late tertiary syphilis. Other diseases, e.g. autoimmune disease and malignancy, may give false positive results. *T. pallidum* haemagglutination assay (TPHA) and the fluorescent treponemal antibody test are positive in most patients in primary disease, and remain positive in spite of treatment. They do not distinguish between syphilis and other treponemes, e.g. yaws.

Management

Intramuscular procaine penicillin for 10 days is given for primary and secondary syphilis. For tertiary syphilis treatment is continued for 4 weeks. The Jarisch–Herxheimer reaction, characterized by malaise, fever and headache, occurs most commonly in secondary syphilis and is the result of release of tumour necrosis factor when organisms are killed by antibiotics. Symptoms may be ameliorated by giving prednisolone for 24 hours before penicillin.

HIV AND AIDS

Human immunodeficiency virus (HIV) infection was identified as the causative organism of acquired immuno-deficiency syndrome (AIDS) in 1983. It is estimated that 24 million adults are infected worldwide.

Epidemiology

Transmission is by:

- Sexual intercourse: worldwide, heterosexual intercourse accounts for the vast majority of infections. Homosexual transmission accounts for the majority of infections in Europe, the USA and Australia.
- Mother to child: transmission can occur in utero, during childbirth and via breast milk.
- Contaminated blood, blood products and organ donations: the risk is now minimal in developed countries since the introduction of screening blood products in 1985.
- Contaminated needles: intravenous drug addicts, needlestick injuries in healthcare workers.

HIV infection is not spread by ordinary social or household contact.

Pathogenesis of HIV infection

The virus consists of an outer envelope and an inner core. The core contains RNA and the enzyme reverse transcriptase, which allows viral RNA to be transcribed into DNA and then incorporated into the host cell genome. The rapid emergence of viral quasispecies (closely related but genetically distinct variants) is due to the high mutation rate of reverse transcriptase and the high rate of viral turnover. This genetic diversification has important implications for the evolution of viral variants with resistance to antiviral drugs.

HIV enters T cells by binding to the CD4 receptor and utilizing one or more entry cofactors on T-helper cells (CD4 cells). Other cells of the immune system bearing the CD4 receptor are also affected. There is a progressive and severe depletion of infected CD4 lymphocytes which results in host susceptibility to infections with intracellular bacteria and mycobacteria. The coexisting antibody abnormalities predispose to infections with capsulated bacteria, e.g. *strep. pneumoniae* and *H. influenzae*. The clinical illness associated with HIV infection is due to this immune dysfunction, and also to a direct effect of HIV on certain tissues.

Natural history and clinical features

The typical pattern of HIV infection is shown in Figure 1.2. Throughout the course of HIV infection viral load and immunodeficiency progress steadily, despite the absence of observed disease during the latency period.

The spectrum of illness associated with HIV infection is broad. Several classification systems exist, the most widely used being the Centers for Disease Control (CDC):

- Acute seroconversion illness: a self-limiting non-specific illness occurs 4–8 weeks after exposure in some patients. Symptoms include fever, myalgia, oral ulceration, generalized lymphadenopathy and a maculopapular rash. An 'aseptic meningitis' picture is common.
- Asymptomatic infection (clinical latency): the number of HIV-infected lymphocytes gradually increases, and although the patients remain well, they remain infectious. This stage may last up to 10 years. A subgroup of patients with asymptomatic infection have persistent generalized lymphadenopathy, defined as

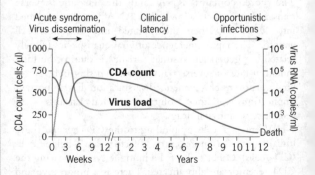

Figure 1.2
Schematic representation of the course of HIV-1 infection in vivo.

nodes more than 1 cm in diameter at two or more extrainguinal sites for more than 3 months in the absence of causes other than HIV infection.
• Symptomatic HIV infection: the clinical picture is the result of direct HIV effects and of the associated immunosuppression.

The clinical findings resulting from direct HIV infection are summarized in Table 1.9. In addition, drugs used in the treatment of HIV infection may have side effects which may present similarly to clinical features of HIV infection, e.g. myelosuppression may be due to HIV infection or zidovudine; renal failure to infection or drugs such as foscarnet and amphotericin B.

Immunosuppression associated with HIV infection allows the development of opportunistic infections, and tumours that may have an oncogenic viral aetiology. Presentation of

Table 1.9 Direct HIV effects

Neurological disease	AIDS dementia complex Distal sensory peripheral neuropathy Autonomic neuropathy causing diarrhoea and postural hypotension
Eye	Retinal cottonwool spots – rarely troublesome
Mucocutaneous	Dry, itchy flaky skin Pruritic papular eruption Aphthous ulceration in the mouth
Haematological	Anaemia of chronic disease Neutropenia Autoimmune thrombocytopenia
Gastrointestinal	Anorexia leading to weight loss in advanced disease HIV enteropathy leading to diarrhoea and malabsorption
Renal	Renal impairment Nephrotic syndrome
Respiratory	Chronic sinusitis and otitis media Lymphoid interstitial pneumonitis – lymphocytic infiltration of the lung, causing dyspnoea and a dry cough
Endocrine	Reduced adrenal function – infection may precipitate clear adrenal insufficiency
Cardiac	Myocarditis and cardiomyopathy

infections may differ from that seen in immunocompetent patients:

- Atypical or lack of typical signs, as the inflammatory response is impaired
- Multiple pathogens may coexist
- Indirect serological tests are frequently unreliable.

These factors mean that serological tests may be unreliable and, in many cases, to make the correct diagnosis material must be obtained from the appropriate site for examination and culture.

Protozoal infections

Toxoplasmosis gondii most commonly causes encephalitis and cerebral abscess in AIDS patients. Clinical features include focal neurological signs, fits, fever, headache and possible confusion. Eye involvement with chorioretinitis may also be present. Diagnosis is made on the basis of positive toxoplasmosis serology and multiple ring-enhancing lesions on CT scan. Treatment is with pyrimethamine, sulphadiazine and folinic acid; lifelong maintenance is required to prevent relapse. *Cryptosporidium parvum* causes severe chronic watery diarrhoea and sclerosing cholangitis. Diagnosis is made by demonstrating cysts on stool microscopy or on small bowel biopsy specimens obtained at endoscopy. Treatment is supportive. Microsporidia infection (usually *Enterocytozoon bieneusi*) causes a diarrhoeal illness. Diagnosis is made by demonstrating spores in the stools. Treatment is with albendazole.

Viruses

Cytomegalovirus (CMV) causes:

- Retinitis with floaters, loss of visual acuity and orbital pain. Fundoscopy shows a characteristic appearance of the retina with haemorrhages and exudate. Treatment is with intravenous ganciclovir or foscarnet, continued long-term to prevent reactivation. Oral and topical forms of ganciclovir have been developed for maintenance treatment and avoid the hazards of intravenous catheter sepsis
- Colitis, which presents with bloody diarrhoea and abdominal pain. Diagnosis is made by demonstrating

characteristic 'cytomegalic cells' (large cells containing an intranuclear inclusion and sometimes intracytoplasmic inclusions) on light-microscopic examination of mucosal biopsy specimens. Treatment is with intravenous ganciclovir or foscarnet

- Oesophageal ulceration, causing painful dysphagia
- Less commonly, polyradiculopathy, encephalitis and pneumonitis.

Herpes simplex virus infection causes genital and oral ulceration, and systemic infection. Varicella zoster occurs at any stages of HIV infection, but may be more aggressive and longer lasting than in immunocompetent patients. Herpes virus 8 is associated with Kaposi's sarcoma. Infection usually responds to acyclovir. Epstein–Barr virus (EBV) causes oral hairy leukoplakia, presenting as a pale ridged lesion on the side of the tongue. Treatment is with acyclovir. Human papilloma virus (HPV) produces genital and plantar warts. HPV infection is associated with the more rapid development of squamous cell cancer of the cervix and anal cancer. Papovavirus causes progressive multifocal leucoencephalopathy, which presents with intellectual impairment and often hemiparesis and aphasia.

Fungi

Pneumocystis carinii causes pneumonia in severely immunocompromised patients (CD4 count $<200/mm^3$). There is an insidious onset of breathlessness, a non-productive cough, fever and malaise. The chest X-ray may be normal or show bilateral perihilar interstitial infiltrates, which can progress to more diffuse shadowing. Definitive diagnosis is made by demonstrating the organisms in specimens obtained at bronchoalveolar lavage. Treatment is with intravenous co-trimoxazole, intravenous pentamidine or dapsone and trimethoprim. Systemic corticosteroids reduce mortality in severe cases (P_aO_2 <9.5 kPa). Recurrence is largely prevented (secondary prophylaxis) by the use of low-dose co-trimoxazole (960 mg three times weekly) or nebulized pentamidine (300 mg monthly). Prophylaxis is also offered (primary prophylaxis) to those at high risk of infection (CD4 cell count $<200/mm^3$).

Cryptococcus most commonly causes meningitis in AIDS patients. There is an insidious onset of fever, nausea and headache, eventually with impaired consciousness and change in affect. Diagnosis is made by CSF microscopy (Indian ink staining shows the organisms directly) and culture. Treatment is with intravenous amphotericin B or fluconazole, and oral fluconazole continued long term to suppress infection.

Mucosal infection with candida (usually *Candida albicans*) is very common in HIV-infected patients and presents as creamy plaques in the mouth, vulvovaginal region and oesophagus (producing dysphagia and retrosternal pain). Infection usually responds to treatment with fluconazole or itraconazole. Disseminated infection with *Aspergillus fumigatus* occurs in advanced HIV infection. The prognosis is poor, with amphotericin B being the mainstay of therapy.

Bacterial infection

This may present early in HIV infection, is often disseminated and frequently recurs. *Mycobacterium tuberculosis* (TB) can cause disease at all stages of HIV infection, but extrapulmonary TB is more common with advanced disease. *Mycobacterium avium intracellulare* (MAI) occurs in patients with advanced AIDS. Clinical features include fever, anorexia, weight loss, diarrhoea and anaemia with bone marrow involvement. MAI is typically resistant to standard antituberculous therapies. A combination of ethambutol, rifabutin and clarithromycin reduces the burden of organisms and provides symptomatic benefit. Other infections include *Strep. pneumoniae, H. influenzae*, staphylococcal skin infection and salmonella.

Neoplasia

The commonest tumours are Kaposi's sarcoma and non-Hodgkin's lymphoma.

- Kaposi's sarcoma is a vascular tumour which appears as red–purple, raised, well circumscribed lesions on the skin, hard palate and conjunctivae, and in the gastrointestinal tract. The lungs and lymph nodes may also be involved. Human herpes virus 8 is implicated in the pathogenesis. Localized disease is treated with radiotherapy; systemic disease is treated with chemotherapy.

- Non-Hodgkin's lymphoma occurs in the brain, gut and lung. It is an aggressive tumour with a poor prognosis.
- Squamous cell carcinoma of the cervix and anus is associated with HIV. Human papillomavirus may play a part in the pathogenesis.

Diagnosis and monitoring

Testing for HIV infection must only be undertaken with informed consent and the patient should receive advice from a trained counsellor about the implications of a positive test (e.g. difficulties in obtaining life insurance, mortgages).

HIV infection is diagnosed by the following tests:

- IgG antibodies in the serum may not appear for up to 3 months after infection. They are the most commonly used marker of HIV infection
- Measurement of HIV RNA (viral load) in plasma
- Measurement of viral p24 antigen (p24 Ag) in plasma if RNA assay is unavailable. Antigen disappears 8–10 weeks after exposure.

Following a diagnosis of HIV infection the number of circulating CD4 lymphocytes are measured 3-monthly; patients with counts below $200/mm^3$ are at greatest risk of HIV-related pathology. Plasma levels of HIV RNA ('viral load', measured in copies of RNA per ml) is a measure of viral replication. The viral load is the best indicator of long-term prognosis, and levels fall with effective antiretroviral medication.

The diagnosis of AIDS is made when an HIV-positive patient develops one or more of a defined list of opportunistic infections, malignancies or HIV-associated illnesses (Table 1.10) in the absence of other causes of immunosuppression, e.g. leukaemia, immunosuppressive drugs.

Management

Management involves treatment with antiretroviral drugs, social and psychological care, prevention of opportunistic infections and prevention of transmission of HIV. HIV infection cannot be cured and the aim of treatment is to suppress viral replication to as low a level as possible for as long as possible. Table 1.11 lists the antiretroviral drugs.

Table 1.10 AIDS-defining diagnoses (1993 classification, Europe*)

Candidiasis of bronchi, trachea, lungs or oesophagus
Cervical carcinoma, invasive
Coccidioidomycosis, disseminated or extrapulmonary
Cryptococcus, extrapulmonary
Cryptosporidiosis, with diarrhoea for > 1 month
Cytomegalovirus disease other than in liver, spleen or nodes
Encephalopathy, HIV related
Herpes simplex ulcers for 1 month or bronchitis, pneumonitis or oesophagitis
Histoplasmosis, disseminated or extrapulmonary
Isosporiasis, with diarrhoea for > 1 month
Kaposi's sarcoma
Lymphoid interstitial pneumonitis
Mycobacterium avium complex or *M. kansasii*, disseminated or extrapulmonary
Mycobacterium tuberculosis
Mycobacterium, other species or unidentified species disseminated or extrapulmonary
Pneumocystis carinii pneumonia
Pneumonia, recurrent
Progressive multifocal leucoencephalopathy
Salmonella (non-typhoid) septicaemia, recurrent
Toxoplasmosis of brain
Wasting syndrome, due to HIV (weight loss > 10% baseline, with no other cause identified)

* USA definition also includes those with a CD4 count <200/mm^3

Table 1.11 Antiretroviral drugs

Nucleoside reverse transcriptase inhibitors	Protease inhibitors	Non-nucleoside reverse transcriptase inhibitors
Zidovudine (ZDV, AZT)	Saquinavir	Nevirapine
Zalcitabine (ddC)	Ritonavir	Delavirdine*
Didanosine (ddI)	Indinavir	Loviride*
Stavudine (d4T)	Nelfinavir	
Lamivudine (3TC)		

* Not yet licensed in Europe.

In the UK indications to consider the initiation of antiretroviral therapy include:

- Symptomatic HIV disease
- CD4 count less than 350/mm^3
- Very rapidly falling CD4 count
- High viral load (>10 000 copies/ml of plasma).

Treatment is usually started with zidovudine in combination with one other nucleoside reverse transcriptase inhibitor. A protease inhibitor may be added at the start of treatment, or after 3 months if the reduction in viral load is inadequate with dual therapy. The disadvantages of initiating treatment with triple therapy is the potential for adverse reactions and drug interactions, and compliance may be more difficult.

Prevention and control

- Health care workers who sustain a needlestick injury with known HIV-infected material should be advised to take triple therapy for 4–6 weeks after exposure
- Screening of blood products
- The use of condoms reduces sexual transmission of HIV
- Advise drug addicts not to share needles; some areas provide free sterile needles.

Prognosis

The rate of progression among patients infected with HIV varies greatly. For example, approximately 5% of infected persons develop AIDS within 3 years of infection and, by contrast, 12% of infected persons remain free of AIDS for more than 20 years. The total CD4 count has until recently provided the best predictor of risk of progression to AIDS or death. More recently plasma HIV-1 RNA concentrations, which reflect the rate of virus replication, have been shown to provide a more powerful predictor of disease progression than CD4 counts alone. For example, approximately 70% of patients with a virus load of >30 000 copies/ml will die within 6 years.

Gastroenterology and nutrition

GASTROENTEROLOGY

....

SYMPTOMS OF GASTROINTESTINAL DISEASE

Dysphagia

Dysphagia is difficulty in swallowing. The causes are listed on page 45.

Heartburn

Heartburn is a retrosternal burning discomfort which spreads up towards the throat and is a common symptom of acid reflux (page 47). The pain can sometimes be difficult to distinguish from the pain of ischaemic heart disease, although a careful history will usually differentiate between the two (page 321).

Dyspepsia

Dyspepsia is a general term often used to describe a range of symptoms referable to the upper gastrointestinal tract, e.g. nausea, heartburn, acidity, pain or distension.

Flatulence

Flatulence is a term used to describe excessive wind, presenting as belching, abdominal distension and the passage of flatus per rectum. It is rarely indicative of serious underlying disease.

Vomiting

Vomiting occurs as a result of stimulation of the vomiting centres in the lateral reticular formation of the medulla. This may result from stimulation of the chemoreceptor trigger zones in the floor of the fourth ventricle or from vagal afferents from the gut. It is associated with many gastrointestinal conditions, but nausea and vomiting without pain are frequently non-gastrointestinal in origin.

Constipation

Constipation is difficult to define because there is considerable individual variation, but it is usually taken to mean infrequent passage of stool or the difficult passage of hard stools.

Diarrhoea

Diarrhoea implies the passage of increased amounts of loose stool (>300 g/24 h) (page 80). This must be differentiated from the frequent passage of small amounts of stool (which patients often refer to as diarrhoea), which is commonly seen in functional bowel disease.

Steatorrhoea

Steatorrhoea is the passage of pale bulky stools that contain fat (>18 mmol/24 h) and indicates fat malabsorption as a result of small bowel, pancreatic or biliary disease. The stools often float because of increased air content and are difficult to flush away.

THE MOUTH

Problems in the mouth are common and often trivial, although they can cause severe symptoms.

Mouth ulcers

Non-infective

- Recurrent aphthous ulceration is the most common cause of mouth ulcers and affects at least 20% of the population; in most cases the aetiology is unknown. The history is of recurrent self-limiting episodes of painful oral ulcers (rarely on the palate). Topical corticosteroids are used for symptomatic relief but they have no effect on the natural history. In a few cases ulcers are associated with trauma or gastrointestinal and systemic diseases, e.g. anaemia, inflammatory bowel disease, coeliac disease, Behçet's syndrome, Reiter's disease, systemic lupus erythematosus, pemphigus, pemphigoid, and fixed drug reactions.
- Squamous cell carcinoma presents as an indolent ulcer, usually on the tongue or floor of the mouth. Aetiological factors include tobacco (smoking and

chewing) and alcohol. Treatment is with surgery, radiotherapy or a combination of both.

Infective

Many infections can affect the mouth, though the most common are viral and include:

- Herpes simplex virus type 1
- Coxsackie A virus
- Herpes zoster virus.

Oral white patches

Oral white patches are associated with smoking, candida infection, lichen planus, trauma and syphilis. Leukoplakia is the term used to describe oral white patches or plaques that cannot be diagnosed clinically or pathologically as any other disease (i.e. a diagnosis of exclusion). Leukoplakia is occasionally a premalignant lesion and thus oral white patches must be biopsied to exclude malignancy. Hairy leukoplakia is an Epstein–Barr-related white patch on the side of the tongue, which may indicate severe immunodeficiency, e.g. AIDS; it is not premalignant.

Atrophic glossitis

A smooth sore tongue with loss of filliform papillae may occur in patients with iron, vitamin B_{12} or folate deficiency.

Geographical tongue

This affects up to 10% of the population and describes discrete areas of depapillation on the dorsum of the tongue. This may be asymptomatic or produce a sore tongue. The aetiology is unknown and there is no specific treatment.

Periodontal disorders

Gum bleeding is most commonly caused by gingivitis, an inflammatory condition of the gums associated with dental plaque. Bleeding may also be associated with generalized conditions such as bleeding disorders and leukaemia. Acute ulcerative gingivitis (Vincent's infection) is characterized by the development of crater-like ulcers, with bleeding, involving the interdental papillae, followed by lateral spread along the gingival margins. It is thought to be the result of spirochaetal infection occurring in the malnourished and immunocompromised. Treatment is with oral metronidazole and good oral hygiene.

Salivary gland disorders

Xerostomia (mouth dryness) may be caused by anxiety, drugs, Sjögren's syndrome and dehydration.

Infection (parotitis) may be viral, i.e. mumps virus, or bacterial (staphylococci or streptococci).

Sarcoidosis produces enlargement of the parotid glands and, if combined with lacrimal gland enlargement, is known as Mikulicz's syndrome.

Calculus formation usually involves the duct of the submandibular gland, and causes painful swelling of the gland before or during mastication.

Tumours most commonly affect the parotid gland and are usually benign, e.g. pleomorphic adenoma. Treatment is with surgical resection. Involvement of the VIIth nerve raises the suspicion of malignancy.

THE OESOPHAGUS

The main oesophageal symptoms are dysphagia, heartburn and painful swallowing.

- Dysphagia (difficulty in swallowing) is usually investigated with a barium swallow, followed by endoscopy where appropriate. The causes are listed in Table 2.1, although the commonest causes are peptic or malignant strictures and bulbar palsies. Typically, mechanical narrowing of the oesophagus, particularly in oesophageal malignancy, produces progressive dysphagia, initially for solids and eventually for liquids. Motor disorders, e.g. achalasia and scleroderma, produce dysphagia for both solids and liquids together.
- Heartburn is a retrosternal or epigastric burning sensation produced by the reflux of gastric acid into the oesophagus. The pain may radiate up to the throat and be confused with chest pain of cardiac origin. It is often aggravated by bending or lying down.
- Painful swallowing occurs with infections of the oesophagus or in gastro-oesophageal reflux disease, particularly with alcohol and hot liquids (see later).

Table 2.1 Causes of dysphagia

Intrinsic lesion
Foreign body
Benign (peptic) stricture
Malignant stricture
Oesophageal ring or web
Pharyngeal pouch

Neuromuscular disorders
Bulbar palsy
Pharyngeal disorders
Myasthenia gravis

Motility disorders
Achalasia
Scleroderma
Diffuse oesophageal spasm
Presbyoesophagus (oesophagus of old age)
Diabetes
Chagas' disease

Extrinsic pressure
Goitre
Mediastinal glands
Enlarged left atrium in mitral valve disease

Achalasia

Achalasia is a disease of unknown aetiology, characterized by either aperistalsis or non-propulsive tertiary contractions in the body of the oesophagus, and the failure of relaxation of the lower oesophageal sphincter (LOS) on initiation of swallowing.

Pathology

There is a decrease in ganglionic cells in the nerve plexus of the oesophageal wall and degeneration in the vagus nerve.

Clinical features

The disease can present at any age but is rare in childhood. There is usually a long history of dysphagia for both liquids and solids, which may be associated with regurgitation. Severe retrosternal chest pain may occur, particularly in younger patients.

Investigations

- Barium swallow will show dilatation of the oesophagus, lack of peristalsis, a gradually tapering lower end (beak deformity) and asynchronous contractions of the oesophagus.
- Oesophagoscopy may be necessary to exclude a carcinoma.
- Manometry demonstrates aperistalsis and failure of LOS relaxation.
- Chest radiographs may show a dilated oesophagus with a fluid level behind the heart. The fundal gas shadow is not present.

Management

Endoscopic pneumatic dilatation of the LOS, under radiographic screening, is currently the procedure of choice and is successful in 80% of cases. Endoscopic injection of botulinum toxin into the LOS has been advocated, with variable success rates. Surgical division of the sphincter (Heller's cardiomyotomy) is used in resistant cases and is now being performed via the laparoscope. Reflux oesophagitis is a complication of treatment, particularly following surgical intervention.

Complications

There is a slight increase in the incidence of carcinoma of the oesophagus in patients with achalasia, regardless of the treatment undertaken.

Systemic sclerosis

There is oesophageal involvement in over 90% of patients with systemic sclerosis. The smooth muscle layer is replaced by fibrous tissue. The LOS pressure is reduced, thereby permitting reflux. Patients may be asymptomatic or complain of reflux and dysphagia. Dysphagia is caused by stricture formation complicating reflux. Treatment is as for reflux and stricture formation.

Diffuse oesophageal spasm

This is a severe form of abnormal oesophageal motility which most commonly presents in middle age, and can produce chest pain and dysphagia. A 'corkscrew' appearance may be seen on barium swallow. 'Nutcracker oesophagus' is a variant characterized by high-amplitude peristaltic waves in the oesophagus. Treatment of these disorders is difficult, but calcium channel blockers may be helpful.

Hiatus hernia

On its own a hiatus hernia is not responsible for symptoms unless there is associated reflux. There are two main forms:

- Sliding: the gastro-oesophageal junction slides through the hiatus and lies above the diaphragm.
- Paraoesophageal: a part of the stomach rolls up through the hiatus alongside the oesophagus, the sphincter remaining below the diaphragm.

Gastro-oesophageal reflux disease

Reflux of gastric contents into the oesophagus is a normal event and clinical symptoms occur only when there is prolonged contact of gastric contents with the oesophageal mucosa.

Pathophysiology

There is low oesophageal sphincter tone, with reduced mucosal resistance to acid and reduced oesophageal clearance of acid. Delayed gastric emptying and prolonged postprandial and nocturnal reflux also contribute. Mechanical or functional aberrations associated with a hiatus hernia may contribute to reflux disease in some patients, but patients may also have reflux in the absence of a hiatus hernia.

Clinical features

Heartburn is the major symptom of reflux oesophagitis. The burning is aggravated by bending, stooping and lying down, and may be relieved by antacids. There may be pain on drinking hot drinks. Cough and nocturnal asthma can occur from aspiration of gastric contents into the lungs. Symptoms do not correlate well with the severity of oesophagitis.

Investigations

Barium swallow This may show an ulcerated lower oesophagus and/or reflux of barium at the time of the examination.

Oesophagoscopy shows the presence of oesophagitis. The mucosa can, however, be normal in patients with symptoms of reflux.

24-hour intraluminal pH monitoring Insertion of a pH probe into the lower oesophagus via the nose allows continual monitoring of acid reflux over 24 hours. This is not performed routinely but is used in difficult diagnostic cases or where there is a poor response to treatment [CM page 228].

Management

Conservative measures with simple antacids, raising the head of the bed, losing weight, a reduction in alcohol intake and cessation of smoking are often sufficient for mild symptoms.

Alginate – containing antacids prevent reflux by forming a 'foam raft' on gastric contents.

H2-receptor antagonists (e.g. ranitidine) improve the symptoms of heartburn.

Prokinetic agents, such as metoclopramide and cisapride, enhance peristalsis and may be of value, particularly as maintenance treatment.

Proton pump inhibitors (e.g. omeprazole, lansoprazole, pantoprazole) inhibit hydrogen-potassium ATPase and block the luminal secretion of gastric acid. They are potent acid blockers and the drugs of choice for all but mild cases.

Surgery may be necessary for the few patients who continue to have symptoms in spite of full medical therapy, or in young people whose symptoms return rapidly on stopping treatment. The fundus of the stomach is sutured around the lower oesophagus to produce an antireflux valve (Nissen fundoplication). This procedure is performed laparoscopically which reduces length of hospital stay and the time taken to return to work, compared to open operation.

Complications

Oesophageal stricture formation is the major complication of reflux and presents with intermittent dysphagia. It is treated with endoscopic dilatation. Long-standing acid reflux may cause metaplasia from squamous to columnar epithelium in the lower oesophagus, a change known as

Barrett's oesophagus. This is premalignant for adenocarcinoma of the oesophagus.

Malignant oesophageal tumours
Pathology

- Squamous cell, usually of the middle third of oesophagus
- Adenocarcinoma
- Kaposi's sarcoma is seen in patients with AIDS, but is rarely symptomatic.

Epidemiology

Squamous carcinoma The incidence is 5–10 per 100 000 in the UK, although it varies greatly throughout the world, being particularly high in China and parts of Africa and Iran. It is most common in the 60–70-year age group. It is associated with heavy alcohol intake, heavy smoking and a high intake of salted fish and pickled vegetables. Other predisposing factors include the Plummer–Vinson syndrome (iron deficiency anaemia and oesophageal web causing dysphagia), tylosis (an autosomal dominant condition with hyperkeratosis of palms and soles), achalasia and coeliac disease.

Adenocarcinoma This arises from the columnar-lined epithelium of the lower oesophagus which results from long-standing reflux (Barrett's oesophagus).

Clinical features

Symptoms include progressive dysphagia (initially for solids and later for liquids), weight loss, and chest pain, which may be due to bolus food impaction or local infiltration. Physical signs are usually absent.

Investigations

- Barium swallow or endoscopy are the initial investigations.
- CT, MRI and endoscopic ultrasonography may be helpful in staging the lesion for surgery.

Management

In many patients only symptomatic treatment to relieve the dysphagia is possible. This is usually done endoscopically:

- Dilatation and insertion of a plastic or expanding metal stent to keep the oesophagus open
- Laser to photocoagulate the tumour
- Alcohol injections into the tumour to cause local necrosis.

Surgical resection may be carried out in the few patients with localized disease (25% 5-year survival). Radiation and chemotherapy have provided limited success with both squamous cell carcinoma and adenocarcinoma.

Prognosis

The prognosis overall is poor (2% 5-year survival) as most patients can only be treated palliatively.

Benign oesophageal tumours

Leiomyomas are the most common benign tumours. They are usually discovered incidentally and do not often produce symptoms.

Oesophageal perforation

The commonest cause of oesophageal perforation is iatrogenic and occurs after endoscopic dilatation of oesophageal strictures (usually malignant) or achalasia. It may also occur after forceful vomiting (Boerhaaeve's syndrome), when there is also usually severe chest pain and collapse. On examination there may be fever, hypotension and surgical emphysema. Diagnosis is by chest X-ray, which may be normal or show air in the mediastinum and neck, and a pleural effusion. A gastrografin swallow (not barium) will confirm the diagnosis. Treatment is with intravenous antibiotics, nil by mouth and intravenous fluids. Surgical repair is needed for patients with large tears or who fail to settle with conservative management.

THE STOMACH AND DUODENUM
Acute gastritis, acute ulceration and erosions

There is no universally accepted classification for these conditions, partly because there is a poor correlation among clinical, pathological and endoscopic findings.

Aetiology

The most common cause is aspirin or other non-steroidal anti-inflammatory drugs (NSAIDs), resulting, in part, from depletion of mucosal prostaglandins. Other causes include infections, e.g. cytomegalovirus and herpes simplex virus, and alcohol in high concentrations. Acute ulcers may be seen after severe stress (stress ulcer), burns (Curling's ulcer), and in renal and liver disease.

Pathology

There is an acute inflammatory cell infiltrate in the superficial gastric mucosa, predominantly with neutrophils. Multiple erosions (small superficial mucosal breaks) are described as acute erosive gastritis. Acute gastric ulceration occurs in the same setting as erosions but the ulcers are larger.

Clinical features

Common symptoms include indigestion, vomiting and haemorrhage, although these correlate poorly with endoscopic and pathological findings.

Investigations

Symptoms often settle spontaneously, although endoscopy and biopsy are sometimes required to clarify the diagnosis.

Management

Treatment is symptomatic, with removal of the offending cause if possible.

Chronic gastritis

This is commonly found in patients being investigated for dyspepsia.

Aetiology

The most common cause of chronic gastritis is *Helicobacter pylori* infection (see below). Other causes are autoimmune gastritis (the cause of pernicious anaemia associated with antibodies to gastric parietal cells and intrinsic factor) and biliary reflux.

Pathology

There is infiltration of the lamina propria with lymphocytes and plasma cells, which over a long period may lead to gastritis with atrophy and subsequent metaplasia.

Clinical features

Chronic gastritis is usually asymptomatic and discovered incidentally, although gastritis may be responsible for dyspepsia in some people.

Management

No specific treatment is usually required.

Helicobacter pylori and the upper gastrointestinal tract

Helicobacter pylori is a Gram-negative urease-producing spiral-shaped bacterium found predominantly in the gastric antrum and in areas of gastric metaplasia in the duodenum. It is closely associated with chronic active gastritis, peptic ulcer disease, and gastric cancer and gastric B-cell lymphoma. Evidence now suggests that some strains of *H. pylori* (CagA-positive strains) may be particularly associated with gastroduodenal disease.

Epidemiology

The incidence of *H. pylori* infection is higher in the older age groups and associated with lower socioeconomic status. Most cases of infection probably occur in childhood, and transmission is most likely via the oral–oral or faecal–oral routes.

Clinicopathological features

Initially *H. pylori* infection produces an acute gastritis which rapidly becomes chronic active gastritis, and in some cases peptic ulcer disease may develop. Long-standing chronic active gastritis leads to atrophy, intestinal metaplasia and an increased risk of gastric carcinoma.

Investigations

Invasive tests (endoscopic antral biopsy)

- Rapid urease test (an antral biopsy which contains *H. pylori* when added to a urea-containing solution breaks

down urea to release ammonia and produces a pH-
dependent colour change in the indicator present)
- Gram stain and culture
- Histology with direct visualization of the organism.

Non-invasive tests

- Urea breath test. ^{13}C (or ^{14}C) labelled urea is given by
  mouth; the detection of ^{13}C in expired air indicates
  infection with urease-producing *H. pylori*. The breath
  test is particularly useful to confirm eradication of the
  organism after appropriate treatment.
- Serological tests detect IgG antibodies to *H. pylori*. They
  are used to diagnose infection but are not useful for
  confirming eradication because patients may have
  antibodies for years after eradication of the organism.

Management

Eradication of *H. pylori* is indicated for all patients with
proven peptic disease. Recurrence is very uncommon in
those in whom the infection is successfully eradicated.
Treatment regimens are evolving, although proton-pump
inhibitor (PPI)-based triple therapy regimens are currently
favoured, e.g.

- PPI (e.g. omeprazole 20 mg) twice daily for 1 week
  Metronidazole 400 mg twice daily for 1 week
  Clarithromycin 250 mg twice daily for 1 week
- PPI (e.g. omeprazole 20 mg) twice daily for 1 week
  Amoxycillin 1 g twice daily for 1 week
  Clarithromycin 500 mg twice daily for 1 week.

Peptic ulcer disease

A peptic ulcer is an ulcer of the mucosa in or adjacent to an
acid-bearing area. Most occur in the stomach or proximal
duodenum.

Epidemiology

Duodenal ulcers are three to four times more common than
gastric ulcers and occur in 15% of the population at some
time. They are more common in men than in women (4:1)
and both are more common in elderly people. There is a
significant geographical variation.

Aetiology

There is an imbalance between acid and pepsin and mucosal defences (mucus, bicarbonate and prostaglandins). *H. pylori* plays a central role, although the mechanisms are unclear (Table 2.2). Genetic factors may have a role to play. NSAIDs are an important cause of gastric ulceration, though less commonly duodenal ulcers. Peptic ulceration is also seen in hyperparathyroidism and the Zollinger–Ellison syndrome.

Table 2.2 Proposed pathogenic mechanisms of *H. pylori*

Increased fasting and meal-stimulated serum gastrin
Decreased somatostatin (D) cells in the antrum
Increased parietal cell mass
Increased pepsinogen-1
Disruption of mucous protective layer
Cytotoxin release

Clinical features

Epigastric pain is the most common presenting symptom. This is typically relieved by antacids but has a variable relationship to food. Duodenal ulcer pain, however, often occurs when the subject is hungry and classically occurs at night. Other symptoms, such as nausea, heartburn and flatulence, may occur. Occasionally ulcers may present with the complications of perforation or painless upper gastrointestinal haemorrhage.

Investigations

Young patients (<45 years) with ulcer type symptoms should undergo screening for *H. pylori* infection by either serology or a breath test; upper gastrointestinal endoscopy is not usually necessary (see management of dyspepsia on page 56). Older patients should undergo endoscopy. In patients found to have a gastric ulcer at endoscopy, multiple biopsies from the centre and edge of the ulcer must be taken, because it is often impossible to distinguish by naked eye a benign from malignant gastric ulcer.

A barium meal is useful if gastric outlet obstruction is suspected.

Management

Ulcers associated with H. pylori Treatment regimens that successfully eradicate *H. pylori* from the gastric antrum result in healing rates of over 90% and prevent recurrence unless reinfection occurs, which is unusual. This approach to treatment is indicated in all patients with *H. pylori*-associated peptic disease.

H. pylori–negative peptic ulcers Most *H. pylori*-negative peptic ulcers are associated with NSAID ingestion. Treatment involves the use of acid-suppressing drugs and stopping the NSAID if at all possible. H_2-receptor antagonists (ranitidine, cimetidine) will heal over 80% of ulcers with a 2-month course of treatment.

Proton pump inhibitors (omeprazole, lansoprazole, pantoprazole) inhibit hydrogen-potassium ATPase (H+/K+ATPase), producing 80–90% inhibition of 24-hour intragastric acidity and almost 100% healing rates after 4 weeks of treatment. Antacids are now usually only prescribed for symptomatic relief of mild episodes of indigestion. If NSAIDs must be continued after ulcer healing, prophylaxis with a PPI or misoprostil (a prostaglandin agonist) is indicated to prevent recurrence.

Follow-up endoscopy plus biopsy should be performed for all gastric ulcers to demonstrate healing and exclude malignancy (initial biopsies may be false negatives).

Surgery With the introduction of modern drugs surgery is rarely performed for peptic ulceration but is reserved for the treatment of complications, namely recurrent haemorrhage, perforation and outflow obstruction.

Complications

Perforation This is becoming less common, partly as a result of the introduction of H_2-receptor antagonists. Duodenal ulcers perforate more commonly than gastric ulcers, usually into the peritoneal cavity. Management is initially surgical, with closure of the perforation and drainage of the abdomen. *H. pylori* should subsequently be eradicated. Conservative treatment with intravenous fluids and antibiotics may be indicated in elderly or very ill patients.

Gastric outlet obstruction Outflow obstruction occurs because of surrounding oedema or scarring following healing. Copious projectile vomiting is the main symptom, and a succussion splash may be detectable clinically. Metabolic alkalosis may develop as a result of loss of acid. Management is initially with nasogastric suction and replacement of fluids and electrolytes. In some cases oedema may settle with conservative management, but treatment with surgery or balloon dilatation is often required.

Haemorrhage – *see below*

Management of dyspepsia in the community

Because significant GI pathology is relatively uncommon in most young people with dyspepsia, and because of the close association of *H. pylori* with peptic disease, most would agree that investigation with endoscopy is not necessary in all patients. Older patients (>45 yr) with persistent dyspepsia should be investigated with a gastroscopy or a barium meal to rule out significant disease, as should all patients with 'alarm symptoms' such as dysphagia, weight loss or gastrointestinal bleeding. In other patients *H. pylori* status should be assessed serologically and, if positive, eradication therapy instituted. Further investigation can then be reserved for those who remain symptomatic or who are *H. pylori* negative on initial testing.

Malignant gastric tumours
Epidemiology

Gastric cancer is the sixth most common fatal cancer in the UK. The incidence increases with age and is more common in men. The frequency varies throughout the world, being more common in Japan and Chile, and relatively less common in the USA. Although the incidence overall is decreasing worldwide, proximal gastric cancers are increasing in frequency.

Aetiology

This is unknown, although there is increasing evidence that *H. pylori* infection plays an important part. Dietary factors, such as alcohol, spiced, salted or pickled foods, and nitrate ingestion may also have a role. Smoking and achlorhydria (e.g. pernicious anaemia) are also significantly associated with gastric cancer.

Pathology

Tumours most commonly occur in the antrum and are almost always adenocarcinomas. They may be localized ulcerated lesions with rolled edges (intestinal type), or more diffuse with extensive submucosal spread, giving the picture of linitus plastica (diffuse type).

Clinical features

Pain similar to peptic ulcer pain is the most common symptom. With more advanced disease, nausea, anorexia and weight loss are common. Vomiting with outflow obstruction occurs if the tumour is near the pylorus, or dysphagia can occur with lesions in the cardia. Almost 50% have a palpable epigastric mass, and a lymph node is sometimes felt in the supraclavicular fossa (Virchow's node). In patients with advanced disease there may be evidence of metastatic spread to the peritoneum and liver, with ascites and hepatomegaly. Skin manifestations of malignancy, such as dermatomyositis and acanthosis nigricans, are occasionally associated.

Investigations

Barium meal or gastroscopy and biopsy are the investigations of choice, biopsy providing histological confirmation. CT, MRI and endoscopic ultrasonography may be useful in staging the tumour and guiding operability.

Management

Surgery is the best form of treatment if the tumour is operable. Chemotherapy has had little impact and is not usually given outside clinical trials.

Prognosis

The overall survival is poor (10% 5-year survival). Those patients undergoing curative operations, however, have a 5-year survival of 50%. In Japan, where the incidence of the disease is high and there is an active screening programme, earlier diagnosis and an aggressive surgical approach have resulted in a 5-year survival of 90%.

Benign gastric tumours

The most common is a leiomyoma, which is usually asymptomatic although it can ulcerate and bleed. Gastric polyps are uncommon and usually regenerative. Adenomatous polyps can occur but are rare.

··

GASTROINTESTINAL BLEEDING

Acute upper gastrointestinal bleeding

Haematemesis is the vomiting of blood. Melaena is the passage of black tarry stools, which is the result of altered blood from the upper intestine (50 ml or more is required to produce melaena).

Aetiology

Chronic peptic ulceration is still the most common cause of upper gastrointestinal bleeding (Figure 2.1). Relative incidences vary according to patient population. Aspirin and NSAIDs may be responsible for bleeding from both duodenal and gastric ulcers, particularly in elderly people. Corticosteroids have been implicated, but in the usual

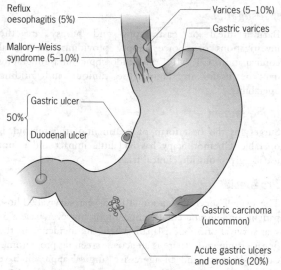

Reflux oesophagitis (5%)

Varices (5–10%)

Gastric varices

Mallory–Weiss syndrome (5–10%)

Gastric ulcer

50% {

Duodenal ulcer

Gastric carcinoma (uncommon)

Acute gastric ulcers and erosions (20%)

Other uncommon causes
Hereditary telangiectasia (Osler–Weber–Rendu syndrome)
Pseudoxanthoma elasticum
Blood dyscrasias
Dieulafoy gastric vascular abnormality

Figure 2.1
Causes of acute upper gastrointestinal haemorrhage.

therapeutic dosage they probably have no relationship to gastrointestinal bleeding.

Management

Resuscitate In many patients no specific treatment is required, bleeding stops spontaneously and the patient remains well compensated. In patients with large bleeds or clinical signs of shock, urgent transfusion, ideally with whole blood, is required (page 442). Monitoring pulse rate and venous pressure will guide transfusion requirements.

Determine site of bleeding This may be evident from the history, e.g. bleeding from a peptic ulcer is suggested by a history of NSAID ingestion or previous peptic ulceration. Mallory–Weiss syndrome (haematemesis from a tear in the oesophagus) is suggested by a history of vomiting preceding the haematemesis. Endoscopy should be performed as soon as possible, and preferably within 24 hours. More urgent endoscopy may be indicated if varices are strongly suspected from the history. Endoscopy can detect the site of haemorrhage in 80% or more of cases.

Specific management A stepwise approach to the management of upper gastrointestinal bleeding is illustrated in Emergency Box 2.1.

At endoscopy varices should be treated with sclerotherapy (injection of a sclerosant, e.g. ethanolamine, directly into or next to the varix) or banding. Ulcers that are actively bleeding or demonstrate stigmata of recent bleeding (a visible vessel or overlying clot) should be treated by injection of dilute adrenaline or coagulated with the heater probe or laser. If no stigmata of recent hemorrhage are present and the patient is haemodynamically stable, confinement in hospital is usually unnecessary. The role of acid-suppressing agents, such as proton pump inhibitors, in the setting of acute peptic bleeding is controversial, although recent data suggest that PPIs may reduce rebleeding rates and transfusion requirements. Surgery may be required for persistent or recurrent bleeding from ulcers. Further management of bleeding varices is described on page 114.

Prognosis

The overall mortality rate is 5–10%. The following are associated with a poor prognosis:

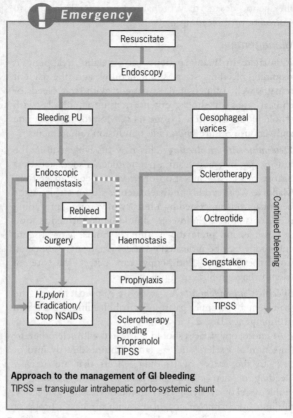

Emergency

Resuscitate

Endoscopy

Bleeding PU   Oesophageal varices

Endoscopic haemostasis

Rebleed   Sclerotherapy

Surgery   Haemostasis   Octreotide

Prophylaxis   Sengstaken

H.pylori Eradication/ Stop NSAIDs

Sclerotherapy Banding Propranolol TIPSS   TIPSS

Continued bleeding

Approach to the management of GI bleeding
TIPSS = transjugular intrahepatic porto-systemic shunt

Emergency Box 2.1
Approach to the management of GI bleeding.

- Old age (>65 years)
- Shock
- Continued bleeding or rebleeding
- Presence of chronic liver disease.

Lower gastrointestinal bleeding

Massive bleeding is rare and usually the result of diverticular disease or ischaemic colitis. Minor bleeds from haemorrhoids are common. The causes are listed in Table 2.3.

Table 2.3 Causes of lower GI bleeding

Haemorrhoids
Carcinoma
Colitis: ulcerative colitis, Crohn's, infective
Angiodysplasia
Colonic diverticulae
Polyps
Meckel's diverticulum
Ischaemic colitis
Anal fissure

Management

With large bleeds resuscitation with intravenous fluids/whole blood may be required. The site of bleeding must then be determined using the following investigations as appropriate:

- Rectal examination, e.g. carcinoma
- Proctoscopy, e.g. haemorrhoids
- Sigmoidoscopy, e.g. inflammatory bowel disease
- Barium enema – any mucosal lesion
- Colonoscopy – diagnosis and removal of polyps
- Angiography – vascular abnormality, e.g. angiodysplasia

Specific management

Lesions should be treated as appropriate.

Chronic gastrointestinal bleeding

Chronic gastrointestinal bleeding usually presents with iron deficiency anaemia and chronic blood loss. Blood loss producing anaemia in all men, and in women after the menopause, is always the result of bleeding from the gastrointestinal tract. The causes of chronic blood loss are those that cause acute bleeding (see Figure 2.1 and Table 2.3). However, oesophageal varices, duodenal ulcers and diverticular disease very rarely bleed chronically.

Investigations

Initial investigations are a 'top and tail', performed at the same endoscopic session, i.e. gastroscopy and colonoscopy.

Further investigations are reserved for difficult cases where the above tests have not identified a source of bleeding:

- Small bowel barium follow-through
- Angiography
- Technetium-labelled red cell scan
- Small bowel enteroscopy.

THE SMALL INTESTINE

The small intestine has a number of functions, many of which are concerned with the digestion and absorption of nutrients. Nutrients are absorbed throughout the small intestine, with the exception of vitamin B_{12} and bile salts, which have specific receptors in the terminal ileum. [CM pages 246–249].

The presenting features of small bowel disease are diarrhoea, steatorrhoea (pale, bulky stools that contain fat), abdominal pain or discomfort, and weight loss, which is the result of accompanying anorexia. The two most common causes of small bowel disease in developed countries are coeliac disease and Crohn's disease. In many small bowel diseases malabsorption of specific substances occurs, but these deficiencies do not dominate the clinical picture. An example is Crohn's disease, in which malabsorption of vitamin B_{12} can be demonstrated, but this is not usually a clinical problem. The major disorders of the small intestine that cause malabsorption are shown in Table 2.4.

Table 2.4 Disorders of the small intestine causing malabsorption

Coeliac disease
Dermatitis herpetiformis
Tropical sprue
Bacterial overgrowth
Intestinal resection
Whipple's disease
Radiation enteritis
Parasite infection, e.g. *Giardia intestinalis*
Crohn's disease

Coeliac disease (gluten-sensitive enteropathy)

Coeliac disease is a condition in which there is an abnormal jejunal mucosa that improves morphologically when the patient is treated with a gluten-free diet and relapses when gluten is reintroduced. Gluten is contained in wheat, rye, barley and possibly oats.

Epidemiology

Worldwide distribution, but it is rare in African people and more common in Ireland (incidence 1 in 300; 1 in 1500 in UK).

Aetiology

The toxic portion of gluten is the peptide gliadin. The exact mechanism by which gluten causes damage to the intestinal mucosa is not known. The strong association with the haplotypes HLA-A1, -B8, -DR3 -DR7 and -DQW2 suggests a possible immunological origin.

Pathology

There are absent small intestinal villi with elongation of crypts (subtotal villous atrophy). There is a chronic inflammatory cell infiltrate in the lamina propria, with an increase in intraepithelial cell lymphocytes [CM page 254].

Clinical features

Coeliac disease can present at any age but there are two peaks in incidence: in infancy, after weaning on to gluten-containing foods, and in adults at 30–40 years. It often presents with non-specific symptoms of tiredness and malaise, or symptoms of small intestinal disease (see above).

Physical signs are usually few and non-specific, and related to anaemia and nutritional deficiency. There is an increased incidence of atopy and autoimmune disease.

Investigations

Jejunal mucosal biopsy obtained via the endoscope. The mucosa shows the histological features described above. Other causes of a flat mucosa (Table 2.5) are rare in adults.

Table 2.5 Causes of villous atrophy in adults

Coeliac disease
Dermatitis herpetiformis
Giardiasis
Malnutrition
Ischaemia
Lymphoma
Whipple's disease
Tropical sprue

Serum antibodies Antigliadin, antireticulin, and antiendo-mysial antibodies are present in most cases.

Blood count A mild anaemia is present in 50% of cases. There is almost always folate deficiency, commonly iron deficiency and, rarely, vitamin B_{12} deficiency.

Radiology Small bowel follow-through may show a dilated bowel with thickened folds.

Management

Treatment is with a gluten-free diet, which should be continued lifelong. A repeat biopsy after treatment shows morphological improvement in the mucosa and confirms the diagnosis.

Complications

There is an increased incidence of malignancy, particularly intestinal lymphoma, small bowel cancer and oesophageal cancer.

Dermatitis herpetiformis

Dermatitis herpetiformis is an itchy, symmetrical eruption of vesicles and crusts over the extensor surfaces of the body. Most patients also have a gluten-sensitive enteropathy, which is usually asymptomatic. The skin condition responds to dapsone, but both the gut and the skin will improve on a gluten-free diet.

Tropical sprue

Tropical sprue is a chronic, progressive small intestinal disorder presenting with malabsorption which occurs in residents or visitors to a tropical area where the disease is endemic (Asia, some Caribbean islands, Puerto Rico, parts of South America).

Aetiology

The aetiology is unknown but the disease occurs in epidemics and improves with antibiotics, suggesting an infectious aetiology.

Clinical features

The disease may present many years after being in the tropics. There is diarrhoea, anorexia and abdominal distension. Nutritional deficiencies develop over a variable period of time.

Investigations

Malabsorption should be demonstrated, particularly of fat and vitamin B_{12} The intestinal mucosa shows villous atrophy affecting the whole small bowel. It is necessary to exclude infective causes of diarrhoea, particularly *Giardia intestinalis*.

Management

Treatment is with a combination of folic acid and tetracycline, which may be required for up to 6 months. Nutritional deficiencies must also be corrected.

Bacterial overgrowth

The upper small intestine is almost sterile. Bacterial overgrowth may occur when there is stasis of intestinal contents as a result of abnormal motility, e.g. systemic sclerosis or a structural abnormality, e.g. diverticulum.

Clinical features

There may be diarrhoea and/or steatorrhoea caused by the deconjugation of bile salts by bacteria. Vitamin B_{12} deficiency, resulting from its metabolism by bacteria, can also occur.

Diagnosis

Breath tests The hydrogen or ^{14}C breath tests are the investigations of choice. These depend on the ability of the organisms to metabolize either glucose or labelled bile salts, given by mouth, with the production of either hydrogen (from glucose) or $^{14}CO_2$ (from bile salts), which are then absorbed and can be measured in the exhaled air.

Proximal small intestinal aspirates Proximal small intestinal aspirates (obtained via the endoscope or by a peroral tube) will reveal high numbers of coliforms and *Bacteroides* sp.

Management

If possible the underlying cause should be corrected. This may not be possible and rotating courses of antibiotics are then necessary, such as tetracycline and metronidazole.

Whipple's disease

Whipple's disease is a rare systemic disease which almost always involves the small intestine. Common clinical features include steatorrhoea, abdominal pain, fever, lymphadenopathy, arthritis and neurological involvement. Intestinal biopsy shows PAS-positive macrophages. On electron microscopy the macrophages are seen to contain bacteria called *Tropheryma whippei*. Treatment of the disease is with antibiotics.

Intestinal resection

The effects of small intestinal resection depend on the extent and the area involved. Resection of the terminal ileum leads to malabsorption of:

- Vitamin B_{12}, leading to megaloblastic anaemia
- Bile salts, which overflow into the colon and interfere with salt and water absorption, producing diarrhoea. Bile salts in the colon also increase oxalate absorption, which may result in renal oxalate stones (page 291).

If there is extensive resection increased hepatic bile salt synthesis cannot compensate for faecal loss and there is steatorrhoea secondary to bile salt deficiency. After massive intestinal resection there is severe loss of water and electrolytes, with malnutrition.

Miscellaneous intestinal conditions [CM page 258].

Tuberculosis (TB)

This results from reactivation of the primary disease caused by *Mycobacterium tuberculosis* (page 418) and is most commonly seen in Asian immigrants. The ileocaecal valve is the most common site affected.

Clinical features

There is abdominal pain, diarrhoea, anorexia, weight loss and fever. A mass may be palpable. The symptoms, signs and radiology (see below) can be similar to those of Crohn's disease, and TB must always be considered in the differential diagnosis of Asians presenting with apparent Crohn's disease.

Diagnosis

Radiology The chest radiograph will show evidence of pulmonary tuberculosis in 50% of cases. The small bowel follow-through may show features similar to those of

Crohn's disease (page 72). Abdominal ultrasonography shows mesenteric thickening and lymphadenopathy.

Endoscopy Colonoscopy with terminal ileal biopsies is usually performed. It is not always possible to obtain bacteriological confirmation on tissue culture, and treatment is started if there is a high degree of suspicion.

Surgery Laparotomy is rarely needed for diagnosis.

Management

Treatment is similar to that for pulmonary tuberculosis, i.e. isoniazid, rifampicin and pyrazinamide, although 1 year's treatment is required.

Protein-losing enteropathy

This involves increased protein loss across an abnormal intestinal mucosa. If there is inadequate hepatic synthesis of albumin to compensate for the intestinal loss, patients develop hypoalbuminaemia and oedema. Causes include Crohn's disease, Ménétrièr's disease (thickening and enlargement of gastric folds), coeliac disease and lymphatic disorders, e.g. lymphangiectasia.

Meckel's diverticulum

This is a congenital abnormality affecting 2–3% of the population. A diverticulum projects from the wall of the ileum approximately 60 cm from the ileocaecal valve. About half will contain gastric mucosa which secretes acid, and peptic ulceration may occur, with complications of bleeding or perforation. Diverticula may also become inflamed and present similar to appendicitis. Treatment is surgical removal.

Chronic intestinal ischaemia

This is rare and results from atheromatous occlusion of mesenteric vessels in elderly people. The characteristic symptom is abdominal pain occurring after food. Diagnosis is made using angiography.

Malignant small intestinal tumours

These are rare and present with abdominal pain, diarrhoea, anorexia and anaemia. Carcinoid tumours have additional clinical features, described below.

Carcinoid tumours

Pathology

These originate from argentaffin cells (serotonin producing) of the intestine. The most common sites are the appendix, terminal ileum and rectum. Carcinoid tumours produce serotonin (5-hydroxytryptamine, or 5-HT), kinins, histamine and a variety of other hormones that are metabolized by the liver.

Clinical features

In the presence of liver metastases tumour products are able to drain directly into the hepatic vein (without being metabolized) and then into the systemic circulation, where they produce a variety of effects resulting in the carcinoid syndrome: flushing, wheezing, diarrhoea and abdominal pain, and right-sided cardiac valvular fibrosis causing stenosis and regurgitation.

Investigations

A high level of 5-hydroxyindole acetic acid (5-HIAA), the breakdown product of serotonin, is found in the urine and this is useful in diagnosing carcinoid syndrome. Ultrasonography examination of the liver confirms the presence of secondary deposits.

Management

Treatment is symptomatic and aimed at:

- Reducing tumour mass through surgical resection, hepatic artery embolization or chemotherapy
- Inhibition of tumour products with 5-HT antagonists, e.g. cyproheptadine or octreotide (a long-acting somatostatin analogue).

Adenocarcinoma

Adenocarcinoma accounts for 50% of malignant small bowel tumours; there is an increased incidence in coeliac disease and Crohn's disease.

Lymphoma

Non-Hodgkin's lymphoma constitutes 15% of malignant small bowel tumours and may be B cell or T cell in origin.

The latter occur with increased frequency in coeliac disease.

Benign small bowel tumours

- The Peutz–Jegher syndrome is an autosomal dominant condition with mucocutaneous pigmentation (circumoral, hands and feet) and hamartomatous gastrointestinal polyps. Polyps may occur anywhere in the gastrointestinal tract, but are most common in the small bowel. They may bleed or cause intussusception, and virtually never become malignant.
- Adenomas, leiomyomas and lipomas are rare. They are usually asymptomatic and discovered incidentally.
- Familial adenomatous polyposis (page 78).

INFLAMMATORY BOWEL DISEASE

Two main forms are recognized: Crohn's disease, which affects any part of the gastrointestinal tract, and ulcerative colitis (UC), which affects the large bowel only.

Epidemiology

Inflammatory bowel disease (IBD) is more common in the western world, occurring at any age but most commonly between the ages of 20 and 40 years. Both sexes are affected, but UC is more common in women. In western populations the prevalence of UC is approximately 1 in 1000 and of Crohn's disease 1 in 1500 of the population.

Aetiology

It is probable that environmental factors operate in a genetically predisposed individual.

Environmental

- *Infective agents* Measles virus and *Mycobacterium paratuberculosis* have been put forward as possible causes of Crohn's disease, but a causal relationship has not been established.
- *Smoking* Crohn's disease is more common in smokers and UC less common. In Crohn's disease smoking doubles the risk of postoperative recurrence.

- *Other factors*, such as oral contraceptive use and ingestion of refined sugar, have been associated with IBD in some studies.

Genetic There is a familial tendency in both UC and Crohn's disease; twin studies suggest a stronger genetic influence in Crohn's disease than UC. A susceptibility locus on chromosome 16 has been demonstrated for Crohn's disease, but this is likely to be one of many genes that confer susceptibility. There is an increased incidence of HLA-B27 in inflammatory bowel disease with ankylosing spondylitis.

Pathology

UC and Crohn's disease have important differences both macroscopically and microscopically (Table 2.6).

Table 2.6 Histological differences between Crohn's disease and ulcerative colitis

	Crohn's disease	Ulcerative colitis
Macroscopic	Affects any part of the gut from mouth to anus	Affects only the colon. Begins in the rectum and extends proximally in varying degrees
	Discontinuous involvement ('skip lesions')	Continuous involvement
	Deep ulcers and fissures in the mucosa: 'cobblestone appearance'	Red mucosa which bleeds easily Ulcers and pseudopolyps (regenerating mucosa) in severe disease
Microscopic	Transmural inflammation Granulomata ++	Mucosal inflammation No granulomata but goblet cell depletion and crypt abscesses

Clinical features

Crohn's disease is a progressive chronic disease with symptomatology depending on the region(s) of involved bowel; the commonest site is ileocaecal (in 40% of patients). The main feature in patients with small bowel disease is abdominal pain, usually with weight loss. Less commonly terminal ileal disease presents as an acute abdomen with right iliac fossa pain mimicking appendicitis. Colonic disease presents with diarrhoea, bleeding and pain related to defecation. In perianal disease there are anal tags, fissures, fistulae and abscess formation.

UC presents with diarrhoea, often containing blood and mucus. The clinical course may be one of persistent diarrhoea, relapses and remissions, or severe fulminating colitis (Table 2.7).

Patients with inflammatory bowel disease, particularly Crohn's disease, may have one or more extraintestinal manifestations, and these are listed in Table 2.8.

Table 2.7 Definition of a severe attack of ulcerative colitis

Bloody diarrhoea	>6/day
Fever	>37.5°C
Tachycardia	>90/min
ESR	>30 mm/h
Anaemia	Hb <10 g/dl
Serum albumin	<30 g/l

Table 2.8 Extragastrointestinal manifestations of inflammatory bowel disease

Eyes	Uveitis, episcleritis, conjunctivitis
Joints	Monoarticular arthritis (knees and ankles), ankylosing spondylitis,* sacroileitis
Skin	Erythema nodosum, pyoderma gangrenosum (necrotizing ulceration of the skin, commonly on the lower legs)
Liver*†	Fatty change, sclerosing cholangitis, chronic hepatitis, cirrhosis
Calculi*	Increased incidence of gallbladder and renal calculi
Vasculitis	(Rare)
Amyloidosis	(Rare)

* These manifestations are not related to disease activity.
† Biochemical abnormalities are common; clinically overt disease is uncommon.

Investigations

The purpose of investigations is to define the nature of the disease and the extent and severity of bowel involvement.

Blood count Anaemia is common and usually the normochromic/normocytic anaemia of chronic disease, although iron deficiency anaemia may occur. The platelet count, ESR and C-reactive protein are often raised, and the serum albumin may be low in severe disease.

Radiology In Crohn's disease a small bowel follow-through shows an asymmetrical alteration in the mucosal pattern, with deep ulceration and areas of narrowing (string sign) largely confined to the ileum. Skip lesions may be seen. A barium enema may demonstrate aphthous ulceration or deeper ulceration in the colon. Ultrasonography and CT scanning are particularly helpful in delineating abscesses, and will show thickened bowel in involved areas. MRI may be useful in perianal disease.

In UC a barium enema shows the extent of disease, and in long-standing disease the colon is shortened and narrowed. A plain radiograph should be performed during a severe attack to look for toxic dilatation of the colon.

Endoscopy Rigid or flexible sigmoidoscopy will establish the diagnosis of UC and, less commonly, Crohn's disease. A rectal biopsy can be taken for histological examination to determine the nature of the inflammation. Colonoscopy allows the exact extent and severity of colonic and terminal ileal inflammation to be determined, and biopsies can be taken.

Differential diagnosis

Crohn's disease must be differentiated from other causes of chronic diarrhoea, malabsorption and malnutrition. In children it is a cause of short stature. Other causes of terminal ileitis are TB and *Yersinia enterocolitica* infection (causing an acute illness). Inflammatory bowel disease affecting the colon must be differentiated from other causes of colitis: infection (page 24), ischaemia and microscopic colitis (macroscopically normal mucosa but inflammation detected histologically).

Management (Table 2.9)

Medical
Patients with Crohn's disease who smoke should be advised to stop, as this will decrease the number of relapses and reduce postoperative recurrence.

- 5-aminosalicylic acid (5-ASA) preparations (mesalazine, olsalazine, balsalazide) will induce a remission in mild

Table 2.9 Summary of treatments used in IBD

Treatment of the acute attack
5-aminosalicyclic acid preparations*
Corticosteroids
Elemental diet
Metronidazole*
Methotrexate
Cyclosporin
Azathioprine*

* Also used to maintain a remission

attacks of UC and in colonic Crohn's disease. In lower doses they are useful as a maintenance treatment to reduce the number of relapses. 5-ASA preparations can also be administered as an enema or suppository to treat proctosigmoiditis (i.e. inflammation of the rectum and sigmoid colon).

- Corticosteroids: oral steroids are used to treat acute attacks and the dose is tailed off as symptoms improve. In severe attacks intravenous steroids are necessary (Emergency Box 2.2). Proctosigmoiditis can be treated locally with steroid enemas and suppositories. Budesonide is a topically acting steroid which is poorly absorbed from the gastrointestinal tract and has fewer systemic effects than other steroids. A coated preparation

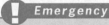 **Emergency**

Admit to hospital

Investigations
Full blood count, C-reactive protein
Serum albumin
Serum urea and electrolytes
Blood cultures (Gram-negative sepsis is common)
Plain abdominal radiograph looking for toxic dilatation (diameter, colon >5 cm) mucosal islands, and/or perforation
Stool cultures (×3) to exclude coincidental infection

Treatment
Intravenous steroids: hydrocortisone 100 mg 6-hourly
Correct electrolyte and fluid imbalance
Consider i.v. cyclosporin in patients not responding to steroids

Emergency box 2.2
Management of acute severe colitis

allows delayed release of the drug after oral administration, and is used in the treatment of mild/moderate ileocaecal Crohn's disease.

- Azathioprine is used in patients with Crohn's disease and UC who continue to have frequent relapses despite taking an adequate dose of 5-ASAs.
- An elemental diet (liquid preparation of amino acids, glucose and fatty acids) will induce a remission in a relapse of small bowel Crohn's disease. The exact mode of action is not known. These diets are unpalatable and often have to be given via a nasogastric tube.
- Metronidazole is useful in severe perianal Crohn's disease resulting from its antibacterial action.
- Methotrexate is used in the minority of patients with active Crohn's disease which is resistant to conventional treatment with steroids. The long-term efficacy of this treatment is not known.
- Cyclosporin is occasionally used in patients with severe acute UC who fail to improve after treatment with intravenous steroids. The management of severe colitis is summarized in Emergency Box 2.2. Management should be in conjunction with the appropriate surgical team because patients not responding to medical therapy will need to undergo colectomy.

Surgery
Surgery is indicated for:

- Failure of medical therapy
- Complications (Table 2.10)
- Failure to grow in children.

In Crohn's disease resections are kept to a minimum as recurrence is almost inevitable in the remaining bowel. In some patients with small bowel disease, strictures can be widened (strictuloplasty) without resection. Mesalazine, commenced postoperatively and continued as prophylaxis, has been shown to reduce the recurrence rate after surgery
The surgical options in ulcerative colitis are:

- Ileoanal anastomosis, in which the terminal ileum is used to form a reservoir (a 'pouch') and the patient is continent with a few bowel motions per day. The pouch may become inflamed ('pouchitis'), leading to bloody diarrhoea which is treated initially with metronidazole.

- Panproctocolectomy with ileostomy (the whole colon and rectum is removed and the ileum brought out on to the abdominal wall as a stoma).
- Colectomy with an ileorectal anastomosis (diseased rectum left in situ and diarrhoea may still occur).

Table 2.10 Complications of inflammatory bowel disease

Toxic dilatation + perforation
Stricture formation
Abscess formation (Crohn's disease)
Fistulae and fissures (Crohn's)
Cancer: in UC the risk of colon cancer increases with extent and duration of disease (30% after 30 years of total colitis). The risk of colon cancer is also increased in patients with colonic Crohn's disease

Prognosis

Both diseases are characterized by relapses and remissions. Almost all patients with Crohn's disease have a significant relapse over a 20-year period. The mortality rate is twice as high as that of the general population. The prognosis of ulcerative colitis is variable. Only 10% of patients with proctitis develop more extensive disease, but with severe fulminant disease the mortality rate is 15–25%.

THE COLON AND RECTUM

Diverticular disease

Pouches of mucosa extrude through the muscular wall through weakened areas near blood vessels to form diverticula. The term diverticulosis means the presence of diverticula. Diverticulitis implies inflammation, which occurs when faeces obstruct the neck of the diverticulum. Diverticula are common, affecting 50% of the population over 50 years of age.

Aetiology

The precise cause of diverticular disease is unknown, although it appears to be related to the low-fibre diet eaten in western populations. It is thought that insufficient dietary fibre leads to increased intracolonic pressure, which causes herniation of the mucosa at sites of weakness.

Clinical features

It is asymptomatic in 90% and usually discovered incidentally when a barium enema or colonoscopy is performed for other reasons. Symptoms are usually the result of bleeding or acute diverticulitis (left iliac fossa pain, fever, nausea, vomiting). Complications include abscess formation, perforation, fistula formation and intestinal obstruction. Acute diverticulitis is diagnosed by CT scan or in some cases by ultrasound.

Management

Acute attacks are treated with antibiotics (ciprofloxacin and metronidazole). Surgery is indicated rarely for complications and for frequent attacks of diverticulitis.

Constipation (Table 2.11)

This is a very common problem in the general population, and often requires no more than dietary advice and reassurance. It is particularly common in elderly people, in whom it is often associated with immobility and poor diet, and in young women in whom it may be associated with slow colonic transit or postpartum pelvic floor abnormalities. Most have simple constipation associated with low fibre intake. Colorectal cancer should always be excluded in middle-aged and elderly people.

Table 2.11 Causes of constipation

Simple
Bowel obstruction e.g. by colon cancer
Painful anal conditions
Drugs, e.g. opiates, aluminium antacids
Hypothyroidism
Depression
Immobility
Hirschsprung's disease

Management

A high-fibre diet and bulking agents should be the first line of treatment. Laxatives should only be used as a short-term treatment.

Miscellaneous conditions

Megacolon

This term describes a number of conditions in which the colon is dilated. The most common cause is chronic constipation. Other causes are Chagas' disease and Hirschsprung's disease (congenital aganglionic segment in the rectum). Treatment is similar to that for simple constipation, although Hirschsprung's disease responds to surgical resection.

Ischaemic colitis

This usually presents in the older age groups, with abdominal pain and rectal bleeding, and occasionally shock. Sigmoidoscopy is often normal apart from blood. Treatment is symptomatic, although surgery may be required for gangrene, perforation or stricture formation.

Colon polyps and the polyposis syndromes

A polyp is an elevation above the mucosal surface. They may be single or multiple, are usually asymptomatic and are almost always adenomas (70–80%). In the polyposis syndromes hundreds of polyps may be present.

Hamartomatous polyps Hamartomas are benign tumours composed of an overgrowth of mature cells and tissues that normally occur in the affected part, in this case the colon. They may be one of two types:

- *Juvenile polyps* These are dominantly inherited polyps which occur in children and teenagers, and present early with diarrhoea, bleeding or intussusception.
- *Peutz–Jeghers polyps* Peutz–Jeghers syndrome is a dominantly inherited condition consisting of mucocutaneous pigmentation, and multiple polyps in the large and small bowel, which rarely undergo malignant change.

Adenomatous polyps Adenomatous polyps are tumours of benign neoplastic epithelium. They are common, occurring in about 10% of the population. The aetiology is unknown, although genetic and environmental factors have been implicated. They rarely produce symptoms, although large polyps can bleed or cause anaemia, and villous adenomas can occasionally present with diarrhoea and hypokalaemia. Adenomatous polyps carry a malignant risk which increases with polyp size. Treatment is by endoscopic removal.

Familial adenomatous polyposis (FAP) This is an autosomal dominantly inherited condition in which individuals usually develop hundreds of adenomatous polyps throughout the gastrointestinal tract at an early age, resulting inevitably in colon cancer unless the large bowel is removed. The gene responsible for FAP, known as the APC gene, is located on the long arm of chromosome 5. Gene testing is offered to unaffected members of FAP families to establish whether or not they carry the gene. Many of these patients have congenital hypertrophy of the retinal pigment epithelium (CHRPE) and this, along with genetic analysis, facilitates screening of young patients. Carriers of the gene are counselled and offered prophylactic colectomy in young adulthood. After colectomy these patients remain at risk of small bowel cancer, particularly of the duodenum.

Colorectal cancer

Most colorectal cancers occur sporadically. In 5–10% of patients they occur in patients with HNPCC (see page 80) or FAP. Colorectal cancer may also occur on a background of long-standing UC or colonic Crohn's disease.

Sporadic colorectal cancer

Epidemiology

This is the second most common tumour in the UK, and the incidence increases with age: most patients are over 50. Colon cancer is rare in Africa and Asia, largely because of environmental differences. A diet high in meat and animal fat and low in fibre is thought to be an important aetiological factor. In the west, the lifetime risk is 1 in 50, increasing to 1 in 20 in those with one affected first-degree relative.

Inheritance

Multiple molecular genetic abnormalities are now thought to be involved in the development of sporadic colon cancer.

These include the activation of tumour-promoting genes or oncogenes (c-*Ki-ras*, c-*myc*) and the inactivation of tumour suppressor genes (*MCC, DCC, p53*). The risk of a tumour developing increases with increasing number of genetic abnormalities.

Pathology

It is likely that most carcinomas (other than on a background of IBD) start as a benign adenoma, the so-called 'adenoma–carcinoma' sequence. Spread is by direct invasion through the bowel wall, with later invasion of blood vessels and lymphatics and spread to the liver. The mortality of colorectal cancer is directly related to the stage at presentation, and the stage is most commonly classified according to the modified Dukes' classification (Table 2.12). Synchronous (i.e. more than one tumour) tumours are present in 2% of cases.

Table 2.12 Modified Dukes' grading of colon cancer

Dukes' A	Tumour confined to the bowel wall
Dukes' B	Tumour extending through the bowel wall
Dukes' C	Regional lymph nodes involved
Dukes' D	Distant metastases

Clinical features

Most tumours are in the left side of the colon. They cause rectal bleeding and stenosis, with symptoms of increasing intestinal obstruction such as an alteration in bowel habit and colicky abdominal pain. Carcinoma of the caecum and ascending colon often presents with iron deficiency anaemia or a right iliac fossa mass. Clinical examination is usually unhelpful, although a mass may be palpable transabdominally or in the rectum. Hepatomegaly may be present with liver metastases.

Investigation

Examination of the colon is performed with a double-contrast barium enema or colonoscopy. A full blood count may show anaemia, and abnormal serum liver biochemistry suggests the presence of liver secondaries. Faecal occult blood tests have been used in population screening studies but are not of value diagnostically.

Management

Treatment is surgical, with tumour resection and end-to-end anastomosis of bowel if possible. Adjuvant chemotherapy with 5-fluorouracil and levamisole increases survival in Dukes' grade C cases, and in some cases with Dukes' B cancer. Patients with up to two or three liver metastases confined to one lobe of the liver may be offered hepatic resection. Patients who have multiple hepatic metastases which cannot be resected may benefit from chemotherapy, which increases median survival and improves quality of life.

Prognosis

The overall 5-year survival rate is 40%, but is over 95% in tumours confined to the bowel wall (Dukes' grade A).

Screening

High-risk individuals should be offered screening colonoscopy. Mass population screening of the over-50s with faecal occult blood tests or sigmoidoscopy has been shown to reduce the mortality from colon cancer, but this strategy has not yet been widely adopted because of the cost implications and the relatively poor uptake by healthy individuals.

Hereditary non-polyposis colorectal cancer (HNPCC)

HNPCC has an autosomal dominant mode of transmission with incomplete penetrance. It results from a mutation in one of the four known DNA mismatch repair genes located on chromosomes 2, 3 and 7, which in turn leads to widespread genomic instability. These patients have an increased risk of developing tumours at an early age, and more often develop right-sided tumours. Many of these patients also have an increased incidence of gynaecological and other malignancies.

....

DIARRHOEA

True diarrhoea is defined as an increase in stool weight to more than 300 g in 24 hours. This must be differentiated from the frequent passage of small amounts of stool (usually functional), and this is achieved with a 3-day stool collection for faecal weight. Acute diarrhoea is usually due to infection or dietary indiscretion; chronic diarrhoea is defined as diarrhoea persisting for more than 14 days.

There are four main mechanisms: osmotic, secretory, abnormal motility.

Osmotic diarrhoea

This occurs when there are large quantities of non-absorbed hypertonic substances in the bowel lumen. The diarrhoea stops when the patient stops eating or the malabsorptive substance is discontinued. The causes of osmotic diarrhoea are as follows:

- Ingestion of non-absorbable substance, e.g. magnesium sulphate
- Generalized malabsorption
- Specific malabsorptive defect, e.g. disaccharidase deficiency.

Secretory diarrhoea

Secretory diarrhoea results from the net secretion of fluid and electrolytes into the bowel lumen, and continues when the patient fasts. The causes are:
- Inflammation, e.g. ulcerative colitis, Crohn's disease
- Infection, e.g. shigella, salmonella
- Enterotoxins, e.g. from *E. coli*, cholera toxin
- Hormone-secreting tumours, e.g. VIPoma (page 140)
- Bile salts (in the colon) following ileal resection
- Fatty acids (in the colon) following ileal resection
- Some laxatives.

Motility related

Abnormal motility often produces frequency rather than true diarrhoea. Causes are thyrotoxicosis, diabetic autonomic neuropathy and post-vagotomy.

Investigation

Acute diarrhoea lasting a few days is the result of dietary indiscretion or an infection. Investigation is not needed and treatment is symptomatic to maintain hydration. Chronic diarrhoea always requires investigation. Figure 2.2 outlines an approach to the investigation of a patient with chronic diarrhoea. Laxative abuse, usually seen in young females, must be excluded as a cause of chronic diarrhoea. Patients taking anthraquinone purgatives, e.g. Senokot, develop pigmentation of the colonic mucosa (melanosis coli) which may be seen at sigmoidoscopy. Other laxatives may be detected in the stool or urine.

Diarrhoea is a common problem in patients with AIDS, resulting either from a specific AIDS enteropathy or from an infection (cryptosporidia, microsporidia, cytomegalo-virus infection).

FUNCTIONAL BOWEL DISEASE

This is a general term used to embrace two syndromes:

• Non-ulcer dyspepsia
• Irritable bowel syndrome.

These conditions are extremely common worldwide, accounting for 60–70% of patients seen in the gastroenterology clinic. The two conditions overlap, with some symptoms being common to both.

Non-ulcer dyspepsia
Clinical features
There are a variety of symptoms, which are usually stress related. Common symptoms include indigestion, wind, nausea, early satiety and heartburn. Symptoms are sometimes very similar to peptic ulceration.

Investigation

This is frequently unnecessary, particularly in young people, but may be necessary to exclude peptic disease (see page 53).

Management

This is mainly by reassurance. Antacids and H_2-receptor antagonists are rarely of benefit. The prokinetic agents cisapride and metaclopramide are sometimes helpful, particularly in those with fullness and bloating.

An Approach to the Investigation of Chronic Diarrhoea

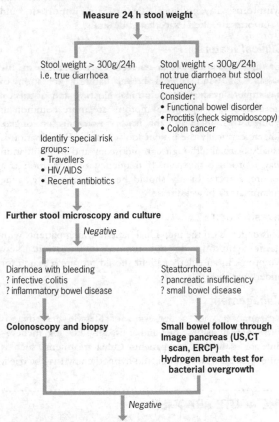

Perform outpatient sigmoidoscopy & biopsy, stool cultures.
If negative: Does the patient have 'true' diarrhoea?

Measure 24 h stool weight

Stool weight > 300g/24h
i.e. true diarrhoea

Stool weight < 300g/24h
not true diarrhoea but stool
frequency
Consider:
• Functional bowel disorder
• Proctitis (check sigmoidoscopy)
• Colon cancer

Identify special risk
groups:
• Travellers
• HIV/AIDS
• Recent antibiotics

Further stool microscopy and culture

Negative

Diarrhoea with bleeding
? infective colitis
? inflammatory bowel disease

Steattorrhoea
? pancreatic insufficiency
? small bowel disease

Colonoscopy and biopsy

**Small bowel follow through
Image pancreas (US,CT
scan, ERCP)
Hydrogen breath test for
bacterial overgrowth**

Negative

**Neuroendocrine evaluation: Serum gastrin, VIP, calcitonin,
urine 5-HIAA**
Consider factitious diarrhoea: e.g. ingestion of laxatives
**Determine if diarrhoea decreases with fasting (i.e. suggests
osmotic diarrhoea) and iv fluid replacement**

VIP = vasoactive intestinal polypeptide
5-HIAA = 5-hydroxyindoleacetic acid

Figure 2.2
An approach to the investigation of chronic diarrhoea.

Irritable bowel syndrome

Aetiology

The aetiology is unknown. Abnormalities in gut motility have been found but these do not always correlate with symptoms. Psychological factors are important, and symptoms are often exacerbated by stress.

Clinical features

Crampy abdominal pain relieved by defecation or the passage of wind, altered bowel habit, a sensation of incomplete evacuation, abdominal bloating and distension are common symptoms. Symptoms are more common in women than men, and the history is usually prolonged. Characteristically the patient looks healthy. Examination is usually normal, although sigmoidoscopy and air insufflation may reproduce the pain. If frequency of defecation is a feature, a rectal biopsy should be performed to exclude inflammatory bowel disease.

Investigation

This depends on the individual patient. Young patients with classic symptoms do not require investigation. New symptoms in an elderly patient should prompt a search for underlying disease.

Management

Reassurance, with a discussion of lifestyle and diet, is valuable. A high-fibre diet and antispasmodics, e.g. mebeverine, are useful in some patients. Other treatments, such as antidepressants, biofeedback and hypnotherapy, may be tried.

....

THE ACUTE ABDOMEN

This section deals with acute abdominal conditions that cause patients to be hospitalized within a few hours of the onset of their pain. Most are admitted under the care of the surgical team, and some will need a laparotomy. Medical conditions that may present as an acute abdomen include diabetic ketoacidosis, myocardial infarction and pneumonia. The irritable bowel syndrome may also present with acute severe abdominal pain.

History

A detailed history, which should include gynaecological symptoms, will often point to the cause of the pain.

- Acute abdominal pain may be intermittent or continuous. Intermittent (colicky) pain describes pain that occurs for a short period (usually a few minutes) and is interspersed with pain-free periods lasting a few minutes or up to half an hour. This is characteristic of mechanical obstruction of a hollow viscus, e.g. ureteric calculus or bowel obstruction (Table 2.13). Additional symptoms of bowel obstruction, which may or may not be present, are abdominal distension, vomiting and absolute constipation (i.e. failure to pass flatus or stool). Biliary pain (previously called biliary colic) resulting from obstruction of the gallbladder or bile duct is not colicky but usually a constant upper abdominal pain.

Table 2.13 Causes of mechanical intestinal obstruction

Constriction from the outside	Bowel entrapped in a hernia
	Adhesions
	Volvulus, particularly of the sigmoid
Disease of the bowel wall	Crohn's disease
	Carcinoma
	Diverticular disease
Intraluminal obstruction	Foreign body
	Gallstones

Continuous pain is constant with no periods of complete relief. It occurs in many abdominal conditions.

- The onset of pain may be sudden or gradual. Sudden onset suggests perforation of a viscus (e.g. duodenal ulcer), rupture of an organ (e.g. aortic aneurysm) or torsion (e.g. ovarian cyst). The pain of acute pancreatitis often begins suddenly.
- The site of the pain must be noted. In general, upper abdominal pain is produced by pathology of either the upper abdominal viscera – e.g. acute cholecystitis, acute pancreatitis – or the stomach and duodenum. The pain of small bowel obstruction is often in the centre of the

abdomen. A common cause of acute right iliac fossa pain is acute appendicitis.

- Radiation of pain to the back suggests acute pancreatitis, rupture of an aortic aneurysm or renal tract disease.

Examination

A general physical examination should be made and the following points noted:

- The presence of shock (pale cool peripheries, tachycardia, hypotension) suggests rupture of an organ, e.g aortic aneurysm, ruptured ectopic pregnancy. It may also occur in the later stages of generalized peritonitis resulting from bowel perforation (see below).
- Fever is common in acute inflammatory conditions.
- Peritonitis and bowel obstruction produce specific signs on abdominal examination.

The signs of peritonitis are tenderness, guarding and rigidity on palpation. Guarding is an involuntary contraction of the abdominal muscles when the abdomen is palpated. Peritonitis may be localized or generalized (see below). Bowel sounds are absent with generalized peritonitis.

Mechanical bowel obstruction produces distension and active 'tinkling' bowel sounds. A strangulated hernia may produce obstruction, and the hernial orifices must always be examined.

In most cases a rectal and pelvic examination should be performed.

Investigations

- Blood tests. The white cell count may be raised in inflammatory conditions. The serum amylase may be raised in any acute abdomen, but levels greater than five times normal indicate acute pancreatitis.
- Radiology. An erect chest radiograph may show air under the diaphragm with a perforated viscus. A plain abdominal radiograph shows dilated loops of bowel and fluid levels in obstruction. Ultrasound examination is

useful in the diagnosis of acute cholangitis, appendicitis and gynaecological conditions.
• Surgery. Laparoscopy or laparotomy may often be required, depending on the diagnosis.

Acute appendicitis

Acute appendicitis occurs when the lumen of the appendix becomes obstructed by a faecolith.

Epidemiology

It affects all age groups but is rare in the very young and very old.

Clinical features

The typical clinical presentation is the onset of central abdominal pain which then becomes localized to the right iliac fossa (RIF), accompanied by anorexia and sometimes vomiting and diarrhoea. The patient is pyrexial, with tenderness and guarding in the RIF.

Investigations

In many cases the diagnosis is clinical. There is a raised white cell count and ultrasonography may show an inflamed appendix. CT is being used more frequently to make the diagnosis.

Management

The treatment is surgical, with removal of the appendix. This is now sometimes performed via the laparoscope.

Complications

These arise from gangrene and perforation, leading to localized abscess formation or generalized peritonitis.

Acute peritonitis

Localized peritonitis occurs with all acute inflammatory conditions of the gastrointestinal tract, and management depends on the underlying condition, e.g. acute appendicitis, acute cholecystitis.

Generalized peritonitis occurs as a result of rupture of an abdominal viscus, e.g. perforated duodenal ulcer, perforated appendix. There is a sudden onset of abdominal pain which rapidly becomes generalized. The patient is shocked and lies still, as movement exacerbates the pain. A plain abdominal radiograph shows air under the diaphragm; serum amylase must be checked to exclude acute pancreatitis.

Intestinal obstruction

Intestinal obstruction is either mechanical or functional.

Mechanical (Table 2.13) The bowel above the level of the obstruction is dilated, with increased secretion of fluid into the lumen. The patient complains of colicky abdominal pain, associated with vomiting and absolute constipation. On examination there is distension and 'tinkling' bowel sounds. Small bowel obstruction may settle with conservative management (i.e. nasogastric suction and intravenous fluids to maintain hydration). Large bowel obstruction is treated surgically.

Functional This occurs with a paralytic ileus, which is often seen in the postoperative stage of peritonitis or of major abdominal surgery. It also occurs when the nerves or muscles of the intestine are damaged, causing intestinal pseudo-obstruction. Unlike mechanical obstruction, pain is often not present and bowel sounds may be decreased. Gas is seen throughout the bowel on a plain abdominal radiograph. Management is conservative.

....

THE PERITONEUM

The peritoneal cavity is a closed sac lined by mesothelium. It contains a little fluid to allow the abdominal contents to move freely. Conditions which affect the peritoneum are listed below.

- Infective (peritonitis)   Secondary to gut disease, e.g. appendicitis, perforation
                             Chronic peritoneal dialysis
                             Spontaneous (associated with ascites)
                             Tuberculous
- Neoplasia   Secondary deposits, e.g. from ovary
                             Primary mesothelioma
- Vasculitis   Connective tissue disease.

NUTRITION

....

DIETARY REQUIREMENTS

Food is necessary to provide the body with energy. The average daily requirement (Table 2.14) of a middle-aged adult female in the UK is 8100 kJ (1940 kcal), and for a man is 10 600 kJ (2550 kcal). This is made up of 50% carbohydrate, 35% fat and 15% protein, plus or minus 5% alcohol. Energy requirements increase during periods of rapid growth, such as adolescence, pregnancy and lactation, and with sepsis.

Body weight is maintained at a 'set point' by a precise balance of energy intake and total energy expenditure (the sum of the resting metabolic rate, activity energy expenditure and the thermic effect of food eaten). Weight gain is almost always due solely to an increase in energy intake which exceeds the total energy expenditure. Occasionally weight gain is due to a decrease in energy expenditure, e.g. hypothyroidism, or to fluid retention, e.g. heart failure or ascites. On the other hand, weight loss associated with cancer and chronic diseases is due to a reduction in energy intake secondary to a loss of appetite (anorexia). In a few conditions, such as sepsis and severe trauma, there is an increase in energy requirements (hypercatabolic or hypermetabolic) which will result in a negative energy balance if there is no compensatory increase in energy intake.

A balanced diet also requires sufficient amounts of minerals and vitamins (Table 2.14). In the western world vitamin deficiency is rare except in specific groups, e.g.

Table 2.14 Protein, energy and water requirement of normal and hypercatabolic adults

| | Nutritional requirements | |
Metabolic state	Normal	Hypercatabolic
Protein (g/kg)	1	2–3
Nitrogen (g/kg)	0.17	0.3–0.45
Energy (kcal/kg)	25–30	35–50
Water (ml/kg)	30–35	30–35

alcoholics and patients with small bowel disease, who may have multiple vitamin deficiencies, and patients with liver and biliary tract disease who are susceptible to deficiency of the fat-soluble vitamins (A, D, E, K). Deficiencies of the B vitamins, riboflavin and biotin, are rare in all patient groups and are not discussed further. Dietary deficiency of vitamin B_6 (pyridoxine, pyridoxal and pyridoxamine) is also extremely rare, but drugs (e.g isoniazid and penicillamine) that interact with pyridoxal phosphate may cause B_6 deficiency and a polyneuropathy. Vitamin B_{12} and folate deficiency is discussed on page 146 and vitamin D deficiency on page 238.

There is recent evidence from epidemiological studies that β-carotene (a precursor of vitamin A) and vitamin E supplementation of western diets may protect against cancer and ischaemic heart disease by virtue of their antioxidant properties. However, randomized controlled trials using β-carotene supplements did not show any protective effect. There is some evidence that vitamin E may protect against the development of ischaemic heart disease, and one controlled trial has shown a reduction in the risk of non-fatal myocardial infarction when supplements were given to patients with advanced ischaemic heart disease.

NUTRITIONAL SUPPORT

Patients should be screened for nutritional status on admission to hospital and during their hospital stay. Current recommendations suggest that:

- Patients should be asked simple questions about recent weight loss, their usual weight and whether they have been eating less than usual.
- Their weight and height should be recorded and body mass index (BMI) calculated (weight [kg]/ height [m]^2).

Some form of nutritional supplementation is required in those patients who cannot eat, should not eat, will not eat or cannot eat enough. It is necessary to provide nutritional support for:

- All severely malnourished patients on admission to hospital. Severe malnutrition is indicated by a BMI of less than 15
- Moderately malnourished patients (BMI 15–19) who, because of their physical illness, are not expected to eat for 3–5 days
- Normally nourished patients not expected to eat for 7–10 days.

Enteral nutrition is cheaper, more physiological and has fewer complications than parenteral (intravenous) nutrition, and should be used if the gastrointestinal tract is functioning normally. With both parenteral and parenteral nutrition a complete feeding regimen consisting of fat, carbohydrates, protein, vitamins, minerals and trace elements can be provided to provide the nutritional requirements of the individual (Table 2.14). Ideally a multidisciplinary nutrition support team should supervise the provision of artificial nutritional support.

Enteral nutrition

Foods can be given by:

- Mouth
- Fine-bore nasogastric tube for short-term enteral nutrition
- Percutaneous endoscopic gastrostomy (PEG): this is useful for patients who need feeding for longer than 2 weeks
- Needle catheter jejunostomy: a fine catheter is inserted into the jejunum at laparotomy and brought out through the abdominal wall.

A polymeric diet with whole protein, carbohydrate and fat is usually used; sometimes an elemental diet composed of amino acids, glucose and fatty acids is used for patients with Crohn's disease (page 74).

Total parenteral nutrition (TPN)

Parenteral nutrition may be given via a feeding catheter placed in a peripheral vein or a silicone catheter placed in the subclavian vein. Central catheters must only be placed by experienced clinicians under strict aseptic conditions in a sterile environment. The risk of introducing infection is reduced if these catheters are only used for feeding purposes, and not the administration of drugs or blood. Peripheral feeding lines usually only last for about 5 days and are reserved for when feeding is necessary for a short period. Central lines may last for months to years. Complications of TPN are given in Table 2.15.

Table 2.15 Complications of TPN

Catheter related: sepsis, thrombosis, embolism and pneumothorax
Metabolic, e.g. hyperglycaemia
Electrolyte disturbances
Hypercalcaemia
Liver dysfunction

Monitoring of artificial nutrition

Patients receiving nutritional support should be weighed twice weekly: they require regular clinical examination to check for evidence of fluid overload or depletion. Patients receiving nutritional support in hospital initially require daily measurements of urea and electrolytes and blood glucose. More frequent measurement of blood glucose with BM stix is indicated in patients beginning TPN. Liver biochemistry, calcium and phosphate are measured twice weekly. Serum magnesium, zinc and nitrogen balance (see below) is measured weekly. The frequency of biochemical monitoring is adjusted according to the patient's clinical and metabolic status.

It is necessary to give 40–50 g of protein per 24 hours to maintain nitrogen balance, which represents the balance between protein breakdown and synthesis. The aim of any regimen is to achieve a positive nitrogen balance, which can usually be obtained by giving 3–5 g of nitrogen in excess of output. The amount of protein required to maintain nitrogen balance in a particular individual can be calculated from the amount of urinary nitrogen loss using the formula:

$$N_2 \text{ loss (g/24 h)} = \text{urinary urea (mmol/24 h)} \times 0.028 + 2$$

Urinary nitrogen $\times$ 6.25 = grams of protein required (most proteins contain about 16% nitrogen).

Most patients require about 12 g of nitrogen per 24 hours, but hypercatabolic patients require more, about 15 g/day.

ɣ Glutamyl transpeptidase

Bilirubin <17μmol/L

Aminotransferases (enzymes in hepatocytes)

Aspartate aminotransferase (AST) 10-40u/L

Alanine aminotransferase (ALT) 5-40u/L

More specific to liver

Alkaline phosphatase (25-115u/L)
- cholestasis
- bone disease

Liver, biliary tract and pancreatic diseases

3

SYMPTOMS OF LIVER DISEASE

Acute liver disease, e.g. viral hepatitis, may be asymptomatic or present with generalized symptoms of lethargy, anorexia and malaise in the early stages, with jaundice developing later (page 95).

Chronic liver disease may also be asymptomatic and discovered from an incidental finding of abnormal liver biochemistry. Some patients with chronic liver disease may present at a late stage with complications of cirrhosis, causing:

- Ascites with abdominal swelling and discomfort (page 116).
- Haematemesis and melaena from (often massive) gastrointestinal bleeding (page 114)
- Confusion and drowsiness (page 118).

Patients presenting in this way are often extremely unwell and a detailed history may not be obtained. However, physical examination will often reveal the signs of chronic liver disease (page 112) and thus point to liver disease as the cause of the presenting illness.

Pruritus (itching) occurs in cholestatic jaundice from any cause (page 97), but is particularly common in primary biliary cirrhosis, when it may be the only symptom (without jaundice) at presentation. Pruritus may occur in association with other systemic diseases (e.g. hyperthyroidism, polycythaemia, renal failure, malignant disease) and skin diseases (e.g. scabies, eczema), but in these cases there are usually additional symptoms or signs that suggest the diagnosis.

INTERPRETING LIVER BIOCHEMISTRY AND LIVER FUNCTION TESTS

A routine blood sample sent to the laboratory for liver biochemistry will be processed by an automated multichannel analyser to produce serum levels of bilirubin, aminotransferases, alkaline phosphatase, γ-glutamyl transpeptidase and serum proteins. Liver synthetic function is determined by measuring the serum albumin and the prothrombin time (clotting factors are synthesized in the liver). A prolonged prothrombin time may also occur as a result of vitamin K deficiency in biliary obstruction (low concentration of intestinal bile salts results in poor absorption of vitamin K); however, unlike liver disease, clotting is corrected by giving parenteral vitamin K.

- *Bilirubin* (normal range <17 µmol/l) A small or moderate rise in the serum bilirubin without other abnormalities of liver enzymes is usually the result of Gilbert's syndrome, haemolysis or ineffective erythropoiesis. Hyperbilirubinaemia caused by hepatobiliary disease is almost always accompanied by other abnormalities of liver biochemistry; very high levels occur most frequently in biliary tract obstruction. Serial measurements are useful in following the progress of some diseases, e.g. primary biliary cirrhosis, or the response to treatment, e.g. after placement of a stent in cancer of the head of the pancreas.
- *Aminotransferases.* These enzymes are present in hepatocytes and leak into the blood with liver cell damage. Very high levels may occur with acute hepatitis (20–50 times normal). Aspartate aminotransferase (AST) (normal range 10–40 U/l) is also present in heart and skeletal muscle, and raised serum concentrations are seen with myocardial infarction and skeletal muscle damage. Alanine aminotransferase (ALT) (normal range 5–40 U/l) is more specific to the liver than AST.
- *Alkaline phosphatase* (normal range 25–115 U/l) is situated in the canalicular and sinusoidal membranes of the liver. Raised serum alkaline phosphatase concentrations are seen in cholestasis from any cause, whether intra- or extrahepatic disease. Circulating alkaline phosphatase is also derived from bone, and raised serum levels occur in

Paget's disease, osteomalacia, growing children, and bony metastases. In these cases differentiation from cholestasis is made by the absence of a rise in serum γ-glutamyl transferase (γGT) (see below). The placenta secretes its own isoenzyme and its level is raised in pregnancy.

- *γ-Glutamyl transpeptidase* (normal range, male <50 U/l, female <32 U/l) is a liver microsomal enzyme which may be induced by alcohol and enzyme-inducing drugs, e.g. phenytoin. A raised serum concentration is a useful screen for alcohol abuse. In cholestasis the γGT rises in parallel with the serum alkaline phosphatase because it has a similar pathway of excretion.

JAUNDICE

Jaundice (icterus) is a yellow discoloration of the sclerae and skin as a result of a raised serum bilirubin, and is usually detectable when the bilirubin is greater than 30–60 μmol/l (normal range <17 μmol/l).

Bilirubin is derived predominantly from the breakdown of haemoglobin in the spleen, and is carried in the blood bound to albumin. Unconjugated bilirubin is conjugated in the liver by glucuronyl transferase to bilirubin glucuronide, and this is excreted into the small intestine in bile. In the terminal ileum conjugated bilirubin is converted to urobilinogen and excreted in the faeces (as stercobilinogen) or reabsorbed and excreted by the kidneys (Figure 3.1).

The usual division of jaundice into prehepatic, hepatocellular and obstructive is an oversimplification, because in hepatocellular jaundice there is invariably cholestasis and the clinical problem is whether the cholestasis is intrahepatic or extrahepatic. Jaundice is therefore considered under the following headings:

- Haemolytic jaundice
- Congenital hyperbilirubinaemias
- Cholestatic jaundice.

Haemolytic jaundice

Increased breakdown of red cells leads to increased production of bilirubin, which may result in mild jaundice only, as the liver can usually handle the increased bilirubin

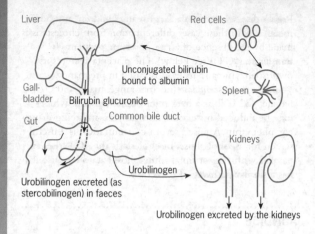

Figure 3.1
Pathways in bilirubin metabolism.

derived from haemolysis. The unconjugated bilirubin is not water soluble and therefore does not pass into the urine, unlike the conjugated hyperbilirubinaemia of cholestatic jaundice. The urinary urobilinogen is increased. The causes are those of haemolytic anaemia (page 153), with the clinical features dependent on the cause (e.g. anaemia, splenomegaly, jaundice). Investigations show features of haemolysis (page 154), with raised serum unconjugated bilirubin and normal alkaline phosphatase and transferases.

Congenital hyperbilirubinaemia

The most common is Gilbert's syndrome, which affects 2–5% of the population. It is asymptomatic and is usually picked up as an incidental finding of a slightly raised serum bilirubin (up to 70 μmol/l) which is caused by an increase in unconjugated bilirubin. There are no signs of liver disease and the other liver enzymes are normal. Many abnormalities in bilirubin handling have been demonstrated, though most patients have reduced levels of UDP-glucuronyl transferase activity which conjugates bilirubin with glucuronic acid.

The other congenital abnormalities of bilirubin metabolism (Crigler–Najjar, Dubin–Johnson and Rotor syndromes) are rare.

Cholestatic jaundice

This can be divided into the following (Table 3.1):

Table 3.1 Causes of cholestatic jaundice

Intrahepatic
Hepatitis – acute and chronic
Drugs
Cirrhosis
Pregnancy

Extrahepatic
Common bile duct stone
Carcinoma of head of pancreas/ampulla/bile duct
Iatrogenic biliary stricture following surgery
Pancreatitis
Sclerosing cholangitis

- Intrahepatic cholestasis, caused by hepatocellular swelling in parenchymal liver disease or abnormalities at a cellular level of bile excretion.
- Extrahepatic cholestasis resulting from obstruction of bile flow at any point distal to the bile canaliculi.

Investigation

An outline of the approach to the investigation of jaundice is shown in Figure 3.2

- Serum liver biochemistry will confirm the jaundice. The AST tends to be high early in the course of hepatitis, with a smaller rise in alkaline phosphatase. Conversely, in extrahepatic obstruction the alkaline phosphatase is elevated, with a smaller rise in the AST.
- Ultrasonography examination will show dilated bile ducts in extrahepatic cholestasis and identify the level of obstruction. Mass lesions may also be identified.
- Serum viral markers for hepatitis A and hepatitis B may be present. Antibodies to hepatitis C virus develop late in the course of acute infection.

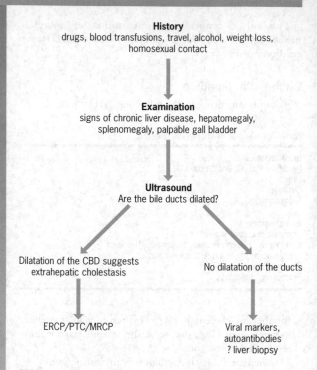

History
drugs, blood transfusions, travel, alcohol, weight loss,
homosexual contact

Examination
signs of chronic liver disease, hepatomegaly,
splenomegaly, palpable gall bladder

Ultrasound
Are the bile ducts dilated?

Dilatation of the CBD suggests
extrahepatic cholestasis

No dilatation of the ducts

ERCP/PTC/MRCP

Viral markers,
autoantibodies
? liver biopsy

ERCP = endoscopic retrograde cholangiopancreatography
PTC = percutaneous transhepatic cholangiogram
MRCP = magnetic resonance cholangiopancreatography

Figure 3.2
Approach to the investigation of cholestatic jaundice. The order of
investigation is influenced by the age of the patient and hence the likely
cause of jaundice, A young person is most likely to have intrinsic liver
disease, e.g. viral hepatitis and it may be more appropriate to organize tests
to exclude these conditions before proceeding to ultrasound.

- Other tests Cholestasis impairs the absorption of fat-
  soluble vitamins. Malabsorption of vitamin K often
  results in a prolonged prothrombin time, which is
  reversed by the parenteral administration of vitamin K.
  Impairment of liver synthethic function in advanced
  liver disease also results in a prolonged prothrombin
  time and a low serum albumin.

Serum autoantibodies are present in autoimmune liver disease (see later).

HEPATITIS

The pathological features of hepatitis are liver cell necrosis and inflammatory cell infiltration. Clinically the liver may be enlarged and tender, jaundice may be evident, and laboratory evidence of hepatocellular damage is invariably found in the form of elevated serum transferase levels. Hepatitis is divided into acute and chronic types (Table 3.2) on the basis of clinical and pathological criteria. Acute hepatitis is most commonly caused by one of the hepatitis viruses. Usually there is complete resolution of the liver cell damage, with a return to normal structure and function. Occasionally there is progression to massive liver cell necrosis, which may result in death. Chronic hepatitis is defined as sustained inflammatory disease of the liver lasting for more than 6 months.

Table 3.2 The causes of acute and chronic hepatitis

Acute	Chronic
Viruses Hepatitis A, B, C, D and E Epstein–Barr virus Cytomegalovirus	Viruses Hepatitis B, C and D
Non-viral infections *Leptospira icterohaemorrhagica* *Toxoplasma gondii* *Coxiella burnetii* (Q fever)	Autoimmune hepatitis
Alcohol	Alcohol
Drugs Anti-TB, e.g. isoniazid Halothane Paracetamol poisoning	Drugs Methyldopa Nitrofurantoin
Others Pregnancy Poisons, e.g. carbon tetrachloride Wilson's disease	Metabolic disorders Wilson's disease α_1-Antitrypsin deficiency

Viral hepatitis ND

The most important causes of viral hepatitis are the well-characterized hepatotrophic viruses named hepatitis A, B and C. Hepatitis D and E are infrequent causes in the UK. Important features of these viruses are summarized in Table 3.3. All cases of viral hepatitis must be notified to the appropriate public health authority. This allows contacts to be traced and provides data on disease incidence.

Hepatitis A ND

Epidemiology

Hepatitis A is the most common type of viral hepatitis, responsible for 20–40% of clinically apparent acute hepatitis. It occurs worldwide and affects particularly children and young adults. Spread is mainly faecal–oral and arises from the ingestion of contaminated food (e.g. shellfish, clams) or water. The virus is excreted in the faeces of infected individuals for about 2 weeks before, and 7 days after, the onset of the illness. It is most infectious just before the onset of the jaundice.

Clinical features

The incubation period is about 15–40 days. A preicteric phase, lasting about 2 weeks, is characterized by nausea, vomiting, diarrhoea, malaise, abdominal discomfort and mild fever. This is followed by the development of jaundice, with dark urine and pale stools, at which stage the patient often begins to feel better. Some patients, however, remain anicteric. There is moderate hepatomegaly and the spleen is enlarged in 10% of cases. Occasionally lymphadenopathy and a skin rash are present. The illness is self-limiting and usually over in 3–6 weeks. Rarely the disease is very severe, with fulminant hepatitis (page 108), liver coma and death.

Investigations

- Liver biochemistry shows a raised serum AST and raised bilirubin when jaundice develops.
- The blood count may show a leucopenia with relative lymphocytosis and a high ESR.
- Serum antibodies to hepatitis A virus (HAV) are present, with anti-HAV IgM indicating an acute infection.

Table 3.3 Some features of the hepatitis viruses

Feature	Hepatitis				
Virus	**A**	**B**	**C**	**D**	**E**
	RNA	DNA	RNA	RNA	RNA
Transmission	Faecal–oral	Parenteral Sexual Vertical	Parenteral	Parenteral	Faecal–oral
Incubation	Short (2–3 weeks)	Long (1–5 months)	Long	Intermediate	Short
Chronicity	No	Yes	Yes	Yes	No
Mortality rate (%) (acute)	<0.5	<1	<1	(Only with B)	1–2 (10% in pregnancy)

Management

No specific treatment is required. Hospital admission is not usually necessary and avoidance of alcohol advised only when the patient is ill.

Prophylaxis

Active immunization with an inactivated HAV vaccine is recommended for people travelling frequently to areas of high prevalence (Africa, Asia, South America, Eastern Europe and the Middle East), for individuals such as homosexuals who engage in high-risk behaviour, and in patients with chronic liver disease in whom the disease may be more severe. Passive immunization with human normal immunoglobulin gives immediate protection for about 2–3 months. This should be offered to people making a brief single visit to a high-risk area and to close contacts or family members of an index case. Control of hepatitis also depends on good hygiene. Travellers to high-risk areas should drink only boiled or bottled water and avoid risky foods.

Hepatitis B ND

Epidemiology

Hepatitis B virus (HBV) is present worldwide but is particularly prevalent in parts of Africa, the Middle East and the Far East. It is spread through the intravenous route (infected blood products, contaminated needles of intravenous drug abusers and tattooists) and through sexual intercourse, particularly in male homosexuals. Vertical transmission from mother to child during parturition is the most important means of transmission worldwide.

Viral structure

The whole virus is the Dane particle (Figure 3.3) which consists of an inner core and an outer surface coat, the hepatitis B surface antigen (HBsAg). The inner core contains double-stranded DNA, DNA polymerase, the core antigen (HBcAg) and e antigen (HBeAg). HBeAg is produced in excess during active viral replication, and its detection in the serum indicates a high degree of infectivity.

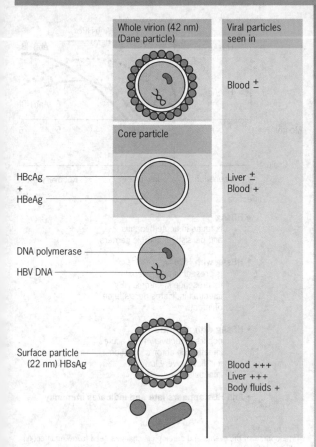

| Whole virion (42 nm) (Dane particle) | Viral particles seen in |

Whole virion (42 nm)
(Dane particle)

Blood ±

Core particle

HBcAg
+
HBeAg

Liver ±
Blood +

DNA polymerase
HBV DNA

Surface particle
(22 nm) HBsAg

Blood +++
Liver +++
Body fluids +

Figure 3.3
Hepatitis B virus: the antigenic components.

Acute infection

Acute infection with HBV may be asymptomatic or produce symptoms and signs similar to those seen in hepatitis A. Occasionally it is associated with a rash or polyarthritis affecting the small joints. The sequence of events following acute infection is depicted in Figure 3.4

Investigation is generally the same as for hepatitis A. The viral markers for HBV are shown in Figure 3.4. If HBsAg

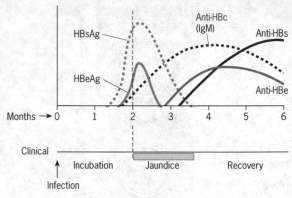

- **HBsAg**
    is found in acute hepatitis
    and persists in chronic carriers.

- **HBsAg with HBeAg**
    is present in acute hepatitis
    its presence in chronic HBV
    infection indicates persistence
    of infectivity

- **HBsAg with anti-HBe**
    occurs in recovery from acute
    infection. In chronic infection
    it indicates very low
    infectivity

- **Anti-HBs appears late and indicates immunity**

Figure 3.4
Time course of the events and serological changes seen following infection with hepatitis B virus.

is present, a full viral profile is performed. There is no specific therapy for acute HBV infection and management is supportive.

Most patients recover completely. This is marked by the disappearance of HBsAg from the serum, the development of antibodies to surface antigen (anti-HBs) and immunity to subsequent infection (Figure 3.4). One per cent of patients with acute hepatitis develop fulminant liver failure.

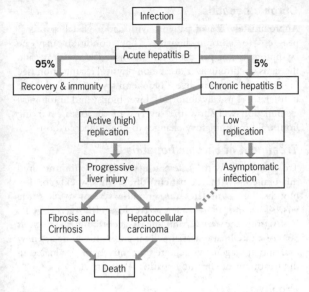

Figure 3.5
The natural history of hepatitis B infection in adults.

A minority of patients do not clear HBsAg from the serum and become chronic carriers. The risk of developing chronic HBV infection is inversely related to age at the time of infection. Ninety per cent of infants infected at birth will become chronically infected with HBV, but only about 5% of adults (Figure 3.5).

Chronic carriers

The persistence of HBsAg in the serum for more than 6 months after acute infection defines the carrier status. Carriers who, in addition, have HBeAg or viral DNA in the serum (i.e. have active viral replication) are highly infectious and are at greatest risk of developing chronic hepatitis (see below) and cirrhosis, with the attendant increased risk of hepatocellular carcinoma. Patients with only HBsAg (low replication) are usually asymptomatic with normal liver biochemistry, and are of relatively low infective risk.

Chronic hepatitis

Approximately 3% of patients with acute viral hepatitis B progress to chronic hepatitis. The condition may be asymptomatic, or present with established liver disease and the signs of chronic liver disease on physical examination (see Figure 3.6). Serum liver biochemistry, particularly the transferases, is usually abnormal. Liver biopsy and histological examination will show the severity of the disease varying from mild inflammatory changes to established cirrhosis.

Treatment of chronic hepatitis B

Treatment is with interferon-α (IF-α) administered subcutaneously (by the patient) three times weekly for 4–6 months. This stimulates the immune system to clear the virus. The aim of treatment is to clear HBeAg and HBV DNA from the serum, and this is accomplished in about 50% of treated patients. Famiclovir and lamivudine are new oval antiviral agents which are currently being evaluated in the treatment of chronic hepatitis B infection.

Prophylaxis

The avoidance of high-risk factors (needle sharing, prostitutes and multiple male homosexual partners) and counselling patients who are potentially infective are important aspects of prevention. Active immunization is available with a recombinant yeast vaccine and is recommended for those at increased risk, e.g. healthcare workers, homosexuals, intravenous drug abusers and haemodialysis patients.

Combined prophylaxis (i.e. active immunization and passive immunization with specific antihepatitis B immunoglobulin) is given to non-immune individuals after high-risk exposure, e.g. a needle-stick injury from a carrier, newborn babies of HBsAg-positive mothers and HBV-negative sexual partners of HBsAg-positive patients.

Hepatitis D (delta or δ agent) ND

Hepatitis D virus is an incomplete RNA virus enclosed in a shell of HBsAg. It is unable to replicate on its own, but is activated by the presence of HBV. It can affect all risk groups for HBV infection, but is seen particularly in intravenous drug abusers. HDV infection can occur as a coinfection with HBV or as a superinfection in an HBsAg-positive patient, and thus presents as an illness indistinguishable from acute HBV infection or as a flare-up of previously quiescent chronic HBV infection. Diagnosis is by finding IgM anti-D in the serum.

Hepatitis C ND

Epidemiology

Hepatitis C virus (HCV) is an RNA virus that was discovered in 1988 and found to be responsible for most of the post-transfusion hepatitides before screening for HCV in donated blood. It is present worldwide, but is more common in southern Europe and Japan. It is transmitted by blood products and perhaps also by sexual intercourse. Ten to 20% of patients do not have identifiable risk factors for HCV infection.

Clinical features

Acute infection is usually mild, with jaundice developing in less than 20% of cases. At least 80% of patients go on to develop chronic liver disease. However, chronic liver disease is often silent and is sometimes discovered only by routine serologic or biochemical testing, such as occurs during blood donation or health screening. Furthermore, a proportion of patients with chronic hepatitis C have normal aminotransferases and are diagnosed when they present with chronic liver disease and cirrhosis. Patients with cirrhosis secondary to chronic HCV are at increased risk for the development for hepatocellular carcinoma. In addition to liver disease, there are two important extrahepatic manifestations of chronic HCV infection: essential mixed cryoglobulinaemia and membranoproliferative glomerulonephritis (page 278).

Diagnosis

Serum antibodies to HCV are found with both past and present infection. Negative serology excludes HCV infection and is thus the initial screening test in a patient with chronic liver disease of undetermined cause. However, antibodies may take 3 months to appear after acute infection, and thus a negative result does not exclude acute HCV infection.

Patients with antibodies to hepatitis C should undergo further tests to look for the presence of HCV RNA (detected by the polymerase chain reaction) in the serum. A positive result indicates ongoing infection, and a liver biopsy is usually then performed to detect the presence or absence of chronic hepatitis and cirrhosis.

Management

It is unclear which patients will progress to chronic liver disease and cirrhosis, and therefore who should be treated in an attempt to prevent progression of the disease, or the development of hepatocellular carcinoma. Currently interferon-α is used in most patients with elevated aminotransferases and histological evidence of active hepatitis. Response rates are variable, but at best liver biochemistry improves in 50% of treated patients, and of these 50% relapse on discontinuation of the treatment. Recently, clinical trials have shown a higher rate of long term response when the antiviral agent, ribavirin, is given in combination with interferon.

Hepatitis E ND

This is an RNA virus which causes enteral (epidemic or waterborne) hepatitis, particularly in developing countries. There is no chronic carrier state and it does not progress to chronic liver disease, but the mortality rate from fulminant hepatic failure is about 1–2%, rising to 20% in pregnant women.

Hepatitis G

This is a recently recognized RNA virus which is transmitted via the parenteral route. Although high prevalence rates have been recorded in patients exposed to blood and blood products, and in drug addicts, there is little evidence that this virus induces hepatic damage.

Fulminant hepatic failure

Fulminant hepatic failure is defined as hepatic failure with encephalopathy developing in less than 2 weeks in a patient with a previously normal liver, or in patients with an acute exacerbation of underlying liver disease. It is an infrequent complication of acute hepatitis (from any cause) and occurs as a result of massive liver cell necrosis. In the UK, viral hepatitis and paracetamol overdose are the most common causes. Presentation is with hepatic encephalopathy of varying severity (Table 3.4), accompanied by severe jaundice and a marked coagulopathy. The complications include cerebral oedema, hypoglycaemia, severe bacterial and fungal infections, hypotension and renal failure (hepatorenal syndrome). Fulminant hepatic failure is managed with supportive treatment in a specialist liver unit. Emergency liver transplantation has become a useful treatment for the very severe cases (grade IV encephalopathy), of which 80% might otherwise die.

Table 3.4 Grading of hepatic encephalopathy

Grade I	Daytime somnolence, asterixis (flapping tremor of outstretched hands)
Grade II	Confusion, disorientation, agitation and impaired coordination
Grade III	Increasing drowsiness, stupor, no communication possible
Grade IV	Coma, increased rigidity, extensor plantar response

Autoimmune hepatitis

Autoimmune hepatitis is a chronic, usually progressive liver disease which is often associated with other autoimmune diseases. It is most common in young and middle-aged women but can occur in any age in either sex.

Aetiology

The aetiology is unknown but there are many immunological abnormalities present. These include hypergammaglobulinaemia, with the most pronounced rise in IgG levels, circulating antibodies such as nuclear, smooth muscle and liver kidney microsomal antibodies, and an increased helper/suppressor T-cell ratio.

Clinical features

The onset is often insidious, with anorexia, malaise, nausea and fatigue. Twenty-five per cent present as an acute hepatitis with rapidly progressive liver disease. The signs of chronic liver disease are often present, with palmar erythema, spider naevae, hepatosplenomegaly and jaundice. Features of other autoimmune diseases may be present.

Investigations

Circulating autoantibodies (antinuclear and antismooth muscle antibodies) are the hallmarks of the disease. There is hypergammaglobulinaemia, and the serum bilirubin and aminotransferases are elevated. Liver biopsy will show the changes of chronic hepatitis, with interface hepatitis and often cirrhosis.

Treatment

Prednisolone 30 mg daily is given for 2–3 weeks. A subsequent reduction in the dose depends on clinical response, but maintenance doses of 10–15 mg are usually required. Azathioprine is used as a steroid-sparing agent.

Prognosis

In treated patients the 5-year survival rate is 90%.

Cirrhosis

Cirrhosis is a histological diagnosis. It is a diffuse process that results from necrosis of liver cells followed by fibrosis and nodule formation. The end result is impairment of liver cell function and gross distortion of the liver architecture, leading to portal hypertension.

Aetiology

The causes of cirrhosis are shown in Table 3.5. Alcohol is the most common cause in the western world, but hepatitis B is the most common cause worldwide.

Pathology

Histologically two types of cirrhosis have been described: micronodular and macronodular.

- Micronodular cirrhosis is characterized by uniform, small nodules up to 3 mm in diameter. This type is often caused by alcohol damage.
- In macronodular cirrhosis large nodules up to several centimetres in diameter are present. This type is often seen following hepatitis B infection.

Table 3.5 Causes of cirrhosis

Common
Alcohol
Chronic hepatitis caused by
   Hepatitis B
   Hepatitis C
   ? Other hepatitis viruses

Others
Biliary cirrhosis: primary and secondary
Autoimmune hepatitis
Haemochromatosis
Cystic fibrosis
Budd–Chiari syndrome
Wilson's disease
Drugs, e.g. methotrexate
α_1-Antitrypsin deficiency
Idiopathic

- There is also a mixed picture, with both small and large nodules.

Clinical features

These are secondary to portal hypertension and liver cell failure (Figure 3.6). Cirrhosis with the complications of encephalopathy, ascites or variceal haemorrhage is designated decompensated cirrhosis. Cirrhosis without any of these complications is termed compensated cirrhosis.

Investigations

These are performed to identify the aetiology and assess the severity of liver disease.

Severity

- Liver biochemistry may be normal. In most cases there is at least a slight elevation of the serum alkaline phosphatase and aminotransferase. A low serum albumin reflects reduced hepatic synthetic function and is the best guide to the severity of liver disease.
- Serum electrolytes: a low sodium indicates severe liver disease secondary to either impaired free water clearance or excess diuretic therapy.
- Haematology: the prothrombin time is prolonged as a result of decreased hepatic synthesis of clotting factors.

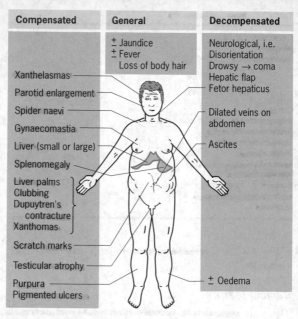

Compensated	General	Decompensated
	± Jaundice ± Fever Loss of body hair	Neurological, i.e. Disorientation Drowsy → coma Hepatic flap Fetor hepaticus
Xanthelasmas		
Parotid enlargement		
Spider naevi		Dilated veins on abdomen
Gynaecomastia		
Liver (small or large)		Ascites
Splenomegaly		
Liver palms Clubbing Dupuytren's contracture Xanthomas		
Scratch marks		
Testicular atrophy		
Purpura Pigmented ulcers		± Oedema

Figure 3.6
Physical signs in chronic liver disease.

- Serum α-fetoprotein (AFP). This is usually undetectable after fetal life, but raised levels may be found in chronic liver disease. Very high levels (>500 U/ml) suggest the complication of hepatocellular carcinoma.

Aetiology

This is determined by the following:

- Hepatitis B and C serology
- Serum autoantibodies
- Miscellaneous: serum copper and serum α_1-antitrypsin should always be measured in young cirrhotic individuals. Serum iron, total iron-binding capacity and ferritin should be measured to exclude haemochromatosis.

Further investigations

A liver biopsy is performed to confirm the severity and type of liver disease. Oesophageal varices are sought with endoscopy. Ultrasonography examination is often performed, its major usefulness being in the early detection of hepatocellular carcinoma.

Management

Cirrhosis is irreversible and frequently progresses. Management is that of the complications seen in decompensated cirrhosis as they arise. The progression of liver disease may be halted by correcting the underlying cause, e.g. venesection for haemochromatosis, abstinence from alcohol for alcoholic cirrhosis. Liver transplantation should be considered in patients with end-stage cirrhosis.

Prognosis

This is very variable and depends on the aetiology and the presence of complications. The severity and prognosis of liver disease can be graded according to five variables: encephalopathy, ascites, prothrombin time, serum bilirubin and albumin (Child's grading, or modifications thereof).

Complications

The complications of cirrhosis are shown in Table 3.6.

Table 3.6 Complications and effects of cirrhosis

Portal hypertension and gastrointestinal haemorrhage
Ascites
Portosystemic encephalopathy
Acute renal failure
Hepatocellular carcinoma (HCC)

Portal hypertension

The portal vein carries blood from the gut and spleen to the liver and accounts for 85% of hepatic vascular inflow (15% is via the hepatic artery). The inflow of portal blood to the liver can be partially or completely obstructed at a number of sites, leading to high pressure proximal to the obstruction and the diversion of blood into portosystemic collaterals. The most important site for collateral formation is at the gastro-oesophageal junction (varices), where they are superficial and liable to rupture, causing massive gastrointestinal haemorrhage.

The main sites of obstruction are:

- Prehepatic, caused by blockage of the portal vein before the liver
- Intrahepatic, resulting from distortion of the liver architecture
- Posthepatic, as a result of obstruction of the hepatic veins.

Aetiology

The causes of portal hypertension are outlined in Table 3.7. In the UK 90% of cases are caused by cirrhosis.

Table 3.7 Causes of portal hypertension

Prehepatic	Portal vein thrombosis
Intrahepatic	Cirrhosis
	Alcoholic hepatitis
	Schistosomiasis
	Granulomata
Posthepatic	Budd–Chiari syndrome
	Veno-occlusive disease
	Right heart failure – rare
	Constrictive pericarditis

Clinical features

The characteristic clinical manifestations of portal hypertension are:

- Gastrointestinal bleeding from oesophageal or gastric varices
- Ascites
- Hepatic encephalopathy.

Only 30% of patients with varices ever bleed from them, and this is most common in those with large varices. Bleeding is often massive and mortality is as high as 50%.

Management

The general management of GI bleeding is discussed on page 59.

Acute bleeding Patients should be resuscitated (see page 442) and undergo urgent gastroscopy to confirm the diagnosis and exclude bleeding from other sites.

- Endoscopic therapy: injection sclerotherapy or banding of varices is the treatment of choice. Bleeding stops in 80% of cases.
- Pharmacological treatment is used as a holding measure if sclerotherapy or banding is not available or unsuccessful. The alternatives are an intravenous infusion of octreotide (a long-acting somatostatin analogue), vasopressin or terlipressin (a long-acting analogue of vasopressin), all of which restrict portal inflow by splanchnic arterial constriction.
- Balloon tamponade with a Sengstaken–Blakemore tube is used if bleeding continues (page 648). It can have serious complications, such as aspiration pneumonia, oesophageal rupture and mucosal ulceration. To reduce complications the tube is only left in situ for up to 24 hours.
- TIPSS (transjugular intrahepatic portosystemic shunting) is at present reserved as a salvage procedure when other methods fail. A metal stent is passed over a guidewire in the internal jugular vein. The stent is then pushed into the liver substance, under radiological guidance, to form a shunt between the portal and hepatic veins, thus lowering portal pressure.
- Surgery (oesophageal transection and ligation of varices) is occasionally necessary if bleeding continues in spite of all the above measures.

Prophylaxis Following an episode of variceal bleeding there is a high risk of recurrence (60–80% over a 2-year period), and therefore treatment is given to prevent further bleeds (secondary prophylaxis). The main options are:

- Injection sclerotherapy or variceal banding until the varices are obliterated
- Oral propranolol, which reduces portal pressure and is as effective as sclerotherapy. This is also given to patients with varices who have never bled (primary prophylaxis)
- Portosystemic shunts (portal vein to vena cava – or splenorenal) are rarely performed. They carry a very low risk of rebleeding but there is a high operative mortality in patients with severe liver disease, and encephalopathy in those surviving the operation. Liver transplantation should always be considered.

Ascites

This is the presence of fluid in the peritoneal cavity and is a common complication of cirrhosis of the liver.

Aetiology

In cirrhosis, peripheral arterial vasodilatation (probably mediated by nitric oxide) leads to a reduction in effective blood volume, with activation of the sympathetic nervous system and renin–angiotensin system, thus promoting salt and water retention. The formation of oedema is encouraged by hypoalbuminaemia and mainly localized to the peritoneal cavity as a result of the portal hypertension.

Clinical features

There is fullness in the flanks, with shifting dullness. Tense ascites is uncomfortable and may produce respiratory distress. A pleural effusion (usually right-sided) and peripheral oedema may be present.

Investigations

A diagnostic paracentesis of 10–20 ml of fluid should be carried out in all patients and the following performed:

- Cell count: a neutrophil count >250 cells/mm^3 indicates underlying (usually spontaneous) bacterial peritonitis
- Gram stain and culture for bacteria and acid-fast bacilli
- Protein: an ascitic protein of 11 g/l or more below the serum albumin level suggests a transudate (exudate <11 g/l)
- Cytology for malignant cells
- Amylase to exclude pancreatic ascites.

The causes of ascites are listed in Table 3.8; the commonest cause is cirrhosis.

Management

Most patients with ascites secondary to cirrhosis are managed with diuretics.

Diuretics The management of ascites resulting from cirrhosis is based on a stepwise approach, starting with bed rest, reduced salt intake (40 mmol/day) and a combination of spirinolactone 100 mg and frusemide 40 mg daily. The rate of fluid loss is best assessed by changes in body weight.

Table 3.8 The causes of ascites

Transudate	Exudate
Cirrhosis	Malignancy
Constrictive pericarditis	Infection, e.g. pyogenic, tuberculous
Cardiac failure	
Hypoalbuminaemia, e.g. nephrotic syndrome	Pancreatitis
	Budd–Chiari syndrome
Meigs' syndrome*	Myxoedema
	Lymphatic obstruction (chylous ascites)

* Meig's syndrome is the combination of an ovarian tumour, ascites and hydrothorax.

The aim of diuretic therapy is to produce weight loss of about 0.5 kg/day, because the maximum rate of transfer of fluid from the ascitic to the vascular compartment is only about 700 ml/day. If there is no response in 2–3 days the dose of diuretics is doubled. Too rapid a diuresis may cause volume depletion and hypokalaemia, and precipitate encephalopathy. In combination with dietary sodium restriction this medical approach is effective in over 90% of patients.

Paracentesis This is used in patients with tense ascites or who are resistant to standard medical therapy. All the ascites can be removed over several hours. There is therefore rapid symptom relief and reduced hospital stay compared to treatment with diuretics. The major danger of this approach is the production of hypovolaemia because the ascites reaccumulates at the expense of the circulating volume. This is largely overcome by the intravenous infusion of plasma expanders (albumin, Dextran-70, gelatin) administered after paracentesis.

Transjugular intrahepatic portosystemic shunt (TIPSS, page 115) is occasionally used for resistant ascites

Complications

Spontaneous bacterial peritonitis occurs in 8% of cirrhotic patients with ascites and has a mortality rate of 50%. The most common infecting organism is *Escherichia coli*. Clinical features may be minimal, but include abdominal pain and fever. Diagnosis is made on the ascitic fluid white cell count, and Gram stain and culture (see above). Empirical therapy, e.g. intravenous ceftazidine or cefotaxime, should be started before the results of culture are available. Spontaneous bacterial peritonitis frequently recurs and indicates a poor prognosis; it is an indication for liver transplantation.

Portosystemic encephalopathy

The term 'portosystemic encephalopathy' (PSE) refers to a chronic neuropsychiatric syndrome which occurs with advanced hepatocellular disease, either chronic (cirrhosis) or acute (fulminant hepatic failure). It is also seen in patients following a portacaval shunt operation.

Pathophysiology

The mechanisms are unclear but are believed to involve 'toxic' substances, normally detoxified by the liver, bypassing the liver via the collaterals and gaining access to the brain. A putative toxin is ammonia produced from the breakdown of dietary protein by gut bacteria. In chronic liver disease there is an acute-on-chronic course, with acute episodes precipitated by a number of possible factors (Table 3.9)

Table 3.9 Factors precipitating portosystemic encephalopathy

Gastrointestinal haemorrhage (i.e. a high protein load)
Infection
Fluid and electrolyte disturbance (spontaneous or diuretic induced)
Sedative drugs, e.g. opiates, diazepam
Development of a hepatoma
Portosystemic shunt operations and TIPSS
Constipation
High dietary protein

Clinical features

The earliest features are lethargy, mild confusion, anorexia and a reversal of the sleep pattern, with the patient sleeping during the day and restless at night. Later there is disorientation, a decreased conscious level and eventually coma (see Table 3.4). The signs are a flapping tremor of the outstretched hand (asterixis), inability to draw a five-pointed star (constructional apraxia) and a prolonged trail-making test (the ability to join numbers and letters within a certain time). Serial attempts are easily compared and used to monitor patient progress.

Investigations

The diagnosis is clinical. An EEG (showing δ waves) and visual evoked potentials may aid diagnosis in difficult cases.

Management

The aims of management are to identify and treat any precipitating factors and to minimize the absorption of nitrogenous material, particularly ammonia, from the gut. This is achieved by the following:

- Laxatives and enemas: lactulose (10–30 ml three times daily) is an osmotic purgative which reduces colonic pH and increases transit. It may be given via a nasogastric tube if the patient is comatose.
- In resistant cases a non-absorbable antibiotic, 1 g 6 hourly is given to reduce the number of bowel organisms and hence production of ammonia.
- Maintenance of nutrition with a high-carbohydrate, low-protein diet.

Once the patient recovers the protein content of the diet may be increased and lactulose continued to produce soft stools but not diarrhoea.

Prognosis

The prognosis is that of the underlying liver disease.

··

TYPES OF CIRRHOSIS

Alcoholic

This is discussed in the section on alcoholic liver disease (page 125).

Primary biliary cirrhosis

Primary biliary cirrhosis (PBC) is a chronic disorder in which there is progressive destruction of intrahepatic bile ducts causing cholestasis, eventually leading to cirrhosis.

Epidemiology

It affects predominantly women aged 40–50 years (female:male ratio 9:1).

Aetiology

The cause of PBC is unknown but most data suggest that it is due to an inherited abnormality of immunoregulation, leading to immune-mediated damage to bile duct epithelial cells. It is thought that disease expression results from an environmental trigger, possibly infective, in a genetically susceptible individual. Antimitochondrial antibodies (AMAs) are present in almost all (>95%) patients, but their role in the pathogenesis of this disorder is unclear.

Clinical features

Pruritus, with or without jaundice, is the single most common presenting complaint. In advanced disease there is, in addition, hepatosplenomegaly and xanthelasma (PBC is a cause of secondary hypercholesterolaemia). Asymptomatic patients may be discovered on routine examination or screening to have hepatomegaly, a raised serum alkaline phosphatase or autoantibodies. Patients with advanced disease may have steatorrhoea and malabsorption of fat-soluble vitamins owing to decreased biliary secretion of bile acids and the resulting low concentrations of bile acids in the small intestine.

Autoimmune disorders, e.g. Sjögren's syndrome, scleroderma and rheumatoid arthritis, are seen with increased frequency.

Investigations

- Liver biochemistry may show only a raised serum alkaline phosphatase, often very high (>1000 U/l).
- Serum AMAs are found in more than 95% of patients and a titre of 1:160 or greater makes the diagnosis very likely. The antibodies are very occasionally found in normal people or in those with autoimmune disease. The M2 subset is specific for PBC and may be useful if there is uncertainty. Other non-specific antibodies, e.g. antinuclear factor, may also be present.
- Serum IgM may be very high.

- Liver biopsy shows loss of bile ducts, lymphocyte infiltration of the portal tracts, granuloma formation and, at a later stage, fibrosis and eventually cirrhosis.
- An ultrasound is sometimes performed in the jaundiced patient to exclude extrahepatic biliary obstruction.

Management

Ursodeoxycholic acid (ursodiol) is the only medical treatment which has been shown to prolong the time before liver transplantation is needed. Its mode of action is to decrease the expression of HLA class 1 antigens on hepatocytes and thus render them less susceptible to immunological attack, in addition to mitigating the toxic effects of naturally occurring bile acids which accumulate in the liver. Pruritus may be helped by cholestyramine, and malabsorption of fat-soluble vitamins (A, D, K) is treated by supplementation. Liver transplantation is indicated for patients with advanced disease.

Prognosis

Asymptomatic patients may show a near-normal life expectancy. In symptomatic patients with jaundice there is a steady downhill course, with death in approximately 5 years without transplantation.

Secondary biliary cirrhosis

Cirrhosis can result from prolonged (i.e. for months) large duct biliary obstruction. Causes include bile duct strictures, gallstones and sclerosing cholangitis. Ultrasonography examination followed by endoscopic retrograde cholangiopancreatography (ERCP) or percutaneous transhepatic cholangiography (PTC) is performed to outline the ducts, and any remediable cause is dealt with.

Hereditary haemochromatosis

Hereditary haemochromatosis (HH) is an inherited disease characterized by excess iron deposition in various organs, leading to eventual fibrosis and functional organ failure. It is one of the most common inherited diseases in those of European descent, occurring in about 1 in 300 people, with approximately 10% of the population being carriers.

Aetiology

Inappropriate and excessive iron absorption from the small bowel leads to overload, with deposition in, and damage to, the cells of the liver, heart, pancreas and pituitary gland. It is inherited as an autosomal recessive, with only homozygotes manifesting the clinical features of the disease. The genetic defect has been localized to the short arm of chromosome 6 and is due to a mutation in the gene designated HFE. HLA-A3, –B7 and –B14 occur with increased frequency compared to the general population.

Clinical features

Most affected individuals present in their 50s. There is a reduced incidence of overt disease in women, presumably because of iron lost in blood during menstruation. The classic triad of bronze skin pigmentation (caused by melanin deposition), hepatomegaly and diabetes mellitus is only present in cases of gross iron overload. Other more common features include gonadal atrophy and loss of libido secondary to pituitary dysfunction. There may be a cardiomyopathy and arthritis resulting from calcium pyrophosphate deposition in both large and small joints.

Investigations

- Serum liver biochemistry is often normal even with cirrhosis.
- Serum iron is elevated and total iron-binding capacity (TIBC) reduced. The transferrin saturation (serum iron/TIBC) is >60%, normally <33%.
- Serum ferritin reflects iron stores and is usually greatly elevated (often >500 µg/l).
- Liver biopsy is performed to measure the extent of tissue damage, to assess tissue iron and to measure the hepatic iron concentration.

Causes of secondary iron overload, such as multiple transfusions, must be excluded. In addition, in alcoholic liver disease hepatic iron stores may increase. The precise reason is unknown, but the hepatic iron concentration does not reach the very high levels seen in haemochromatosis.

Management

The aim of treatment is to remove excess tissue iron and render the patient iron deficient while maintaining a haemoglobin of greater than 11 g/dl. This is best achieved by venesection: 500 ml of blood are removed twice weekly, and this may need to be continued for up to 2 years. Three or four venesections per year are then required to prevent the reaccumulation of iron.

All first-degree relatives are screened with a serum ferritin to detect and treat early disease.

Prognosis

The major complication is the development of hepatocellular carcinoma in patients with cirrhosis. This can be prevented by venesection before cirrhosis develops, and life expectancy is then much the same as for the normal population.

Wilson's disease (hepatolenticular degeneration)

This is a rare, recessively inherited disorder in which there is failure of the normal mechanism to excrete copper in the bile, resulting in accumulation of copper and deposition in various organs to produce cirrhosis and basal ganglia degeneration. Although this is a rare disease it is potentially treatable and therefore all young patients with liver disease must be screened for this condition.

Clinical features

Children usually present with hepatic problems ranging from fulminant hepatic failure to cirrhosis. Young adults have more neurological problems, which start with a mild tremor and speech problems and progress to involuntary movements and eventual dementia. A specific sign is the Kayser–Fleisher ring, which is caused by copper deposition in the cornea. It appears as a greenish-brown pigment at the periphery of the cornea, best seen with a slit-lamp. Additional features are haemolytic anaemia and renal tubular defects.

Investigations

The diagnosis is usually made by demonstrating the following:

123

- Serum copper and ceruloplasmin (the copper-carrying protein) are usually low but can be normal
- Increased 24-hour urinary copper
- Increased hepatic copper concentration in a liver biopsy specimen.

Management

The treatment of choice is lifelong penicillamine, which binds copper and is then excreted in the urine. Liver transplantation may be offered to those with end-stage liver disease. First-degree relatives are screened by slit-lamp examination and serum ceruloplasmin measurements. Asymptomatic homozygotes should be treated.

α_1-Antitrypsin deficiency

This is a rare cause of cirrhosis. α_1-Antitrypsin (α_1-AT) is a glycoprotein and part of a family of protease inhibitors (Pi) which control various inflammatory cascades, e.g. complement and coagulation. The gene is located on chromosome 14. The genetic variants of α_1-AT are characterized by their electrophoretic mobilities as medium (M), slow (S) or very slow (Z). The normal genotype is PiMM, the homozygote for Z is PiZZ and the heterozygotes are PiMZ and PiSZ. S and Z variants are caused by single amino acid substitutions in the polypeptide chain which result in decreased synthesis and secretion of the protein by the liver.

Clinical features

The majority of patients with clinical disease are homozygous with a PiZZ phenotype. They have very low circulating levels of α_1-AT, associated with chronic liver disease and pulmonary emphysema (especially in smokers). The risk of liver disease is much smaller in heterozygotes, e.g. PiSZ or PiMZ.

Investigations

The serum α_1-AT is low. Liver biopsy demonstrates cirrhosis and α_1-AT-containing globules in the hepatocytes.

Management

There is no specific treatment. Patients should be advised to stop smoking.

Alcohol and the liver

Alcohol is the most common cause of chronic liver disease in the western world. Alcoholic liver disease occurs more commonly in men, usually in the fourth and fifth decades, although subjects can present in their 20s with advanced disease. Although alcohol acts as a hepatotoxin, the exact mechanism leading to hepatitis and cirrhosis is unknown. As only 10–20% of people who drink excessively develop cirrhosis, genetic predisposition and immunological mechanisms have been proposed.

There are three major pathological lesions and clinical illnesses associated with excessive alcohol intake: fatty liver, alcoholic hepatitis and cirrhosis.

Fatty liver

This is the most common biopsy finding in alcoholic individuals. Metabolism of alcohol within the liver produces fat, which accumulates within the hepatocyte (steatosis). A similar picture can be seen in obesity, diabetes, starvation and, occasionally, chronic illnesses. Symptoms are usually absent, and on examination there may be tender hepatomegaly. Laboratory tests are often normal, although an elevated mean corpuscular volume (MCV) often indicates heavy drinking. The γGT level is usually elevated. The fat disappears on cessation of alcohol intake but with continued drinking may progress to fibrosis and cirrhosis.

Alcoholic hepatitis

There is necrosis of the liver cells and infiltration of polymorphonuclear leucocytes, with accumulation of dense cytoplasmic material called a Mallory body in the hepatocytes. It may progress to cirrhosis, particularly with continued alcohol consumption. Presentation encompasses a broad spectrum of patients, from those who are asymptomatic to those who are very ill with hepatic failure. Investigations show a leucocytosis with elevated bilirubin and transferases. The albumin may be low and prothrombin time prolonged. Treatment is supportive and adequate nutritional intake must be maintained. Corticosteroids are of benefit in some cases.

Alcoholic cirrhosis

This represents the final stage of liver disease from alcohol abuse. There is destruction and fibrosis, with regenerating nodules producing a classic micronodular cirrhosis. Patients may be asymptomatic, although they often present with one of the complications of cirrhosis and there are usually signs of chronic liver disease. Investigation is as for cirrhosis in general. Management is directed at the complications of cirrhosis, and patients are advised to stop drinking for life. Abstinence from alcohol improves the 5-year survival rate.

LIVER TRANSPLANTATION

This is now an established treatment for end-stage chronic liver disease and, in some circumstances, for acute hepatic failure. Careful selection of patients is crucial. Psychological assessment and education of patients and their families is essential before transplantation. In adults primary biliary cirrhosis is the most common indication and, in these patients where the natural history is well defined, transplantation is offered when the serum bilirubin reaches 100 µmol/l. Absolute contraindications to transplantation are active sepsis outside the liver and biliary tree, HIV positivity and metastatic malignancy. With rare exceptions, patients over 65 years are not transplanted. Graft rejection is reduced by immunosuppression with a cyclosporin or tacrolimus (FK506)-based regimen. Early complications include haemorrhage, sepsis and acute rejection (<6 weeks), which is reversible with intensive immunosuppression. Late complications include recurrence of disease (hepatitis B and C) and chronic rejection, which is not reversible and requires retransplantation. The outcome of liver transplantation is good, with an overall 5-year survival rate of 70–85%.

Budd–Chiari syndrome

Budd–Chiari syndrome is caused by occlusion of the hepatic vein, thereby obstructing venous outflow from the liver.

Aetiology

Budd–Chiari syndrome may occur as a result of obstruction of the hepatic vein by malignancy, radiotherapy, trauma, or hypercoagulability states such as polycythaemia vera, taking the contraceptive pill or leukaemia. The cause is unknown in one-third of cases.

Clinical features

The syndrome presents acutely with abdominal pain, nausea, vomiting, hepatomegaly and ascites, or more insidiously with enlargement of the caudate lobe, splenomegaly, ascites and jaundice.

Investigations

The ascitic fluid shows a high protein content. Ultrasonography or CT scanning will show an enlarged caudate lobe, and Doppler studies will demonstrate abnormalities in the direction of blood flow.

Treatment

This is of the underlying cause, though a portacaval shunt may help; alternatively, liver transplantation may be required.

....

LIVER ABSCESS

Pyogenic liver abscess

Aetiology

The cause of pyogenic liver abscess is often unknown, although biliary sepsis or portal pyaemia from intra-abdominal sepsis may be responsible. Other causes include trauma, bacteraemia or direct extension from, for example, a perinephric abscess. The most common causative organism is *Escherichia coli*, but others include *Streptococcus faecalis*, *Proteus vulgaris* and *Staphylococcus aureus*.

Clinical features

Symptoms can be mild, although abdominal pain, fever, rigors, nausea and vomiting may occur. The patient may be jaundiced and the liver enlarged and tender.

Investigations

- Blood count usually shows a normochromic/normocytic anaemia and the ESR is elevated.
- Liver biochemistry shows a rise in serum alkaline phosphatase and an elevated bilirubin in 25% of cases.
- Ultrasonography and CT are useful for detecting fluid-filled lesions.

Management

Treatment is with broad-spectrum antibiotics and drainage of the abscess, usually under ultrasound guidance.

Amoebic abscess

Aetiology

An amoebic abscess results from spread of the organism *Entamoeba histolytica* from the bowel to the liver via the portal venous system (page 18). Multiple microabscesses develop which coalesce to form single or multiple large abscesses.

Clinical features

The onset is usually gradual with fever, weight loss and malaise, often with no history of dysentery. The patient looks ill, with tender hepatomegaly and sometimes consolidation or an effusion in the right side of the chest.

Investigations

This is as for pyogenic abscess. Serological tests for amoebae, e.g. complement-fixation test or enzyme-linked immunosorbent assay (ELISA), are almost always positive. Aspiration of the abscess yields fluid 'like anchovy sauce'.

Management

Metronidazole 800 mg three times daily is given for 10 days. Surgical drainage is used for large abscesses or those failing to respond to medical treatment.

Hydatid disease

For details of hydatid disease see page 27.

Jaundice in pregnancy

Viral hepatitis is the single most common cause of jaundice in pregnancy. Three types of liver disease are specific to pregnancy: acute fatty liver of pregnancy (a severe fulminating illness with jaundice, vomiting and hepatic coma), recurrent intrahepatic cholestasis (presenting with jaundice and pruritus), and haemolysis (occasionally producing jaundice), which occurs in pre-eclamptic toxaemia. The three conditions present most commonly in the third trimester and resolve with delivery of the baby.

LIVER TUMOURS

The most common malignant liver tumours are metastatic, particularly those from the gastrointestinal tract, breast or bronchus. Primary liver tumours may be either benign or malignant.

Hepatocellular carcinoma (hepatoma)

Hepatocellular carcinoma (HCC) is one of the most common cancers worldwide, although it is rare in the western hemisphere.

Aetiology

Several risk factors have been identified, including cirrhosis, hepatitis B infection and hepatitis C infection. Other suggested aetiological factors include aflatoxin, androgenic steroids and, possibly the contraceptive pill.

Clinical features

Weight loss, anorexia, fever, ascites and abdominal pain occur. The rapid development of these features in a patient with cirrhosis is suggestive of HCC.

Investigations

- Serum α-fetoprotein is raised.
- Ultrasonography or radioisotope scans show large filling defects in 90% of cases.
- Liver biopsy under ultrasound control provides histological confirmation.

Management

Surgical resection is occasionally possible, but chemotherapy and radiotherapy are unhelpful.

Prognosis

Survival is seldom for more than 6 months.

Benign liver tumours

The most common are haemangiomas, usually found incidentally on a liver ultrasonogram or CT scan. They require no treatment. Hepatic adenomas are less common and associated with use of oral contraceptives. Resection is required if there are symptoms (e.g. pain, intraperitoneal bleeding).

....

GALLSTONES

Gallstones are present in 10–20% of the population. They are most common in women and the prevalence increases with age.

Pathophysiology

Gallstones are of two types:

* *Cholesterol gallstones*, composed mainly of cholesterol and accounting for 80% of all gallstones in the western world. Cholesterol, insoluble in water, is held in solution by the detergent action of bile salts and phospholipids, with which it forms micelles and vesicles. Cholesterol gallstones only form in bile which has an excess of cholesterol relative to bile salts and phospholipids (supersaturated or lithogenic bile), thus allowing cholesterol crystals to form and grow as stones (Table 3.10).

Table 3.10 Risk factors for cholesterol gallstones

Risk factor	Mechanism
Increased age	
Sex (F>M)	Increased cholesterol in bile
Obesity	
Rapid weight loss	
Contraceptive pill	
Terminal ileal disease	Decreased bile salts in bile caused by
Terminal ileal resection	interruption of enterohepatic circulation

- *Pigment stones*, consisting of bilirubin polymers and calcium bilirubinate. They are seen in patients with chronic haemolysis, e.g. hereditary spherocytosis and sickle-cell disease, in which bilirubin production is increased, and also in cirrhosis. Pigment stones may also form in the bile ducts after cholecystectomy and with duct strictures.

Clinical presentation

Most gallstones never cause symptoms and cholecystectomy is not indicated in asymptomatic cases. The complications are summarized in Figure 3.7.

Acute cholecystitis

Acute cholecystitis follows the impaction of a stone in the cystic duct or neck of the gallbladder. Very occasionally acute cholecystitis may occur without stones (acalculous cholecystitis).

Clinical features

There is constant severe pain in the epigastrium and right hypochondrium, with radiation to the back and shoulder. There may be nausea, vomiting and jaundice. On examination there is fever and right hypochondrial tenderness, which is worse on inspiration (Murphy's sign).

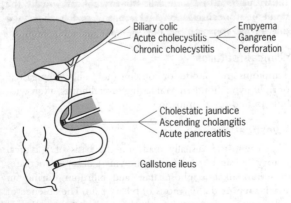

Biliary colic — Empyema
Acute cholecystitis — Gangrene
Chronic cholecystitis — Perforation

Cholestatic jaundice
Ascending cholangitis
Acute pancreatitis

Gallstone ileus

Figure 3.7
The complications of gallstones.

Investigations

- White cell count shows a leucocytosis.
- Serum liver biochemistry may be mildly abnormal.
- Radiology. The diagnosis is made by ultrasonography showing gallstones and a distended gallbladder with a thickened wall. There is focal tenderness directly over the visualized gallbladder (sonographic Murphy's sign).

Management

The initial treatment is conservative, with nil by mouth, intravenous fluids, pain relief and antibiotics, e.g. amoxycillin. Cholecystectomy is usually performed within 48 hours of the acute attack, and always if complications (see above) develop. Alternatively the patient may be readmitted for cholecystectomy 2–3 months later.

Chronic cholecystitis

Chronic inflammation of the gallbladder is often found in association with gallstones. There is no evidence that this produces any symptoms, and cholecystectomy is not indicated. Chronic right hypochondrial pain and fatty food intolerance are likely to be functional in origin and gallstones an incidental finding.

Biliary pain

Biliary pain, at one time called biliary colic, is usually the result of stone impaction in Hartman's pouch, the cystic duct or the common bile duct (CBD).

Clinical features

Symptoms are episodes of constant (not colicky) epigastric or right hypochondrial pain lasting several hours, often with little to find on examination.

Investigations

The diagnosis is usually made on the basis of a typical history and an ultrasonogram showing gallstones. Increases of serum alkaline phosphatase and bilirubin during an attack support the diagnosis of biliary pain. The absence of inflammatory features (fever, white cell count and local peritonism) differentiates this from acute cholecystitis.

Management

The treatment is analgesia and elective cholecystectomy. Abnormal liver biochemistry or a dilated CBD or stone in the CBD on ultrasonography, is an indication for exploration of the CBD at surgery.

Common bile duct stones (cholelithiasis)

Clinical features

CBD stones may be asymptomatic. Usually one or more of the symptoms of pain, jaundice and fever are present. The jaundice is cholestatic in type, and therefore the urine is dark, the stools pale and the skin may itch. High fever and rigors indicate biliary tract infection (cholangitis). Charcot's triad is the three symptoms occurring together, and indicates cholangitis.

Investigations

- White cell count shows a leucocytosis if infection is present.
- Blood cultures are often positive (*E.coli, S. faecalis*) in the presence of cholangitis.
- Liver biochemistry shows a cholestatic picture with a raised serum bilirubin and alkaline phosphatase.
- Radiology. Ultrasonography may show a dilated common bile duct containing a stone. Endoscopic ultrasound is more sensitive than transabdominal ultrasonography and is sometimes performed if there is a high index of suspicion and the latter is negative.
- ERCP confirms the diagnosis and allows stone removal.
- MRCP (magnetic resonance cholangiopancreatography) is a new technique which allows visualization of the biliary tract and pancreas. It may have a role in patients where ERCP is not possible or has failed.

Management

Treatment depends on the clinical situation, but includes analgesia for pain, and antibiotics (amoxicillin, with gentamicin in severe cases) if infection is present. The stone must be removed from the duct either by exploration of the

CBD at the time of cholecystectomy, or at ERCP following sphincterotomy and stone extraction with a Dormia basket or balloon.

Management of gallbladder stones

Cholecystectomy is the treatment of choice for symptomatic gallstones. This is almost always done via the laparoscope or by minilaparotomy.

Dissolution therapy In patients who refuse or are unfit for surgery pure cholesterol gallstones are dissolved by oral bile acids (e.g. ursodeoxycholic acid). Few patients are suitable for this approach because bile acids dissolve only radiolucent stones in a functioning gallbladder. Even after 2 years of treatment many stones have not dissolved, and those that have return when treatment is stopped.

Lithotripsy Shock-wave treatment of gallstones can be carried out using ultrasound guided lithotripters. The indications for treatment are the same as for dissolution therapy.

Primary sclerosing cholangitis

Primary sclerosing cholangitis (PSC) is a chronic cholestatic liver disease characterized by a progressive obliterating fibrosis of the intra- and extrahepatic ducts. Episodes of ascending cholangitis and jaundice are common. PSC is a progressive disease which may eventually lead to secondary biliary cirrhosis and, often, premature death from cholangiocarcinoma (bile duct cancer). It is of unknown cause; 75% or more cases have ulcerative colitis which may be asymptomatic. 80% of patients have myeloperoxidase ANCA antibodies (page 695) and liver biopsy shows fibrosis around the bile ducts (onion skin lesion) and ERCP shows multiple strictures. Extrahepatic strictures may be amenable to dilatation. Treatment is limited to management of the general complications of the disease, such as pruritus, fat malabsorption and complications arising from chronic liver disease. No specific treatment has been shown to retard the rate of disease progression and the only option is eventual liver transplantation. Patients with AIDS have been found to have sclerosing cholangitis that is believed to be infectious in origin.

PANCREATITIS

The classification of pancreatitis is difficult because of the inability to separate acute and chronic forms clearly. By definition, acute pancreatitis, which can occur as isolated or recurrent attacks, is distinguished from chronic pancreatitis by the absence of continuing inflammation, irreversible structural changes and permanent loss of exocrine and endocrine pancreatic function. The causes are shown in Table 3.11

Table 3.11 Causes of pancreatitis

Acute	Chronic
Gallstones	Alcohol (>85% of cases)
Alcohol	Idiopathic
Idiopathic (unknown cause)	Protein–energy
Metabolic: hypercalcaemia, hyperlipidaemia	malnutrition
Iatrogenic: postsurgical, ERCP	Hereditary
Drugs: e.g. azathioprine, corticosteroids	Cystic fibrosis

Acute pancreatitis

This is an acute condition presenting with abdominal pain and raised pancreatic enzymes in the blood or urine, resulting from inflammatory disease of the pancreas.

Pathogenesis

The exact pathophysiology is not well understood. Whatever the initiating event, there is acinar cell injury and release of activated proteases into the pancreatic interstitium. Disruption of acinar cells promotes migration of inflammatory cells from the microcirculation into the interstitium. Release of a variety of mediators and cytokines leads to a local inflammatory response, and sometimes a systemic inflammatory response that can result in single or multiple organ failure.

Clinical features

Epigastric or upper abdominal pain radiating through to the back is the cardinal symptom. There is often nausea and vomiting, and in severe cases multiorgan failure may develop. On examination there is epigastric tenderness, guarding and rigidity. Rarely, ecchymoses around the umbilicus (Cullen's sign) or in the flanks (Grey Turner's sign) may occur.

Diagnosis

A raised serum amylase, in conjunction with an appropriate history and clinical signs, strongly suggests a diagnosis of acute pancreatitis. Serum amylase may also be moderately raised in other abdominal conditions, such as acute cholecystitis and perforated duodenal ulcer, although very high amylase levels (>5 times normal) strongly suggest pancreatitis. In difficult cases peritoneal lavage with estimation of amylase in the peritoneal fluid may be useful. Ultrasonography or contrast enhanced CT scanning may reveal a swollen pancreas, sometimes with peripancreatic fluid collections. The presence of gallstones in the gallbladder or common bile duct suggest these as the aetiological factor.

Management

Nasogastric suction and intravenous hydration are instituted. Nothing is given by mouth, and in severe cases intravenous feeding is required. Analgesics with opiates (other than morphine) are usually required. As yet no specific drug treatment has been shown to be beneficial. The majority of cases are mild without systemic complications and associated only with interstitial inflammation; these patients usually recover uneventfully. Less commonly acute pancreatitis is associated with failure of one or more organ systems, such as renal failure, respiratory failure and impaired coagulation with disseminated intravascular coagulation. These severe attacks are usually associated with pancreatic necrosis, which is identified on CT scanning as focal areas of reduced tissue perfusion. Imipenim and cefuroxime reduce the number of septic complications and improve mortality in some patients with acute necrotizing pancreatitis. Surgical treatment is sometimes required for very severe necrotizing pancreatitis, particularly if it is infected, or if complications such as pancreatic abscesses or pseudocysts occur. Patients with biliary pancreatitis and evidence of cholangitis or progressive jaundice (both of which suggest a stone impacted in the common bile duct) may require urgent ERCP and stone removal.

Complications

General complications include hyperglycaemia, hypocalcaemia, renal failure and shock.

Prognosis

The mortality rate varies from 1% in mild cases to 50% in severe cases. Patients who recover may have recurrent attacks, depending on the aetiology.

Chronic pancreatitis

Chronic pancreatitis is defined as continuing inflammatory disease of the pancreas, characterized by irreversible morphological change and/or permanent impairment of function. Chronic calcifying pancreatitis is the commonest form in most developed countries, and is usually caused by alcohol. The disease is not reversible but it is possible to arrest the disease process, particularly if the patient stops drinking alcohol.

Clinical features

There is central abdominal pain which is located in the epigastrium and characteristically radiates to the back. The pain may be intermittent or constant, and exacerbations are precipitated by an alcoholic binge. The abdominal pain is accompanied by severe weight loss as a result of anorexia, and may be difficult to distinguish from the pain of pancreatic cancer.

Diabetes may develop and steatorrhoea occurs when the secretion of pancreatic lipase is reduced by 90%. Occasionally the patient presents with biliary obstruction, jaundice and cholangitis.

Investigation

The diagnosis of chronic pancreatitis is made by radiological techniques which demonstrate structural changes in the gland, and metabolic studies which demonstrate functional abnormalities.

Radiology. A plain abdominal radiograph will show pancreatic calcification in some cases. ERCP demonstrates dilatation of the pancreatic duct, with stenotic segments. Ultrasonography and CT scanning will show the dilated duct and demonstrate irregular consistency and outline of the gland.

Functional assessment. The serum amylase is of no use in the diagnosis of chronic pancreatitis, but may be raised during an acute episode of pain. A raised blood sugar indicates diabetes mellitus.

- The Lundh test. A tube is passed via the mouth into the duodenum and pancreatic trypsin and lipase are collected from the duodenal lumen after stimulation of secretion with a test meal.
- PABA test. N-benzoyl-L-tyrosyl P-aminobenzoic acid is given by mouth. Pancreatic chymotrypsin releases free P-aminobenzoic acid (PABA), which is absorbed and excreted in the urine. With pancreatic insufficiency there is reduced absorption and the amount measured in the urine is correspondingly low.

Treatment

The patient should be told to stop drinking alcohol. The pain may require opiates for control, with the attendant risk of addiction. Surgical resection combined with drainage of the pancreatic duct into the small bowel (pancreatico-jejunostomy) may be of value for severe disease with intractable pain. Pancreatic supplements (e.g. pancreatin 2–4 g with each meal) are useful for those with steatorrhoea and may reduce the frequency of attacks of pain in those with recurrent symptoms. Diabetes requires appropriate treatment with diet, oral hypoglycaemics or insulin.

Carcinoma of the pancreas

Epidemiology

Pancreatic cancer is the fourth most common cause of cancer death in the western world. Men are affected more commonly than women, and the incidence increases with age (peak in the seventh decade).

Aetiology

The aetiology is unknown but smoking, alcohol, coffee and dietary fats have all been implicated.

Clinical features

Cancer affecting the head of the pancreas presents with painless jaundice as a result of obstruction of the common duct, and weight loss. Cancer of the body or tail presents with abdominal pain, weight loss and anorexia. Diabetes may occur and there is an increased risk of thrombophlebitis. In cancer of the head of the pancreas, examination may reveal jaundice and a distended palpable gallbladder (Courvoisier's law: if, in a case of painless jaundice, the gallbladder is palpable the cause will not be gallstones). In gallstone disease chronic inflammation and fibrosis prevent distension of the gallbladder.

Investigation

The diagnosis is made with ultrasonography and/or CT. Duodenoscopy and ERCP may detect tumour in the head of the pancreas or at the ampulla. Endoscopic ultrasound is being increasingly used for staging and in difficult cases.

Management

Curative resection is not usually possible and treatment is therefore almost always palliative. Bypass of the obstructed common bile duct will relieve jaundice and this is usually performed with endoscopic placement of a stent, surgery being reserved for cases where the duodenum is obstructed. Chemotherapy and radiotherapy are of little value.

Prognosis

The prognosis is appalling: overall the 5-year survival rate is 1%, most patients being dead within a year of diagnosis.

ENDOCRINE TUMOURS

These tumours arise in the pancreas from APUD (amine precursor uptake and decarboxylation) cells, and are sometimes called apudomas. They usually secrete one hormone that produces the clinical effect, although other hormones are often also synthesized. Circulating hormone concentrations can be measured and high levels provide the diagnosis. Most neuroendocrine tumours express large numbers of somatostatin receptors. Intravenous injection of ^{111}In-labelled octreotide is therefore taken up readily by these tumours, and this test is the investigation of choice to localise the tumour and demonstrate the presence of metastases in patients suspected of having a neuroendocrine tumour. Endoscopic ultrasonography is also used in some patients to localize the tumour.

Gastrinomas (Zollinger–Ellison syndrome)

Gastrinomas arise from the G cells of the pancreas and secrete large amounts of gastrin. This stimulates maximal gastric acid secretion, resulting in the development of peptic ulcers, which are often multiple, large and may be resistant to conventional treatment. Diarrhoea may also occur as a result of inhibition of digestive enzymes at low pH in the intestine. Treatment is with omeprazole (which inhibits the H^+/K^+ proton pump necessary for acid secretion). Surgery is reserved for removal of the primary tumour only.

Vipomas

These rare tumours produce vasoactive intestinal polypeptide (VIP), which stimulates intestinal water and electrolyte secretion, causing severe watery diarrhoea and dehydration. Treatment is with surgical resection or octreotide.

Glucagonomas

Glucagonomas arise from the α cells of the pancreas and produce pancreatic glucagon. Patients present with diabetes mellitus and a unique necrolytic migratory erythematous rash.

Diseases of the blood and haematological malignancies

4

ANAEMIA

Anaemia is present when there is a decrease in the level of haemoglobin (Hb) in the blood below the reference range for the age and sex of the individual. Reduction of Hb is usually accompanied by a fall in red cell count (RCC) and packed cell volume (PCV, haematocrit), although an increase in plasma volume (as with massive splenomegaly) may cause anaemia with a normal RCC and PCV ('dilutional anaemia'). The normal values for these indices are given in Table 4.1, all of which are measured using automated cell counters as part of a routine full blood count (FBC).

Table 4.1 Normal values for adult peripheral blood

	Men	Women
Hb (g/dl)	13–18	11.5–15.5
PCV (haematocrit, l/l)	0.42–0.53	0.36–0.45
RCC (10^{12}/l)	4.5–6.0	3.9–5.1
MCV (fl)	80–96	
MCH (pg)	27–33	
MCHC (g/dl)	32–35	
WCC (10^9/l)	4.0–11.0	
Platelets (10^9/l)	150–400	
ESR (mm/h)	<20	
Reticulocytes (%)	0.2–2.0	

ESR, erythrocyte sedimentation rate; Hb, haemoglobin; MCH, mean corpuscular haemoglobin; MCHC, mean corpuscular haemoglobin concentration; MCV, mean corpuscular volume of red cells; PCV, packed cell volume; RCC, red cell count; WCC, white cell count.

Clinical features

Symptoms depend on the severity and speed of onset of anaemia. A very slowly falling level of Hb allows for haemodynamic compensation and enhancement of the oxygen-carrying capacity of the blood. In general elderly people tolerate anaemia less well than young people. The symptoms are non-specific and include fatigue, faintness and breathlessness. Angina pectoris and intermittent claudication may occur in those with coexistent atheromatous arterial disease. On examination the skin and mucous membranes are pale; there may be a tachycardia and a systolic flow murmur. Cardiac failure may occur in elderly people or those with compromised cardiac function.

Classification of anaemias (Table 4.2)

The anaemias are classified in terms of the red cell indices, particularly the mean corpuscular volume (MCV). The mean corpuscular haemoglobin (MCH) provides little additional information. This classification is useful because the type of anaemia then indicates the underlying causes and necessary investigations.

Microcytic anaemia

Iron deficiency

Iron is necessary for the formation of haem and iron deficiency is the most common cause of a microcytic anaemia. Iron is absorbed in the duodenum and jejunum; factors that promote absorption include gastric acid, iron deficiency and active erythropoiesis. Iron is transported in the plasma bound to the protein transferrin, which is synthesized in the liver and normally about one-third saturated with iron (Figure 4.1), and stored in the reticuloendothelial system as ferritin and haemosiderin. A fixed amount of iron, about 1 mg, is lost in sweat, urine and faeces each day. In women there is an additional loss during menses, and premenopausal women may often border on iron deficiency.

Aetiology

The most common cause of iron deficiency is blood loss from the uterus or gastrointestinal tract. Other causes are:

• Increased demands, e.g. during growth and pregnancy
• Decreased absorption with small bowel disease or after gastrectomy
• Poor intake; this is rare in developed countries.

Table 4.2 Classification of the anaemias based on MCV

Microcytic hypochromic	Normocytic/normochromic	Macrocytic
Low MCV and MCH	**Normal MCV and MCH**	**High MCV**
Iron deficiency	Acute blood loss	Megaloblastic
Anaemia of chronic disease	Anaemia of chronic disease	Vitamin B$_{12}$ deficiency
Thalassaemia	Aplastic anaemia	Folate deficiency
Sideroblastic anaemia	Combined deficiency, e.g. iron and folate	
	Haemolytic anaemia	Normoblastic
	Endocrine disorders	Myelodysplasia
	Hypopituitarism	Haemolysis
	Hypothyroidism	Other defects of DNA synthesis,
	Hypoadrenalism	e.g. chemotherapy

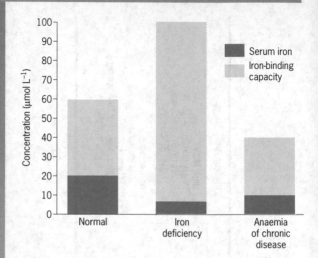

Figure 4.1
Serum iron and total iron-binding capacity in normal subjects and iron deficiency anaemia and anaemia of chronic disease.

Clinical features

Symptoms and signs are the result of anaemia (see earlier) and of decreased epithelial cell iron, which causes brittle hair and nails, atrophic glossitis, angular stomatitis and koilonychia (spoon-shaped nails). Rarely, pharyngeal webs occur which may cause dysphagia (Paterson–Brown–Kelly syndrome).

Investigations

- Blood count shows a low Hb with a low MCV.
- Blood film: the red cells are microcytic and hypochromic, with anisocytosis (variation in size) and poikilocytosis (variation in shape).
- Serum iron is low and the total iron-binding capacity (TIBC) is high (Figure 4.1).
- Serum ferritin reflects iron stores and is low.
- Bone marrow examination is only necessary in complicated cases, and shows erythroid hyperplasia and absence of iron.

Iron deficiency is almost always the result of gastrointestinal blood loss in men and in postmenopausal women, and further investigation is required (see page 61). Mild anaemia in premenopausal women is usually the result of menstrual blood loss.

Differential diagnosis

This is from other causes of a microcytic/hypochromic anaemia (see Table 4.2).

Management

- Treat the underlying cause.
- Oral iron, e.g. ferrous sulphate 200 mg three times daily, is given for about 6 months to correct the anaemia and replace iron stores.
- Parenteral iron injections are rarely necessary and are used only when patients are intolerant or there is a poor response to oral iron, e.g. severe malabsorption.
  Intravenous iron carries a significant risk of anaphylactoid reactions, and is only used when there is no alternative.

Anaemia of chronic disease

This occurs in patients with a variety of chronic diseases, including chronic renal failure, chronic inflammatory diseases such as Crohn's disease and polymyalgia rheumatica, and chronic infections such as tuberculosis and infective endocarditis. Anaemia of chronic disease presents with a normochromic, normocytic or microcytic anaemia which is differentiated from iron deficiency by measurement of iron indices (Figure 4.1). Serum ferritin is elevated or within the normal range. It is the result of decreased release of iron from bone marrow to developing erythroblasts, inadequate erythropoietin response to the anaemia, and decreased red cell survival. Treatment is of the underlying cause.

Sideroblastic anaemia

Sideroblastic anaemia is a rare disorder of haem synthesis characterized by a refractory anaemia with hypochromic cells in the peripheral blood and ring sideroblasts in the bone marrow. Ring sideroblasts are erythroblasts with iron deposited in mitochondria around the nucleus. It may be inherited or acquired (secondary to myelodysplasia, alcohol, lead or isoniazid, or idiopathic). Treatment is to withdraw the causative agents. Some cases respond to pyridoxine (vitamin B$_6$). In many cases anaemia is transfusion dependent and iron overload becomes a problem.

Macrocytic anaemias

Macrocytosis is a rise in mean cell volume of the red cells above the normal range (80–96 fl [fentolitres] in adults). Macrocytic anaemia can be divided into megaloblastic and non-megaloblastic types, depending on the bone marrow findings.

Megaloblastic anaemia

The megaloblastic anaemias are a group of anaemias characterized by the presence in the bone marrow of developing red blood cells with delayed nuclear maturation relative to that of the cytoplasm (*megaloblasts*). The underlying mechanism is defective DNA synthesis, which may also affect the white cells (causing hypersegmented neutrophil nuclei with six lobes, and sometimes leucopenia) and platelets (causing thrombocytopenia). The most common cause (see Table 4.2) of megaloblastic anaemia is deficiency of vitamin B$_{12}$ or folate, which are both necessary to synthesize DNA.

Vitamin B$_{12}$ deficiency

Vitamin B$_{12}$ is obtained from animal sources such as meat, fish, eggs and milk. The daily requirement is 1 μg which is easily supplied by a balanced western diet (containing 10–30 μg daily). Vitamin B$_{12}$ is liberated from protein complexes in food by pancreatic and gastric enzymes and binds to intrinsic factor which is secreted from gastric parietal cells. This complex is delivered to the terminal ileum, where vitamin B$_{12}$ is absorbed and transported to the tissues by the carrier protein transcobalamin II. Vitamin B$_{12}$ is stored in the liver, where there is sufficient supply for 2 or more years. The causes of vitamin B$_{12}$ deficiency are listed in Table 4.3.

Pernicious anaemia

Pernicious anaemia is an autoimmune condition in which there is atrophy of the gastric mucosa with failure of intrinsic factor production and consequent vitamin B$_{12}$ malabsorption. It is the most common cause of vitamin B$_{12}$ deficiency in western countries.

Table 4.3 Vitamin B_{12} deficiency – causes

Low dietary intake
Vegans

Impaired absorption
Stomach
    Pernicious anaemia
    Gastrectomy
Small bowel
    Ileal disease or resection
    Coeliac disease
    Tropical sprue
    Bacterial overgrowth

Transcobalamin deficiency (rare)

Epidemiology

This is a disease of elderly people (1 in 8000 over the age of 60 years affected). It is more common in women and in people with fair hair and blue eyes. There is an association with other autoimmune diseases, e.g. hypothyroidism and vitiligo.

Pathology

There is glandular atrophy of the gastric mucosa causing absent acid and intrinsic factor secretion.

Clinical features

The onset of pernicious anaemia is insidious, with progressively increasing symptoms of anaemia. There may be glossitis (a red sore tongue), angular stomatitis and mild jaundice. Neurological features can occur with very low levels of serum B_{12} and include a polyneuropathy caused by symmetrical damage to the peripheral nerves and posterior and lateral columns of the spinal cord (subacute combined degeneration of the cord). The latter presents with progressive weakness, ataxia and eventually paraplegia if untreated. Dementia and visual disturbances due to optic atrophy may also occur.

Investigations

- Blood count and film: a macrocytic anaemia (MCV often >110 fl) is often seen with hypersegmented neutrophil nuclei and, in severe cases, leucopenia and thrombocytopenia.

- Serum vitamin B_{12} is low, frequently <50 ng/l (normal >160 ng/l).
- Red cell folate may be reduced because vitamin B_{12} is necessary to convert serum folate to the active intracellular form.
- Serum bilirubin is raised as a result of excess breakdown of haemoglobin, owing to ineffective erythropoiesis in the bone marrow.
- Serum autoantibodies: parietal cell antibodies are present in 90% and antibodies to intrinsic factor in 50%.
- The Schilling test (Table 4.4) will differentiate pernicious anaemia from small bowel malabsorption as the cause of vitamin B_{12} deficiency. Defective vitamin B_{12} absorption is corrected by intrinsic factor in the former. In practice the cause is often apparent from the history and auto-antibody screen, and the Schilling test is rarely performed.
- Bone marrow examination shows a hypercellular bone marrow with megaloblastic changes. This is not necessary in straightforward cases.

Table 4.4 Schilling test

Part I
- Give 1 µg ^{58}Co–vitamin B_{12} orally to the fasting patient.
- Give 1000 µg B_{12} (non-radioactive) by intramuscular injection to saturate vitamin B_{12}-binding proteins and to flush out ^{58}Co–vitamin B_{12}.
- Collect urine for 24 h. Normal subjects excrete more than 10% of the radioactive dose.

If abnormal:
Part II
- Repeat part I after giving oral intrinsic factor capsules.

Result
- If excretion still abnormal, lesion is in the terminal ileum or there is bacterial overgrowth.
- If excretion now normal, diagnosis is pernicious anaemia or gastrectomy.

Management

Traditionally, treatment is with intramuscular hydroxycobalamin. Injections (1 mg) are given twice weekly for 3 weeks to replenish body stores, and then

3-monthly injections continued for life. However, gastrointestinal absorption of vitamin B$_{12}$ is not entirely dependent on the presence of intrinsic factor and there has been renewed interest in treatment with high dose (2 mg daily) oral cobalamin.

Complications

There is an increased incidence of gastric carcinoma. However, screening is not routinely recommended and endoscopy or barium meal examination of the stomach is performed only if there are gastric symptoms.

Folate deficiency

Folate is found in green vegetables and offal, and absorbed in the upper small intestine. The daily requirement for folate is 100–200 μg and a normal mixed diet contains 200–300 μg. Body stores are sufficient for about 4 months, but folate deficiency may develop much more rapidly in patients who have a poor intake and excess utilization of folate, for example patients in intensive care. The causes of folate deficiency are shown in Table 4.5. The main cause is poor intake, which may occur alone or in combination with excessive utilization or malabsorption.

Table 4.5 Causes of folate deficiency

Poor intake	Old age, poverty, alcohol excess (also impaired utilization), anorexia
Malabsorption	Coeliac disease, tropical sprue
Excess utilization	
Physiological	Pregnancy, lactation, prematurity
Pathological	Chronic haemolytic anaemia, malignant and inflammatory diseases, dialysis
Drugs	Phenytoin, trimethoprim, sulphasalazine

Clinical features

Symptoms and signs are the result of anaemia.

Investigations

Red cell folate is low (normal range 160–640 μg/ml) and is a more accurate guide of tissue folate than serum folate, which is also low (normal range 4.0–18 μg/l). If the history does not suggest dietary deficiency, further investigations such as a jejunal biopsy should be performed to look for small bowel disease.

Management

The underlying cause must be treated and folate deficiency corrected by giving oral folic acid 5 mg daily for 4 months; higher daily doses may be necessary with malabsorption. In megaloblastic anaemia of undetermined cause, folic acid alone must not be given, as this will aggravate the neuropathy of vitamin B_{12} deficiency. Prophylactic folic acid is given to patients with chronic haemolysis (5 mg weekly) and pregnant women.

Prevention of neural tube defects with folic acid To prevent first occurrence of neural tube defects women who are planning a pregnancy should be advised to take folate supplements (at least 400 µg/day) before conception and during the first 12 weeks of pregnancy. Larger doses (5 mg daily) are recommended for mothers who already have an infant with a neural tube defect.

Differential diagnosis of megaloblastic anaemias

A raised MCV with macrocytosis on the peripheral blood film can occur with a normoblastic rather than a megaloblastic bone marrow (Table 4.6). The most common cause of macrocytosis in the UK is alcohol excess. The exact mechanism for the large red cells in each of these

Table 4.6 Causes of macrocytosis other than megaloblastic anaemia

Physiological
Pregnancy
Newborn

Pathological
Alcohol excess
Liver disease
Reticulocytosis
Hypothyroidism
Haematological disorders
   Myelodysplastic syndrome (a frequent cause in the elderly)
   Sideroblastic anaemia
   Aplastic anaemia
Drugs: hydroxyurea and azathioprine
Cold agglutinins

conditions is uncertain, but in some is thought to be due to excessive lipid deposition on red cell membranes.

Anaemia caused by marrow failure (aplastic anaemia)

Aplastic anaemia is defined as pancytopenia (deficiency of all cell elements of the blood) with *hypocellularity* (aplasia) of the bone marrow. It is an uncommon but serious condition which may be inherited but is more commonly acquired.

Aetiology

A list of the main causes of aplasia is given in Table 4.7. Suppression of bone marrow pluripotential stem cells by cytotoxic T cells is responsible for many cases of idiopathic acquired aplastic anaemia. Many drugs have been associated with the development of aplastic anaemia, and this occurs as a predictable dose-related effect (e.g. chemotherapeutic agents) or as an idiosyncratic reaction (e.g. chloramphenicol).

Table 4.7 Causes of pancytopenia

Hypocellular bone marrow	Cellular bone marrow
Aplastic anaemia	Megaloblastic anaemia
Congenital	Bone marrow infiltration or
Idiopathic acquired (50% of cases)	replacement
Chemicals, e.g. benzene	Lymphoma
Drugs: cytotoxics, chloramphenicol,	Acute leukaemia
gold	Myeloma
Insecticides	Secondary carcinoma
Ionizing radiation	Myelofibrosis
Infections, e.g. viral hepatitis,	
measles, HIV	Hypersplenism
Paroxysmal nocturnal haemoglobinuria	Systemic lupus erythematosus
Overwhelming sepsis	

Clinical features

Symptoms are the result of the deficiency of red blood cells, white blood cells and platelets, and include anaemia, increased susceptibility to infection, and bleeding. Physical findings include bruising, bleeding gums and epistaxis. Mouth infections are common.

Investigations

- Blood count shows pancytopenia with low or absent reticulocytes.
- Bone marrow examination shows a hypocellular marrow with increased fat spaces.

Differential diagnosis

This is from other causes of pancytopenia (Table 4.7). A bone marrow trephine biopsy is essential for assessment of the bone marrow cellularity.

Management

The cause of the aplastic anaemia must be eliminated if possible. Supportive care, including transfusions of red cells and platelets and antibiotic therapy, should be given as necessary. The course of aplastic anaemia is very variable, ranging from a rapid spontaneous remission to a persistent, increasingly severe pancytopenia, which may lead to death through haemorrhage or infection. Bad prognostic features are the following:

- A peripheral blood neutrophil count $<0.5 \times 10^9/l$
- A peripheral blood platelet count $<20 \times 10^9/l$
- A reticulocyte count of $<40 \times 10^9/l$ (0.1%).

In those patients who do not undergo spontaneous recovery the options for treatment are as follows.

- Bone marrow transplantation (BMT) from a histocompatible sibling donor is the treatment of choice for young patients (<20 years).
- Immunosuppressive therapy with antilymphocyte globulin and cyclosporin is used for patients over the age of 45 in whom BMT is not indicated because of the high risk of graft-versus-host disease.

The treatment of patients aged 20–45 varies between different centres, some favouring BMT, whereas others use immunosuppressive therapy.

....

HAEMOLYTIC ANAEMIA

Haemolytic anaemia results from increased destruction of red cells with a reduction of the circulating lifespan (normally 120 days). Haemolysis may be extravascular (within the reticuloendothelial system) or intravascular (within the blood vessels). The causes of haemolytic anaemia in adults are listed in Table 4.8.

Table 4.8 Causes of haemolytic anaemia

Inherited	Acquired
Red cell membrane defect	Immune
Hereditary spherocytosis	Autoimmune haemolytic anaemia
Hereditary elliptocytosis	Haemolytic transfusion reactions
Haemoglobin abnormalities	Non-immune
Thalassaemia	Paroxysmal nocturnal
Sickle-cell disease	haemoglobinuria
	Microangiopathic haemolytic
Metabolic defects	anaemia
Glucose-6-phosphate	March haemoglobinuria
dehydrogenase deficiency	
Pyruvate kinase deficiency	Miscellaneous
	Infections (e.g. malaria)
	Drugs/chemicals
	Hypersplenism

In most haemolytic conditions, red cell destruction is extravascular and cells are removed from the circulation by macrophages in the reticuloendothelial system, particularly the spleen.

When red cells are broken down within the circulation, Hb is released and binds to plasma haptoglobins. When these become saturated, free Hb appears in the urine. Some Hb is broken down in the renal tubular cells and appears as haemosiderin in the urine. Figure 4.2 shows an approach to investigating the patient with suspected haemolytic anaemia.

INHERITED HAEMOLYTIC ANAEMIAS

Membrane defects

Hereditary spherocytosis

Hereditary spherocytosis is the most common inherited haemolytic anaemia in northern Europeans, and is inherited in an autosomal dominant manner. It is the result of a defect in the red cell membrane caused by deficiency of the structural membrane protein *spectrin*. Red cells become

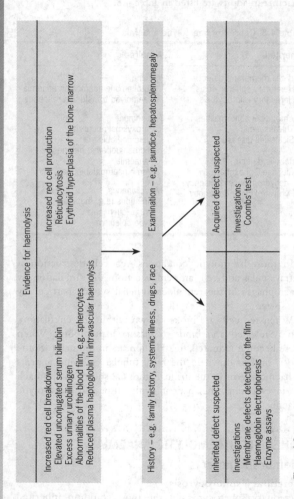

Figure 4.2
An algorithm for investigation of suspected haemolytic anaemia.

Evidence for haemolysis

Increased red cell breakdown
Elevated unconjugated serum bilirubin
Excess urinary urobilinogen
Abnormalities of the blood film, e.g. spherocytes
Reduced plasma haptoglobin in intravascular haemolysis

Increased red cell production
Reticulocytosis
Erythroid hyperplasia of the bone marrow

History – e.g. family history, systemic illness, drugs, race

Examination – e.g. jaundice, hepatosplenomegaly

Inherited defect suspected

Investigations
Membrane defects detected on the film
Haemoglobin electrophoresis
Enzyme assays

Acquired defect suspected

Investigations
Coombs' test

spherical in shape, are more rigid and less deformable than normal red cells, and are thus destroyed prematurely in the spleen.

Clinical features

Hereditary spherocytosis may present with jaundice or be asymptomatic. Patients may develop anaemia, splenomegaly and leg ulcers. As in many haemolytic anaemias, the course of the disease may be interrupted by aplastic, haemolytic and megaloblastic crises. Aplastic anaemia usually occurs after infections, particularly with parvovirus, whereas megaloblastic anaemia is the result of folate depletion caused by hyperactivity of the bone marrow. Chronic haemolysis may lead to the development of pigment gallstones.

Investigations

- Blood count demonstrates reticulocytosis and anaemia, which is usually mild.
- The blood film shows spherocytes (also seen in autoimmune haemolytic anaemia) and reticulocytes.

The diagnosis is made by demonstration of increased red cell osmotic fragility when placed in hypotonic solutions.

Management

Splenectomy should be performed in all but the mildest of cases. This is usually postponed until after childhood, to minimize the risk of overwhelming pneumococcal infection. Following splenectomy, all patients should receive pneumococcal vaccine and long-term prophylactic penicillin.

Hereditary elliptocytosis

Hereditary elliptocytosis is similar to spherocytosis but the red cells are elliptical in shape. It is milder clinically and usually does not require treatment.

Haemoglobin abnormalities

Normal adult Hb is made up of haem and two polypeptide globin chains, α and β. The haemoglobinopathies can be classified into two subgroups: *abnormal chain production* or *abnormal chain structure* of the polypeptide chains (Table 4.9).

Table 4.9 Types of haemoglobin

	Haemoglobin	Structure	Comment
Normal	A	$\alpha_2\beta_2$	92% of adult haemoglobin
	A_{Ic}	$\alpha_2\beta_2$	5% of adult haemoglobin (glycosylated Hb)
	A_2	$\alpha_2\delta_2$	2% of adult haemoglobin; elevated in β-thalassaemia
	F	$\alpha_2\gamma_2$	Normal haemoglobin in fetus from 3rd to 9th month; increased in β-thalassaemia
Abnormal chain production	H	β_4	Found in α-thalassaemia
	Barts	γ_4	Found in homozygous α-thalassaemia
Abnormal chain structure	S	$\alpha_2\beta_2$	Substitution of valine for glutamic acid in position 6 of the β chain
	C	$\alpha_2\beta_2$	Substitution of lysine for glutamic acid in position 6 of the β chain

Thalassaemia

In normal Hb there is a balance (1:1) in the production of α and β chains. The thalassaemias are a group of disorders arising from one or multiple gene defects, resulting in a reduced rate of production of one or more globin chains. The imbalanced globin chain production leads to precipitation of globin chains within red cells or precursors. This results in cell damage, death of red cell precursors in the bone marrow (ineffective erythropoiesis), and haemolysis. The disease was first identified in people living in the Mediterranean region, but is now known to occur worldwide.

There are two main types:

- α-Thalassaemia: reduced α-chain synthesis
- β-Thalassaemia: reduced β-chain synthesis.

β-Thalassaemia In homozygous β-Thalassaemia there is little or no β-chain production, resulting in excess α chains. These combine with whatever δ and γ chains are produced, leading to increased Hb A_2 and Hb F. There are three main clinical forms of β-thalassaemia:

- *β-Thalassaemia trait*: this is the asymptomatic heterozygous carrier state. Anaemia is mild or absent, with a low MCV and MCH. Iron stores are normal.
- *β-Thalassaemia intermedia*: this includes patients with moderate anaemia (Hb 7–10 g/dl) that does not require regular blood transfusions. Splenomegaly, bone deformities, recurrent leg ulcers and gallstones are other features. This may be caused by a combination of homozygous β- and α-thalassaemias.
- *β-Thalassaemia major* (homozygous β-thalassaemia): this presents in the first year of life with severe anaemia (*Cooley's anaemia*), failure to thrive and recurrent infections. Hypertrophy of the ineffective bone marrow leads to bony abnormalities: the thalassaemic facies, with an enlarged maxilla and prominent frontal and parietal bones. Resumption of haemopoiesis in the spleen and liver (extramedullary haemopoiesis), the chief sites of red cell production in fetal life, leads to hepatosplenomegaly.

Investigations

Blood count and film show a hypochromic/microcytic anaemia, raised reticulocyte count and nucleated red cells in the peripheral circulation.

The diagnosis is made by haemoglobin electrophoresis, which shows an increase in Hb F and absent or markedly reduced Hb A.

Management

The mainstay of treatment is blood transfusion, aiming to keep the haemoglobin above 10 g/dl, thus suppressing ineffective erythropoiesis, preventing bony abnormalities and allowing normal development. Iron overload caused by repeated transfusions may lead to damage to endocrine glands, liver, pancreas and heart, with death in the second decade from cardiac failure. Treatment with the iron-chelating agent desferrioxamine may prevent iron loading.

Bone marrow transplantation has been used in some cases of thalassaemia.

α–Thalassaemia

The clinical manifestations of this disorder vary from a mild anaemia with microcytosis to a severe condition incompatible with life. There are four α-globin genes per cell. The manifestations depend on whether one, two, three or all four of the genes are deleted, and thus whether α-chain synthesis is partial or completely absent. In the most severe form, where there is complete absence of α-globin (Hb Barts), infants are stillborn (hydrops fetalis).

Antenatal diagnosis of haemoglobin abnormalities

It is possible to identify a fetus with β–thalassaemia major by DNA analysis of chorionic villous samples taken in the first trimester, or by testing umbilical cord blood in the second trimester. Abortion is offered if the fetus is found to be affected. This examination is appropriate if the mother is found to have a thalassaemia trait during antenatal testing and if on subsequent screening, her partner is also affected.

Sickle–cell disease

Sickle-cell disease is a family of haemoglobin disorders in which the sickle β-globin gene is inherited. The gene for sickle haemoglobin (haemoglobin S) results in the substitution of the amino acid valine for glutamic acid normally present in position 6 of the β chain of haemoglobin. In the homozygous state (*sickle cell anaemia*) both genes are abnormal (HbSS), whereas in the heterozygous state (*sickle cell trait*, Hb AS) only one chromosome carries the abnormal gene. Inheritance of the HbS gene from one parent and HbC from the other parent gives rises to Hb SC disease, which tends to run a milder clinical course than sickle cell disease but with more thromboses.

The sickle β gene is spread widely throughout Africa (25% carry the gene), the Middle East and Mediterranean countries. One of the main factors in this distribution is that patients with sickle-cell trait have a relative resistance to malaria, so are more likely to survive, breed and pass on their genes.

In the deoxygenated state Hb S molecules link to form chains, and this results in increased rigidity of the red cells, causing the classic sickle appearance. Sickling results in premature destruction of red cells (haemolysis) and obstruction of the microcirculation (vaso-occlusion), leading to tissue infarction. As the production of Hb F is normal, the disease is usually not manifest until Hb F decreases to adult levels at about 6 months of age.

Clinical features

In the heterozygous state, Hb AS (sickle-cell trait), there are usually no symptoms unless the patient is exposed to extreme hypoxia, e.g. poor anaesthesia.

Symptoms of the homozygous state, Hb SS (sickle-cell anaemia), are due to haemolysis and vaso-occlusion.

Haemolysis Symptoms vary from mild anaemia to severe haemolysis with recurrent sickle-cell crises. Chronic haemolysis is associated with increased formation of pigment gallstones. Most patients with sickle-cell disease have a steady-state Hb of 6–8 g/dl with a high reticulocyte count (10–20%). Most patients do not have symptoms of anaemia because tissue oxygen delivery is normal owing to a hyperdynamic circulation and the lower oxygen affinity of Hb S, which releases oxygen to the tissues more easily than normal Hb. A rapid fall in the Hb may be due to:

- Aplastic crisis – this is often due to parvovirus infection, which destroys erythrocyte precursors
- Acute sequestration crisis – the liver and spleen become engorged with red cells, leading to a fall in Hb and rapid enlargement of these organs
- Haemolysis due to drugs or infection.

Vaso-occlusion Avascular necrosis of bone marrow results in the bone pain crisis, which may be precipitated by hypoxia, dehydration or infection. In adults bone pain most commonly affects the juxta-articular parts of the long bones, the ribs, spine and pelvis. In early childhood the small bones of the hands and feet are affected (dactylitis), which may result in shortened deformed bones. Most patients with a painful crisis are managed in the community, but hospital admission is necessary (Emergency Box 4.1) when the pain is not controlled by non-opiate analgesia such as paracetamol and NSAIDs. Other complications of vaso-occlusion include:

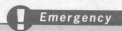

Emergency

- Analgesia:
⇒ diclofenac 1 mg/kg every 8 hours orally
⇒ morphine 10 µg/kg/h by intravenous infusion if no response to diclofenac

- 60% oxygen by face mask if arterial oxygen saturation decreased

- Take blood for FBC, reticulocytes, urea and electrolytes

- Rehydrate with intravenous fluids

- Search for and treat any source of infection

- Check Hb and reticulocyte count at least once daily

- Examine the chest at least once daily and the abdomen for increase in liver or spleen size, which may indicate a sequestration crisis

Emergency Box 4.1
Management of a painful sickle-cell crisis in hospital

- Splenic atrophy, which results in susceptibility to infection with pneumococcus, *Salmonella* species and haemophilus
- Cerebral infarction, causing fits and hemiplegia
- Retinal ischaemia, which may precipitate proliferative sickle retinopathy and visual loss.

Other complications of sickle-cell disease include renal papillary necrosis and chronic renal failure, leg ulcers, and the acute chest syndrome. The latter is a medical emergency characterized by fever, cough dyspnoea and pulmonary infiltrates on the chest X-ray. Sequestration of red cells within the corpora cavernosa causes priapism (prolonged erections) and eventual impotence.

Investigations

- Blood count: in sickle-cell disease there is a low haemoglobin (6–8 g/dl) with a high reticulocyte count. Patients with sickle-cell trait are not anaemic.
- Blood film shows sickled erythrocytes.

Diagnosis is made with Hb electrophoresis showing 80–90% Hb SS and absent Hb A. In addition, sickling can be induced in vitro with sodium metabisulphite.

Treatment and screening

Asymptomatic anaemia requires no treatment. Folic acid is given to patients with severe haemolysis, and to women before conception and during pregnancy. The risk of pneumococcal infection is reduced by prophylaxis with daily oral penicillin and pneumococcal vaccine. Routine vaccination against *Haemophilus influenzae* is given to all children in the UK. Exchange transfusions may be used to reduce the frequency of crises, or as prophylaxis in pregnancy or before surgery.

In clinical trials hydroxyurea has been shown to raise the concentration of fetal Hb and ameliorate the clinical course, but concerns remain over its myelosuppresive side effects. Bone marrow transplantation from an HLA-matched sibling has been used in some patients with severe disease.

People from areas with a high prevalence of sickle-cell disease should be screened before general anaesthesia, and before or during pregnancy.

Prognosis

The median survival is 40–50 years; the commonest cause of death in adult sickle-cell disease is the acute sickle chest syndrome (see above).

Metabolic red cell disorders

A number of red cell enzyme deficiencies may produce haemolytic anaemia, the most common of which is glucose-6-phosphate dehydrogenase (G6PD) deficiency.

Glucose-6-phosphate dehydrogenase deficiency

G6PD is a vital enzyme in the hexose monophosphate shunt, which maintains glutathione in the reduced state. Glutathione is important in combating oxidative stress in the red cell. G6PD deficiency is a common heterogeneous X-linked trait found predominantly in African, Mediterranean and Middle Eastern populations.

G6PD deficiency causes neonatal jaundice, chronic haemolytic anaemia, and acute haemolysis precipitated by the ingestion of fava beans and oxidizing drugs such as quinine, sulphonamides and nitrofurantoin. Diagnosis is by direct measurement of enzyme levels in the red cell. Treatment is the avoidance of precipitating factors, and transfusion if necessary.

ACQUIRED HAEMOLYTIC ANAEMIA

Autoimmune haemolytic anaemia

Autoimmune haemolytic anaemia is classified according to whether the antibody reacts best at body temperature (*warm antibodies*) or at lower temperatures (*cold antibodies*) (Table 4.10). IgG or IgM antibodies attach to the red cell, resulting in extravascular haemolysis through sequestration in the spleen, or in intravascular haemolysis through activation of complement.

Table 4.10 Features of autoimmune haemolytic anaemia

	Warm antibody	Cold antibody
Temperature at which antibody attaches best to red cell	37°C	Lower than 37°C
Type of antibodies	IgG	IgM
Direct Coombs' test	Strongly positive	Positive
Cause of primary condition	Idiopathic	Idiopathic
Cause of secondary condition	Autoimmune disorders, e.g. SLE Lymphomas Drugs, e.g. methyldopa	Infections *Mycoplasma* sp. Infectious mononucleosis Viruses Lymphomas Paroxysmal cold haemoglobinuria (rare)

Warm antibody haemolysis

Clinical features

This anaemia occurs at all ages in both sexes, with a variable clinical picture ranging from mild haemolysis to life-threatening anaemia. About 50% are associated with other autoimmune disorders or lymphoma.

Investigation

There is evidence of haemolysis (page 154) and the direct antiglobulin test (Coombs' test) is positive (Figure 4.3)

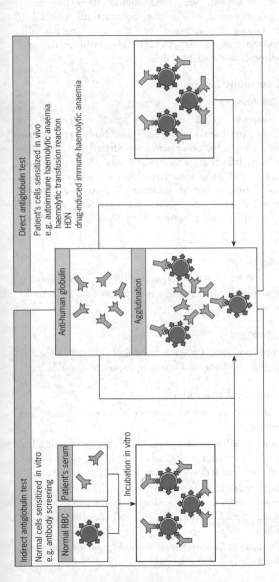

Figure 4.3
Antiglobulin (Coombs') test: the human antiglobulin forms bridges between the sensitized cells causing visible agglutination. The direct test detects patients' cells sensitized in vivo and the indirect test detects normal cells sensitized in vitro.

Indirect antiglobulin test

Normal cells sensitized in vitro
e.g. antibody screening

Normal RBC   Patient's serum

Incubation in vitro

Anti-human globulin

Agglutination

Direct antiglobulin test

Patient's cells sensitized in vivo
e.g. autoimmune haemolytic anaemia
haemolytic transfusion reaction
HDN
drug-induced immune haemolytic anaemia

Management

High–dose steroids (e.g. prednisolone 40–60 mg daily) induce remission in 80% of cases. Splenectomy is useful in those failing to respond to steroids. Occasionally immunosuppressive drugs such as azathioprine and cyclophosphamide are beneficial.

Cold antibody haemolysis

Clinical features

IgM antibodies (cold agglutinins) attach to red cells in the cold peripheral parts of the body and cause agglutination and complement-mediated intravascular haemolysis. Infection with mycoplasma or Epstein–Barr virus may lead to increased synthesis of cold agglutinins (normally produced in insignificant amounts) and produce transient haemolysis. A chronic idiopathic form occurs in elderly people, with recurrent haemolysis and peripheral cyanosis.

Investigation

There is evidence of haemolysis and the direct antiglobulin test is positive. Red cells agglutinate in the cold or at room temperature.

Management

This does not usually require treatment other than for the underlying condition and avoiding exposure to cold.

Drug-induced haemolysis

Drug-induced haemolysis may occur through one of the following mechanisms:

Immune complex A drug–antibody immune complex forms which attaches to the red cell, inducing complement and red cell destruction (e.g. quinine).

Membrane adsorption An antigenic drug–red cell complex is formed, stimulating the adsorption and production of antibodies which results in red cell destruction (e.g. penicillin).

Autoantibody The drug induces production of a red cell autoantibody (e.g. methyldopa).

Non-immune haemolytic anaemia

Paroxysmal nocturnal haemoglobinuria

Paroxysmal nocturnal haemoglobinuria (PNH) is a rare disease in which a clone of red cells is unduly sensitive to complement-mediated lysis in the absence of antibody. There is intravascular haemolysis and episodes of thrombosis. Diagnosis is by Ham's test (in vitro lysis of the red cells in acidified serum). There is no specific treatment for PNH and management is supportive. Bone marrow transplantation has been successful in a small number of patients. The course of the disease is variable, with some cases transforming into aplastic anaemia or leukaemia. The gene defect responsible has recently been characterized, opening the possibility of gene therapy in the future.

Mechanical haemolytic anaemia

Red cells may be injured by physical trauma in the circulation. Examples of this form of haemolysis include the following:

- Prosthetic heart valves: damage to red cells in their passage through heart
- March haemoglobinuria: damage to red cells in the feet from prolonged marching
- Microangiopathic haemolysis: fragmentation of red cells in abnormal microcirculation.

MYELOPROLIFERATIVE AND MYELODYSPLASTIC DISORDERS

Myeloproliferative and myelodysplastic syndromes are both clonal haemopoietic stem cell disorders which arise from a single abnormal multipotential cell in the bone marrow. Both have the potential to transform into acute leukaemia. *Myelodysplastic syndromes* are characterized by ineffective erythropoiesis and peripheral blood cytopenias (see page 170). *Myeloproliferative disorders* are characterized by the overproduction of one or more cell lines (myeloid, erythroid or megakaryocyte), and comprise chronic granulocytic leukaemia (CGL), polycythaemia vera, essential thrombocythaemia and myelofibrosis. These disorders differ from the acute leukaemias (also clonal proliferation of a single cell line), where the cells also do not differentiate normally but where there is progressive accumulation of immature cells.

Polycythaemia

Polycythaemia is defined as an increase in Hb, PCV and red cell count (RCC). The production of red cells by the bone marrow is normally regulated by the hormone erythropoietin, which is produced in the kidney. The stimulus for erythropoietin production is tissue hypoxia. *Absolute polycythaemia* (Figure 4.4) is therefore the result of an appropriate increase in erythropoietin secondary to

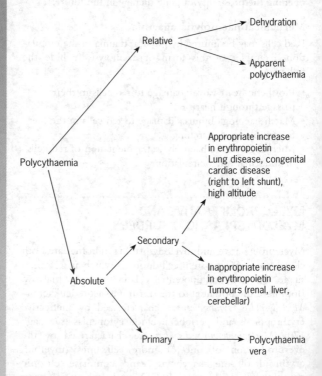

Figure 4.4
The causes of polycythaemia.

hypoxia, an inappropriate increase in erythropoietin resulting from abnormal production by certain tumours, or escape by marrow stem cells from erythropoietin control (polycythaemia vera). Absolute polycythaemia must be differentiated from *apparent polycythaemia* (previously termed stress polycythaemia), where PCV is normal but plasma volume is decreased. Apparent polycythaemia usually affects middle-aged obese men and is associated with smoking, increased alcohol intake and hypertension. The causes of polycythaemia are shown in Figure 4.4.

Primary polycythaemia
Clinical features

Polycythaemia vera, like the other myeloproliferative disorders, occurs principally in middle-aged and elderly people. Symptoms and signs are the result of hypervolaemia and hyperviscosity. Typical symptoms include headache, dizziness, tinnitus, visual disturbance, angina pectoris, intermittent claudication, pruritus and venous thrombosis. Physical signs include a plethoric complexion and hepatosplenomegaly as a result of extramedullary haemopoiesis. Splenomegaly, if present, reliably distinguishes primary polycythaemia from the other polycythaemias. There is an increased risk of haemorrhage as a result of friable haemostatic plugs, and gout caused by increased cell turnover and uric acid production.

Investigations

* Blood count shows a high Hb and PCV. The WCC is raised in 70% and the platelet count in 50% of patients; such abnormalities are rarely present in polycythaemia from other causes.
* Red cell volume, measured with ^{51}Cr-labelled red cells, is increased.
* Plasma volume, measured using ^{131}I-labelled albumin dilution, is normal or increased (compare with relative).
* Bone marrow shows erythroid hyperplasia with increased numbers of megakaryocytes.

Differential diagnosis

This is from secondary and relative polycythaemia. An abdominal ultrasound, arterial P_aO_2 and measurement of serum erythropoietin may be necessary to differentiate. Erythropoietin is low or normal in polycythaemia vera, and usually high in secondary polycythaemia.

Management

There is no cure: treatment is symptomatic.

- Venesection to maintain PCV <0.45 l/l. Regular venesection (e.g. 3-monthly) may be all that is needed in many patients.
- Chemotherapy: hydroxyurea and busulphan are particularly useful to reduce the platelet count.

Radioactive phosphorus (^{32}P) is now used only occasionally because of the risk of inducing malignancies such as acute leukaemia in later life.

Prognosis

Median survival in untreated patients is 1–2 years and may be increased to approximately 14 years with treatment. Thirty per cent will develop myelofibrosis and 5% acute leukaemia. The risk of acute myeloid leukaemia is marginally increased by treatment with busulphan or ^{32}P.

Secondary polycythaemia

Secondary polycythaemia presents with similar clinical features to primary polycythaemia, although the white cell and platelet counts are normal and the spleen is not enlarged. In patients with tumours the primary disease must be treated to lower the level of erythropoietin. In hypoxic patients, oxygen therapy (page 406) may reduce the Hb, and a small-volume phlebotomy (400 ml) may help those with severe symptoms.

Primary (essential) thrombocythaemia

Essential thrombocythaemia is characterized by very high platelet counts (usually >1000 × 10^9/l). Platelet size and function are abnormal, and presentation may be with bleeding or thrombosis. Busulphan and hydroxyurea are used to reduce platelet production. Differential diagnosis is from secondary causes of a raised platelet count and other myeloproliferative disorders (Table 4.11).

Table 4.11 Differential diagnosis of a raised platelet count

Reactive thrombocytosis
    Connective tissue disorders
    Chronic infections
    Inflammatory bowel disease
    Malignancy
    Haemorrhage
    Surgery
    Splenectomy and functional hyposplenism

Primary thrombocythaemia

Primary polycythaemia

Myelofibrosis

Myelodysplasia

Primary myelofibrosis (myelosclerosis)

Myelofibrosis is characterized by haemopoietic stem-cell proliferation associated with marrow fibrosis (abnormal megakaryocyte precursors release growth factors which stimulate fibroblasts).

Clinical features

There are constitutional symptoms of fever, weight loss and lethargy.

Bleeding occurs in the thrombocytopenic patient. There is hepatomegaly and massive splenomegaly caused by extramedullary haemopoiesis.

Investigations

- Blood count shows anaemia. The white cell and platelet counts are high initially, but fall with disease progression as a result of marrow fibrosis.
- Blood film examination shows a leucoerythroblastic picture (immature red cells caused by marrow infiltration) and 'teardrop'-shaped red cells.
- Bone marrow is usually unobtainable by aspiration ('dry tap'); trephine biopsy shows increased fibrosis.

Management

- Transfusions for anaemia.
- Busulphan or hydroxyurea are used to reduce the raised white cell and platelet count.

- Splenic irradiation may be useful to reduce a large painful spleen.
- Splenectomy is performed if the spleen is very large and painful and the transfusion requirements are high.

Prognosis

The median survival is 3 years. Transformation to acute myeloid leukaemia occurs in 10–20%.

Myelodysplasia

Myelodysplasia is a group of acquired bone marrow disorders caused by a defect in stem cells. There is progressive bone marrow failure, which tends to evolve into acute myeloid leukaemia. The myelodysplastic syndromes are predominantly diseases of the elderly, and are increasingly being diagnosed when a routine full blood count shows an unexplained macrocytosis, anaemia, thrombocytopenia or neutropenia. The diagnosis is made on the basis of characteristic blood film and bone marrow appearances.

For most elderly patients with symptomatic disease treatment is supportive, with red cell and platelet transfusions. The possibility of cure applies only to the minority of young patients suitable for an allogeneic bone marrow transplant. Overall median survival is 20 months.

THE SPLEEN

The spleen, situated in the left hypochondrium, is the largest lymphoid organ in the body. Its main functions are phagocytosis of old red blood cells, immunological defence, and to act as a 'pool' of blood from which cells may be rapidly mobilized. Pluripotential stem cells are present in the spleen and proliferate in severe haematological stress (*extramedullary haemopoiesis*), e.g. haemolytic anaemia.

Hypersplenism

Hypersplenism can result from splenomegaly of any cause (Table 4.12). It results in pancytopenia, increased plasma

Table 4.12 Causes of splenomegaly

Sometimes massive (extending into right iliac fossa)	Moderate

Haematological
   Chronic myeloid leukaemia
   Myelofibrosis
	Haematological
	   Lymphomas
	   Leukaemias
	   Myeloproliferative disorders
	   Haemolytic anaemia

Infections
   Chronic malaria
   Schistosomiasis
   Kala-azar
	Infections
	   Septicaemia
	   Infectious mononucleosis
	   Infective endocarditis
	   Tuberculosis
	   Brucellosis

Other
   Tropical splenomegaly
	Inflammation
	   Rheumatoid arthritis
	   Sarcoidosis
	   Systemic lupus erythematosus
	Others
	   Portal hypertension, e.g. cirrhosis
	   Amyloidosis
	   Gaucher's disease

volume and haemolysis caused by increased destruction of red cells.

Splenectomy

This is performed mainly for:

- Trauma
- Idiopathic thrombocytopenic purpura
- Haemolytic anaemias
- Hypersplenism.

The main complications are thrombophilia in the short term and overwhelming infection in the longer term. The main infecting organisms are *Streptococcus pneumoniae*, *H. influenzae* and the meningococci. Vaccines against these three bacteria should be given routinely to patients about to undergo splenectomy. In addition, antibiotic prophylaxis (phenoxymethylpenicillin, twice daily) should be given for the first 2 years after splenectomy, and continued in children up to the age of 16 years. Some authorities recommend lifelong penicillin for all patients after splenectomy.

BLOOD PRODUCTS AND TRANSFUSION

Blood collected from donors is either used 'whole' or processed into blood components and blood products (Figure 4.5).

Blood groups

The blood groups are determined by antigens on the surface of red cells; more than 400 blood groups have been found. The ABO (Table 4.13) and rhesus (Rh) systems are the two most important blood groups, but incompatibilities involving many other blood groups (such as Kell and Duffy) may cause haemolytic transfusion reactions and/or haemolytic disease of the newborn.

Table 4.13 Antigens and antibodies in the ABO system

Blood group	Serum antibody	UK frequency (%)	Comment
O	Anti-A and anti-B	44	'Universal donors' are O Rh negative
A	Anti-B	45	
B	Anti-A	8	
AB	None	3	Universal recipients

Complications of transfusing red blood cells

- ABO incompatibility is the most serious complication and often results from simple clerical errors, leading to the incorrect labelling and identification of blood and patient's blood sample for cross-matching. There is an immediate reaction, starting within minutes of the transfusion, leading to intravascular haemolysis, rigors, lumbar pain, dyspnoea and hypotension. The transfusion must be stopped and the donor units returned to the blood transfusion laboratory for testing with a new blood sample from the patient. Emergency treatment may be needed to maintain the blood pressure (page 442).
- Febrile reactions are usually the result of antileucocyte antibodies in the recipient acting against transfused leucocytes, leading to the release of pyrogens. Typical signs are flushing, fever and tachycardia, which may

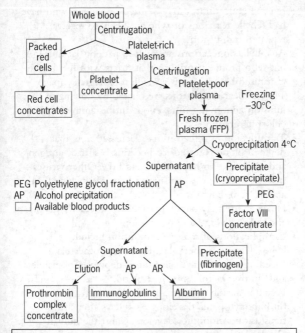

Whole blood is used for the correction of acute massive blood loss.

Packed red cells and red cell concentrates are used for acute bleeds and correction of anaemia.

Platelet concentrates are used to treat or prevent bleeding in patients with severe thrombocytopenia.

Fresh frozen plasma contains all the coagulation factors and is used in acquired coagulation factor deficiencies.

Albumin is sometimes given to patients with acute severe hypoalbuminaemia.

Immunoglobulins are used in patients with hypogammaglobulinaemia to prevent infection and in patients with idiopathic thrombocytopenic purpura. Specific immunoglobulin, e.g. anti-hepatitis B is used after exposure of a non-immune patient to infections.

Figure 4.5
Blood fractionation. (Adapted and reproduced with permission from Hayes, P. and Mackay, T. (1992), Churchill's Pocketbook of Medicine, Edinburgh, Churchill Livingstone.)

respond to slowing of the transfusion. Leucocyte-poor red cell concentrates may be used in patients who have had febrile reactions or who are likely to receive repeated transfusions.

- Anaphylactic reactions are seen in patients lacking IgA but who produce anti-IgA that reacts with IgA in the transfused blood. This is a medical emergency (page 447). Urticarial reactions are treated by slowing of the infusion and giving intravenous antihistamines, e.g. chlorpheniramine.
- Transmission of infection has decreased now that donated blood is tested for hepatitis B surface antigen and antibodies to hepatitis C and HIV. Other viruses that may cause post-transfusion hepatitis include CMV and Epstein–Barr virus.
- Heart failure may occur, particularly in elderly people and those having large transfusions.
- Complications of massive transfusion include hypocalcaemia, hyperkalaemia and hypothermia. Bleeding may occur as a result of depletion of platelets and clotting factors in stored blood.
- Post-transfusion purpura, in which severe thrombocytopenia develops 7–10 days after the transfusion. Antibodies develop against the human platelet antigen 1a, leading to immune destruction of the patient's own platelets

BLEEDING DISORDERS

A bleeding disorder is suggested when the patient has unexplained (i.e. no history of trauma) bruising or bleeding, or prolonged bleeding in response to injury or surgery, e.g. after tooth extraction.

Reactions involved in haemostasis

When a blood vessel is damaged the exposed collagen sets in motion a series of events leading to haemostasis. Haemostasis depends on the interactions of the vessel wall, platelets and coagulation factors.

- Blood vessel damage leads to immediate vasoconstriction, reducing blood flow to the injured area and allowing contact activation of platelets and coagulation factors.

- Platelets adhere to the exposed subendothelial connective tissue; adherence is potentiated by a portion of the factor VIII protein, von Willebrand factor (VIII:vWF). Collagen activates platelet–prostaglandin synthesis, leading to the formation of thromboxane A$_2$ which causes vasoconstriction, and lowers cyclic AMP, thereby initiating the release of platelet granules (Figure 4.6). Aggregation of platelets is facilitated by

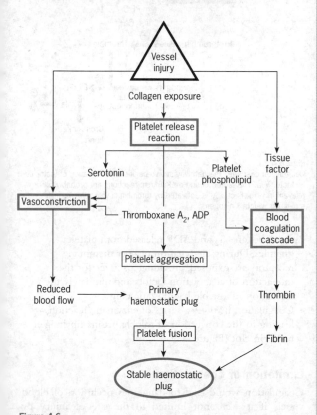

Figure 4.6
Reactions involved in haemostasis. (Adapted from Hoffbrand and Pettit, 1992 Essential Haematology, 2nd edn., Oxford, Blackwell Science.)

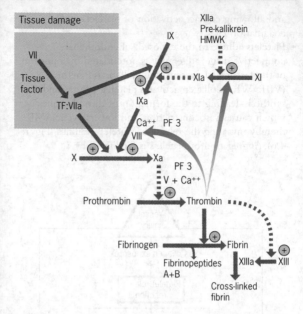

Figure 4.7
Coagulation cascade. The pathway in vivo begins with activation of factor IX by factor VIIa. The factor XII and prekallikrein reactions are probably only relevant in vitro. Factor XI is activated by thrombin in vivo. HMWK, high molecular weight kininogen.

thromboxane A_2 and ADP released from platelet granules. During aggregation platelet membrane receptors are exposed, providing a surface for the interaction of coagulation factors and ultimately the formation of a stable haemostatic plug.

• Coagulation involves a series of enzymatic reactions leading to the conversion of soluble plasma fibrinogen to fibrin clot (Figure 4.7).

Limitation of coagulation

Coagulation would lead to dangerous occlusion of blood vessels if it were not limited to the site of injury by protective mechanisms:

Rapid blood flow Rapid blood flow at the periphery of the damaged area dilutes and removes coagulation factors.

Circulating inhibitors of the coagulation factors

- Antithrombin binds to and forms stable complexes with coagulation factors. Activity is increased by heparin.
- Active protein C destroys factors V and VIII.
- Protein S is a cofactor for protein C.

The fibrinolytic system The plasma protein plasminogen is converted to plasmin by activators present in the tissue and endothelial cells. Plasmin induces lysis of cross-linked (X-linked) fibrin, resulting in the formation of various X-linked fibrin degradation products (FDPs), which include D-dimers which can easily be measured using monoclonal antibodies.

Bleeding disorders are therefore the result of a defect in vessels, platelets or the coagulation pathway (Table 4.14).

Table 4.14 Classification of bleeding disorders

Blood vessel defect
Hereditary
  Hereditary haemorrhagic telangiectasia (rare)
  Connective tissue disorders: Marfan's and Ehlers–Danlos syndromes
Acquired
  Severe infections: meningococcal, typhoid
  Drugs: steroids
  Allergic: Henoch–Schönlein purpura (mainly children)
  Others: scurvy, senile purpura
  Easy bruising syndrome

Platelet defect
Decreased platelet number or decreased function

Coagulation defect
Hereditary
  Haemophilia A or B, von Willebrand's disease
Acquired
  Anticoagulant treatment, liver disease, disseminated intravascular coagulation

Investigation of bleeding disorders

The nature of the defect and therefore the most appropriate initial investigations may be suggested by the history and examination, e.g family history, intercurrent disease, alcohol consumption, drugs. Vascular/platelet bleeding is characterized by bruising of the skin and bleeding from mucosal membranes. The inherited coagulation disorders are typically associated with haemarthroses (bleeding into joints) and muscle haematomas. The most common cause of abnormal bleeding is thrombocytopenia.

- Platelet count and blood film will show the number and morphology of platelets and any blood disorder such as leukaemia.
- Coagulation tests. Coagulation tests are abnormal with deficiencies or inhibitors of the clotting factors. If the abnormal result is corrected by the addition of normal plasma to the patient's plasma in the assay, then the result is abnormal as a result of deficiency and not of inhibitors.

  – The prothrombin time (PT) is prolonged with abnormalities of factors VII, X, V or II, liver disease, or if the patient is on warfarin. The international normalized ratio (INR) is the ratio of the patient's PT to a normal control when using the international reference preparation. The advantage of the INR over the PT, is that it uses international standards and thus anticoagulant control can be compared in different hospitals across the world.

  – Partial thromboplastin time with kaolin (PTTK) is prolonged with deficiencies or inhibitors to one or more of the following factors: XII, XI, IX, VIII, X, V, or I (but not factor VII)

  – Thrombin time (TT) is prolonged with fibrinogen deficiency, dysfibrinogenaemia (normal levels, abnormal function), heparin treatment or disseminated intravascular coagulation.

  The normal ranges of these tests vary from laboratory to laboratory and patient results must be compared with that laboratory reference range.

- The bleeding time is abnormal with von Willebrand's disease, with blood vessel defects, and when there is a decrease in the number or function of platelets.

These tests will localize the site of the problem. Further specialized investigations, e.g. platelet aggregation studies and measurement of individual clotting factors, will be necessary to identify the exact haemostatic defect correctly.

Platelet defects

Platelet defects are the result of thrombocytopenia (Table 4.15) or disorders of platelet function, e.g. those occurring

Table 4.15 Causes of thrombocytopenia

Decreased marrow production
Leukaemia*, myelofibrosis*, aplastic anaemia*, megaloblastic anaemia, alcohol, drugs (e.g. cotrimoxazole), viral infections

Increased destruction
Immune
  Autoimmune, postincompatible transfusion, drugs (heparin, penicillin)
Consumption
  Disseminated intravascular coagulation, hypersplenism, infections
  Haemolytic uraemic syndrome (infection triggering haemolysis, thrombocytopenia and acute renal failure)
  Thrombotic thrombocytopenia purpura (similar to HUS plusneurological disturbance)

Sequestration
Hypersplenism

* Usually also associated with failure of red and white cell production.

with aspirin treatment and uraemia. Congenital abnormalities of platelet number (e.g. Fanconi's anaemia, Wiskott–Aldrich syndrome) or function (e.g. Bernard–Soulier syndrome) are all extremely rare.

Mild thrombocytopenia can be artefactual and due to platelet clumping or a blood clot in the sample, which should be excluded in all cases. Spontaneous bleeding from skin and mucous membranes is unlikely to occur with platelet counts above $20 \times 10^9/l$. Increased destruction or decreased production can be differentiated by bone marrow examination, which will show respectively increased or decreased numbers of megakaryocytes (platelet precursors).

Autoimmune thrombocytopenic purpura

Thrombocytopenia results from immune destruction of platelets. Acute autoimmune thrombocytopenic purpura (AITP) is seen in children, often following a viral infection. There is rapid onset of purpura, which is usually self-limiting and becomes chronic in only about 5% of cases. Chronic AITP is more commonly seen in adults and is associated with platelet autoantibodies in 60–70%.

Aetiology

Chronic AITP is usually idiopathic, but may occur with autoimmune disorders, e.g. SLE, thyroid disease, chronic lymphatic leukaemia and some viral infections, e.g. HIV.

The same drugs that cause autoimmune haemolytic anaemia may also cause thrombocytopenia (and neutropenia).

Clinical features

The condition is characteristically seen in young women. There is a fluctuating course, with easy bruising, epistaxis and menorrhagia. Major haemorrhage is rare.

Investigation

There is thrombocytopenia with normal or increased megakaryocytes on bone marrow examination. The detection of antiplatelet autoantibodies is unnecessary in a straightforward case.

Management

Platelet transfusion and/or high-dose intravenous immunoglobulin produce a rapid but transient rise in the platelet count and may be useful in severe haemorrhage. Prednisolone (60 mg/day) is the initial treatment of choice, and 20% will have a complete and sustained response. Splenectomy, which has a 60% cure rate, is indicated in those with moderate to severe thrombocytopenia who fail medical treatment. Immunosuppressive drugs (e.g. azathioprine) are indicated in refractory cases.

Inherited coagulation disorders

Inherited disorders usually involve a deficiency of only one coagulation factor, whereas acquired disorders involve a deficiency of several factors.

Haemophilia A

This is the result of a deficiency of factor VIII:C, which is one part of the factor VIII molecule. It is inherited as an X-linked recessive, affecting 1 in 5000 males.

Clinical features

Clinical features depend on the factor VIII plasma levels. If more than 5% of the normal level is present the disease is mild, with post-traumatic bleeding only. Levels of less than 1% are associated with frequent spontaneous bleeding into muscles and joints that can lead to a crippling arthropathy. The joints most frequently involved are the knees, elbows, ankles, shoulders and hips.

Investigations

The PTTK is prolonged and plasma factor VIII:C levels are reduced. The PT and bleeding time are normal.

Management

- Intravenous injection of factor VIII concentrates is the mainstay of treatment. They are given as prophylaxis, e.g. before and after surgery, or to treat an acute bleeding episode. Most severely affected patients are now given prophylaxis three times weekly from early childhood to try to prevent permanent joint damage. Many patients also have a supply of factor VIII concentrates at home to inject at the first sign of bleeding. Recombinant factor VIII is now well established as the treatment of choice, though cost constraints have resulted in some patients still being offered treatment with plasma-derived concentrates.
- Desmopressin (DDAVP), which is injected or inhaled, raises the level of factor VIII and may be used to treat patients with mild haemophilia.
- The cloning of the factor VIII gene, and progress in the development of retroviral-vector delivery systems, have led to considerable interest in the possibility that haemophilia A could be 'cured' by gene therapy.

Complications

Recurrent bleeding into joints may lead to deformity and arthritis. In the past, multiple transfusions were associated with an increased risk of acquiring hepatitis C and HIV. This risk has been virtually eliminated because of the exclusion of high-risk blood donors, screening of donors and heat treatment of factor VIII concentrates. Ten per cent of those with severe haemophilia develop antibodies to factor VIII, and may need massive doses to overcome this. Recombinant factor VIIa is used to 'bypass' the inhibitor and shows promise in treating these patients.

Haemophilia B (Christmas disease)

This is the result of a deficiency of factor IX, and affects 1 in 30 000 males. Inheritance and clinical features are the same as for haemophilia B. Treatment is with factor IX concentrates.

Von Willebrand's disease

Von Willebrand's disease is a common bleeding disorder caused by an inherited deficiency of von Willebrand factor, which is an essential cofactor for normal platelet adhesion to damaged subendothelium. This factor also serves as a carrier for factor VIII:C to form the whole VIII complex.

Clinical features

Types I and II are mild forms, with autosomal dominant inheritance and characterized by mucosal bleeding (nose bleeds and gastrointestinal bleeding) and prolonged bleeding after dental treatment or surgery.

Type III patients have more severe bleeding, but rarely experience the joint and muscle bleeds seen in haemophilia A

Investigations

Prolonged bleeding time reflects a defect in platelet adhesion. There is a prolonged PTTK and decreased plasma levels of VIII:C and VIII:vWF.

Management

This depends on the severity of the bleeding, and includes treatment with factor VIII concentrates and desmopressin (DDAVP).

Acquired coagulation disorders

Disseminated intravascular coagulation

There is widespread generation of fibrin within blood vessels, caused by initiation of the coagulation pathway. There is consumption of platelets and coagulation factors, and secondary activation of fibrinolysis leading to production of fibrin degradation products (FDPs), which contribute to coagulation by inhibiting fibrin polymerization.

Aetiology

Intravascular coagulation is initiated by:

- Release of procoagulant substances into the blood (malignancy, amniotic fluid embolism, abruptio placentae and snake bites)

- Contact of blood with an abnormal surface (infection, burns and grafts)
- Generation of procoagulant substances in the blood (promyelocytic leukaemia, haemolytic transfusion reaction).

Clinical features

The presentation varies from no bleeding at all to complete haemostatic failure, with bleeding from venepuncture sites and the nose and mouth. Thrombotic events may occur as a result of vessel occlusion by platelets and fibrin.

Investigations

There is thrombocytopenia, prolonged PT, PTTK and TT, decreased fibrinogen and elevated FDPs. The blood film shows fragmented red cells. In mild cases with compensatory increase of coagulation factors the only abnormality may be an increase in the FDPs, or in the D-dimer fragment.

Management

- Treat the underlying condition.
- Platelets, red cell concentrates and fresh frozen plasma may be necessary in patients who are bleeding.

Vitamin K deficiency

Vitamin K is needed for the formation of active factors II, VII, IX and X. Deficiency which occurs in malabsorption of vitamin K and with warfarin treatment (an inhibitor of vitamin K synthesis) leads to an increase in PT. Treatment, if required, is with parenteral phytomenadione (vitamin K).

Liver disease

Liver disease results in a number of defects of haemostasis: vitamin K deficiency in cholestasis, reduced synthesis of clotting factors, thrombocytopenia and functional abnormalities of platelets. DIC may occur in acute liver failure.

....

THROMBOSIS

A thrombus is defined as a solid mass formed in the circulation from the blood constituents, usually resulting from a complex series of events involving coagulation factors, platelets, red blood cells and the vessel wall.

Arterial thrombosis

Arterial thrombosis is usually the result of atheroma, which forms particularly in areas of turbulent blood flow, such as the bifurcation of arteries. Platelets adhere to the damaged vascular endothelium and aggregate in response to ADP and thromboxane A_2. This may stimulate blood coagulation, leading to complete occlusion of the vessel, or embolization resulting in distal obstruction.

Prevention and treatment of arterial thrombosis

Prevention of thrombosis is with antiplatelet drugs

- Aspirin inhibits cyclo-oxygenase reducing production of thromboxane A2 (page 175). It is the most commonly used antiplatelet drug.
- Dipyridamole potentiates prostacyclin.
- Clopidogrel is a new inhibitor of platelet aggregation induced by ADP.
- Abciximab is a monoclonal antibody against platelet glycoprotein IIb/IIIa receptor. It has been developed as a new strategy for preventing ischaemic complications following coronary angioplasty and has shown promising results in early studies.

Treatment of thrombosis (thrombolytic therapy)

- Streptokinase is a purified fraction of the filtrate obtained from cultures of haemolytic streptococci. It forms a 1:1 complex with plasminogen which activates other plasminogen molecules to form plasmin. The dose in myocardial infarction is 1 500 000 units given by infusion over 1 hour. The main disadvantage of streptokinase is the indiscriminate activation of plasminogen both in clots and in the circulation, leading to an increased risk of haemorrhage. Nevertheless, this is currently the thrombolytic agent of choice.
- Anisoylated plasminogen streptokinase activator complex (APSAC) is a complex of plasminogen and an anisoylated form of streptokinase which has a more sustained duration of action than streptokinase and is more specific for fibrin-bound plasminogen.

- Tissue-type plasminogen activator (tPA) is produced using recombinant gene technology, and was claimed to be more specific for clot-bound plasminogen. However, it has not been shown to produce fewer bleeding episodes than streptokinase.

The use of thrombolytic therapy in myocardial infarction is discussed on page 356. The main risk of thrombolysis is bleeding. Contraindications are a recent major bleed, stroke (within 2 months), uncontrolled hypertension, surgery or other invasive procedure (within 10 days), and bleeding disorders.

Table 4.16 Risk factors for venous thromboembolism

Age
Obesity
Trauma or surgery, especially pelvis or hip
Immobility (bed rest >4 days)
Pregnancy and puerperium
High doses of oestrogens
Previous deep vein thrombosis
Varicose veins
Recent myocardial infarction
Nephrotic syndrome
Inflammatory bowel disease

Inherited deficiency/abnormality of natural anticoagulant proteins (thrombophilia)
    Antithrombin III deficiency
    Protein C deficiency
    Protein S deficiency
    Activated protein C resistance (factor V Leiden mutation)

Acquired
    Antiphospholipid antibody, lupus anticoagulant
    Malignancy
    Myeloproliferative disorder

Venous thrombosis

Unlike arterial thrombosis, venous thrombosis usually occurs in normal vessels, often in the deep veins of the leg. It originates around the valves as red thrombi consisting of red cells and fibrin. Propagation occurs, inducing a risk of embolization to the pulmonary vessels. Chronic venous obstruction in the leg results in a permanently swollen leg which is prone to ulceration (postphlebitic syndrome). Factors predisposing to venous thromboembolism are listed in Table 4.16.

Table 4.17 Anticoagulant treatment

	Heparin	Warfarin
Route of administration	i.v./s.c.	Orally
Half-life	2 hours	2 days
Mode of action	Potentiates antithrombotic effects of antithrombin III	Interferes with vitamin K metabolism
Monitoring	PTTK	PT/INR
Reversal of anticoagulation (usually only if patient is bleeding)	Intravenous protamine (rarely needed)	Stop warfarin, intravenous vitamin K 5 mg, FFP if life-threatening bleed

FFP, fresh frozen plasma.

Prevention and treatment of venous thromboembolism

Heparin and warfarin are the two drugs used most frequently in the prevention and treatment of thromboembolism (Table 4.17). In general, prophylaxis of venous thromboembolism relies on measures that prevent stasis, such as early mobilization, elevation of the legs and compression stockings, with heparin reserved for higher-risk patients. Low molecular weight heparins (e.g. Enoxaparin 20 mg s.c. daily), produced by the enzymatic or chemical breakdown of the heparin molecule, are now preferred to conventional heparin for venous prophylaxis in most cases. These can be administered on a once-daily basis, have greater efficacy than conventional heparin in high-risk patients, and do not require monitoring of clotting times.

In established thromboembolism, full anticoagulation should be undertaken as follows:

- Heparin 5000 units unfractionated is given intravenously as a loading dose.
- Heparin is continued as an intravenous infusion of 1000–2000 units/hour, or as subcutaneous injections of 15 000 units every 12 hours.
- The dose of heparin is adjusted to maintain the PTTK at between 1.5 and 2.5 times the control value.
- Warfarin 5–10 mg orally is started at the same time as the heparin.

Table 4.18. Indications for oral anticoagulation and target INR

Target INR	
2.5	Deep vein thrombosis, pulmonary embolism, symptomatic inherited thrombophillia (page 185), atrial fibrillation, cardioversion, mural thrombus, dilated cardiomyopathy
3.5	Recurrence of venous thromboembolism while on warfarin therapy, antiphospholipid syndrome, mechanical prosthetic heart valve, coronary artery graft thrombosis.

Monitor INR daily or alternate days in early days of treatment and then up to every 8 weeks.

- The dose of warfarin is adjusted to maintain the INR usually at two to three times the control value.
- Heparin can be discontinued when the INR is in the therapeutic range (Table 4.18).

Fixed–dose low molecular weight heparin regimens are increasingly being used for the immediate treatment of established thrombosis. This may allow the treatment of venous thromboembolism without admission to hospital in compliant patients without coexisting risk factors for haemorrhage.

··

THE HAEMATOLOGICAL MALIGNANCIES

The leukaemias

The leukaemias are malignant neoplasms of the haemo-poietic stem cells, characterized by diffuse replacement of the bone marrow by neoplastic cells. In most cases, the leukaemic cells spill over into the blood, where they may be seen in large numbers. The cells may also infiltrate the liver, spleen, lymph nodes and other tissues throughout the body.

Leukaemias are classified on the basis of the cell type involved and the state of maturity of the leukaemic cells. Thus acute leukaemias are characterized by the presence of very immature cells (blast cells) and by a rapidly fatal course in untreated patients. Chronic leukaemias are associated, at least initially, with more mature leucocytes and a relatively indolent course. Acute and chronic leukaemias are further subdivided into the cell type involved:

- Acute myelogenous leukaemia (AML)
- Acute lymphoblastic leukaemia (ALL)

- Chronic myeloid leukaemia (CML)
- Chronic lymphocytic leukaemia (CLL).

Aetiology

In most cases the aetiology is unknown.

Genetic factors Genetic factors are suggested by the increased incidence in patients with chromosomal disorders (e.g. Down's syndrome) and in identical twins of affected patients. Chromosomal abnormalities have been described in patients with leukaemia. The earliest described was the Philadelphia (Ph) chromosome, found in 95% of cases with CML and some patients with ALL. In the Ph chromosome the long arm of chromosome 22 is shortened by reciprocal translocation to the long arm of chromosome 9. It is unclear how these molecular events contribute to the disease process.

Environmental factors

- Chemicals, e.g. benzene compounds used in industry
- Drugs, e.g. chemotherapy using chlorambucil and procarbazine
- Radiation exposure, e.g. nuclear generators and treatment for Hodgkin's disease.

Treatment of haematological malignancies

The treatment of the haematological malignancies is based on the use of chemotherapy and radiotherapy. Surgery and other treatments (e.g. steroids and interferon) are used less often.

Chemotherapeutic agents

There are many chemotherapy drugs in common use. They act in a number of different ways; however, the end result is to inhibit the process of cell division. They therefore affect not only tumour cells, but also the rapidly dividing normal cells of the bone marrow, gastrointestinal tract and germinal epithelium. The principal side effects are:

- Bone marrow suppression, leading to anaemia, thrombocytopenia and infection
- Mucositis, causing mouth ulceration
- Loss of hair (alopecia)
- Sterility, which can be irreversible.

To minimize these side effects, chemotherapy is given at intervals to allow some recovery of normal cell function between cycles. Nausea and vomiting may be severe with some drugs, such as cisplatin, and is related to the direct actions of cytotoxic agents on the brain-stem chemoreceptor trigger zone. Antiemetics such as metoclopramide and domperidone are used initially, but the serotonin 5HT$_3$ antagonists (ondansetron and granisetron) have revolutionized the management of severe vomiting. Finally, chemotherapy drugs may themselves cause cancer, particularly acute leukaemia presenting years after treatment.

Radiotherapy

Radiation damages nuclear DNA and thus impairs the ability of cells to divide. The complications of radiotherapy depend on the radiosensitivity of normal tissue in the path of the radiation field. General side effects are lethargy and loss of energy. There may be damage to the skin (erythema and desquamation), gut (nausea, mucosal ulceration and diarrhoea), testes (sterility) and bone marrow (anaemia, leukopenia).

Acute leukaemia

Epidemiology

Both types of acute leukaemia can occur in all age groups, but ALL is predominantly a disease of childhood, whereas AML is seen most frequently in older adults (middle-aged and elderly).

Clinical features

These are the result of marrow failure: anaemia, bleeding and infection, e.g. sore throat and pneumonia. Sometimes there is peripheral lymphadenopathy and hepatosplenomegaly.

Investigations

A definitive diagnosis is made on the peripheral blood film and a bone marrow aspirate. The various subtypes (Table 4.19) are classified on the basis of morphology and immunophenotyping, and cytogenetic studies of blast cells. If the patient has a fever, blood cultures and chest radiograph are essential.

Table 4.19 The FAB (French, American, British) classification of acute leukaemia

Lymphoblastic

L1	Homogeneous population of small cells (childhood ALL)
L2	Heterogeneous population of cells (more often seen in adults)
L3	Rare – cells such as those seen in Burkitt's lymphoma

Myeloid

M1	Myeloblastic (no maturation)
M2	Myeloblastic (with maturation)
M3	Promyelocytic*
M4	Myelomonocytic†
M5	Monoblastic
M6	Erythroblastic
M7	Megakaryoblastic

* Associated with disseminated intravascular coagulation.
† Characterized by leukaemic skin nodules, gum hypertrophy and CNS infiltration.

- The Blood count shows anaemia and thrombocytopenia. The white cell count is usually raised, but may be normal or low.
- The peripheral blood film shows characteristic leukaemic blast cells.
- Bone marrow aspirate usually shows increased cellularity, with a high percentage of abnormal lymphoid or myeloid blast cells.

Management

The aim of treatment is to achieve complete remission (defined as a normal full blood count and less than 5% of blasts in the bone marrow) and restore the patient to a normal state of health.

General Before starting treatment the following need to be considered:

- Correction of anaemia and thrombocytopenia by administration of blood and platelets
- Treatment of infection with intravenous antibiotics
- Prevention of the acute tumour lysis syndrome (ATLS) with adequate hydration and allopurinol. ATLS results from a massive release of cellular breakdown products consequent upon tumour cell death following effective therapy. The biochemical disturbances include

hyperkalaemia, hyperuricaemia, hyperphosphataemia and hypocalcaemia.

Treatment of AML

This is in two parts: induction of remission and postremission/consolidation.

- Induction of remission is achieved with an aggressive combination of intravenous chemotherapy (e.g. cytosine, arabinoside and daunorubicin) given at intervals to allow marrow recovery in between.
- Postremission therapy. The options are further courses of chemotherapy or myeloablative therapy with allogeneic/autologous bone marrow transplantation (BMT) (see page 197).

Chemotherapy achieves an initial remission rate of 70%, although long-term cure is only around 35% with chemotherapy alone. BMT improves long-term remission to 50%.

Treatment of acute promyelocytic leukaemia (APML)

It has been demonstrated that the use of a differentiating agent, all-*trans*-retinoic acid, given orally, can lead to remission in some patients with APML. It does not appear to be effective in other subtypes of AML. Unfortunately such remissions do not last, and need to be consolidated with conventional chemotherapy.

Treatment of acute lymphoblastic leukaemia (ALL)

The principles of treatment are similar to those for AML; cyclical combination chemotherapy (vincristine, prednisolone and daunorubicin) is given to induce a remission and for postremission therapy. However, ALL has a propensity to involve the CNS, so treatment also includes prophylactic intrathecal drugs (methotrexate or cytosine arabinoside) with or without prophylactic cranial radiotherapy. Most patients also receive oral maintenance chemotherapy for 2–3 years. Relapse may occur in the blood, testes and CNS.

Overall 90% of children with ALL respond to treatment and 50–60% are cured. The results in adults are not so good, with only about 30% being cured.

Chronic myeloid leukaemia

Clinical features

Chronic myeloid leukaemia (CML) occurs most commonly in middle age. There is an insidious onset, with fever, weight loss, sweating and symptoms of anaemia. Massive splenomegaly is characteristic.

Investigations

- Blood count usually shows anaemia and a raised white cell count (often >100×10^9/l). The platelet count may be low, normal or raised.
- Bone marrow aspirate shows a hypercellular marrow with an increase in myeloid progenitors. On cytogenetic analysis the Ph chromosome is present in most patients.

Management

Until recently most people were treated with hydroxyurea. The advent of interferons has changed this, as they induce haematological remission in the majority of patients and cytogenetic remission in about 10%. Side effects such as anergia and fatigue are common with the doses required. Curative treatment with bone marrow transplantation should be considered in younger patients.

Prognosis

The chronic phase described above lasts 3–4 years. This is followed by blast transformation, with the development of acute leukaemia (usually acute myeloid) and, commonly, rapid death. Less frequently, CML transforms into myelofibrosis, death ensuing from bone marrow failure.

Chronic lymphocytic leukaemia

CLL is an incurable disease of older people characterized by an uncontrolled proliferation and accumulation of mature B lymphocytes (although T-cell CLL does occur).

Clinical features

Symptoms are a consequence of bone marrow failure: anaemia, infections and bleeding. An autoimmune haemolysis contributes to the anaemia. Some patients may be asymptomatic, the diagnosis being a chance finding on the basis of a blood count done for a different reason. There may be lymphadenopathy and, in advanced disease, hepatosplenomegaly.

Investigations

- Blood count shows a raised white cell count >15 × 10⁹/l, of which at least 40% are lymphocytes. There may be anaemia and thrombocytopenia.
- Bone marrow aspirate shows infiltration by lymphocytes, with a variable reduction in normal haemopoietic tissue.

Management

Treatment, usually with oral chlorambucil, is indicated only for those with symptomatic disease.

Prognosis

The median survival is 8 years for those with lymphocytosis only. The prognosis is much worse (median survival 2 years) for those patients with marrow failure at presentation.

....

THE LYMPHOMAS

The lymphomas represent abnormal proliferations of B or T cells and are currently classified on the basis of histological appearance into Hodgkin's disease and non-Hodgkin's lymphoma (NHL).

Hodgkin's disease

Clinical features

Hodgkin's disease is primarily a disease of young adults. The most common presentation is painless lymph node enlargement (most often cervical nodes). Systemic symptoms, known as 'B' symptoms, are fever, night sweats and weight loss. Other constitutional symptoms may occur, such as pruritus, fatigue, anorexia and alcohol-induced pain at the site of the enlarged lymph nodes.

On examination enlarged nodes are typically non-tender, discrete and with a rubbery consistency. There may be hepatosplenomegaly.

Investigations

* Blood count often shows a normochromic/normocytic anaemia with a raised ESR.
* Liver biochemistry may be abnormal, with liver involvement.
* Radiology: chest radiography and CT are important for staging and may show mediastinal, intrathoracic or abdominal lymphadenopathy.
* Lymph node biopsy and histological examination are required for a definitive diagnosis. Classically, Sternberg–Reed (binucleate or multinucleate cells) cells are present, with a characteristic admixture of lymphocytes and histiocytes.
* Bone marrow aspirate and trephine biopsy may show involvement in patients with advanced disease.

Table 4.20 Differential diagnosis of lymphadenopathy

Localized	Generalized

Local infection
  Pyogenic infection, e.g. tonsillitis
  Tuberculosis
	Infection
	  Epstein–Barr virus
	  Cytomegalovirus
	  Toxoplasma sp.
	  Tuberculosis
	  HIV infection

Secondary carcinoma	Lymphoma
Lymphoma	Leukaemia

	Systemic disease
	  Systemic lupus
	    erythematosus
	  Sarcoidosis
	  Rheumatoid arthritis

	Drug reaction, e.g. phenytoin

Differential diagnosis

This includes any other cause of lymphadenopathy (Table 4.20).

Management

Treatment is always given with a curative intent and consists of radiotherapy, cyclical combination chemotherapy or both. The choice of treatment depends on:

- Stage (Table 4.21)
- Involved sites
- 'Bulk' of lymph nodes involved
- Presence or absence of 'B' symptoms.

Stage IA and stage IIA disease is treated with radiotherapy.

Table 4.21 Staging classification of Hodgkin's disease*

Stage	Definition
I	Involvement of a single lymph node region or a single extralymphatic organ or site
II	Involvement of two or more lymph node regions on the same side of the diaphragm, or localized involvement of an extralymphatic organ or site and of one or more lymph node regions on the same side of the diaphragm
III	Involvement of lymph node regions on both sides of the diaphragm, which may also be accompanied by involvement of the spleen or by localized involvement of an extralymphatic organ or site or both
IV	Diffuse or disseminated involvement of one or more extralymphatic organs or tissues, with or without associated lymph node involvement

* Each stage is subdivided into A (no systemic symptoms) and B (unexplained fever, night sweats and weight loss > 10% of body weight).

All other stages are usually treated with combination chemotherapy. The prognosis is related to the stage of the disease, with a 5-year survival rate of approximately 90% in stage I. The presence of B symptoms indicates more severe disease with a worse prognosis.

Non-Hodgkin's lymphoma

This is a heterogeneous group of disorders which encompasses many different histological subtypes. Several rather confusing classifications have been suggested, based on parameters such as histological type, rate of cell division or B- or T-cell origin. For example, the subdivision into high-grade or low-grade reflects the rate at which cells are dividing. Ironically, high-grade lymphomas (rapidly dividing cells) are potentially curable, whereas low-grade ones are generally considered incurable (see below). the most commonly used histological classifications are the Kiel classification and the Working classification. However, both may now be replaced by a modified system (REAL, Revised European American Lymphoma Classification) which incorporates cytogenetic abnormalities and recently described entities such as MALT lymphoma (mucosal-associated lymphoid tissue).

Clinical features

Non-Hodgkin's lymphoma (NHL) is rare before the age of 40. The presentation can be very varied and almost any organ in the body can be involved. Peripheral lymph node enlargement is the most common clinical presentation. Systemic symptoms as in Hodgkin's disease may occur. Bone marrow infiltration, leading to anaemia, recurrent infections and bleeding, is often seen in low-grade lymphoma.

Table 4.22 Non-Hodgkin's lymphoma: low grade and high grade

Low grade	High grade
Middle-aged/older people	Any age group
Bone marrow infiltration common	Bone marrow infiltration unusual
Incurable with conventional chemotherapy	Potentially curable

Low- and high-grade lymphomas have a different age distribution and behave differently. They are summarized in Table 4.22.

Investigations

- Blood count may show anaemia. An elevated WCC or thrombocytopenia suggests bone marrow involvement.
- Liver biochemistry may be abnormal if the liver is involved.

- Radiology, such as a chest radiograph and CT, will show involvement of mediastinal, intrathoracic or intra-abdominal lymph nodes.
- Lymph node biopsy is required for definitive diagnosis.
- Bone marrow aspiration and trephine biopsy will confirm marrow involvement.

Management

Treatment depends on the grade and histological subtypes.

- Low-grade disease in general is not curable. However, patients may survive for many years and usually experience several remissions with relatively simple treatment such as chlorambucil, or radiotherapy in localized disease.
- High-grade disease requires combination chemotherapy. Modern regimens, e.g. doxorubicin, cyclophosphamide, vincristine and prednisolone (CHOP), achieve a 60–70% response rate, and cure in about one-third. Some patients with localized disease can be cured with local radiotherapy.

MALT lymphoma

MALT (mucosal-associated lymphoid tissue) lymphoma is an unusual lymphoma affecting the gastrointestinal tract, most commonly the stomach. It has gained increasing recognition because of the close association in the stomach with *Helicobacter pylori* infection. In certain cases, eradication of this organism alone has led to resolution of the lymphoma.

Mycosis fungoides and Sézary's syndrome

These are rare cutaneous T-cell lymphomas that may spread in the later stages to involve lymph nodes and other organs.

Burkitt's lymphoma

This is a form of NHL occurring mainly in African children, and is associated with Epstein–Barr virus infection. Jaw tumours are common, usually with gastrointestinal involvement. Treatment is with radiotherapy and chemotherapy.

MYELOABLATIVE THERAPY WITH BONE MARROW TRANSPLANTATION

Myeloablative therapy is a term used for treatment that employs high-dose chemotherapy or chemotherapy plus radiation, with the aim of clearing the bone marrow completely of both benign and malignant cells. Without bone marrow replacement or 'transplantation', the patient would die of bone marrow failure. Approaches to restore bone marrow function include the following:

- *Allogeneic* bone marrow transplantation: bone marrow *from another individual*, usually an HLA-identical sibling, is infused intravenously following myeloablative therapy. Immunosuppression is required to prevent host rejection and graft-versus-host disease (GVHD). The latter is a syndrome in which donor T lymphocytes infiltrate the skin, gut and liver, causing a maculopapular rash, diarrhoea and liver necrosis. Following allogeneic BMT the blood count usually recovers within 3–4 weeks. The mortality rate is 20–30%, depending on the person's age, and is often a result of infection or GVHD.
- *Autologous* (the patient acts as his or her own source of stem cells) peripheral blood progenitor cells (PBPCs) have virtually replaced autologous BMT as support for myeloablative therapy. With this technique it is possible, by using chemotherapy followed by the growth factor, colony-stimulating factor (G-CSF), to stimulate haemopoietic progenitor cells in the marrow to proliferate so that they can be collected from the peripheral blood. They are stored and reinfused after myeloablative therapy. The main advantage is the short time for blood count recovery because PBPCs are more differentiated. This technique has been used predominantly in patients with Hodgkin's disease, NHL, myeloma and breast cancer. *Allogeneic* PBPCs are currently being evaluated.

THE PARAPROTEINAEMIAS

Multiple myeloma

Multiple myeloma is a neoplastic clonal proliferation of bone marrow plasma cells usually capable of producing monoclonal immunoglobulins (M proteins or paraproteins), which in most cases are IgG or IgA. The paraprotein may be associated with excretion of light chains in the urine, which are either κ or λ; the excess light chains are known as Bence-Jones protein.

Clinical features

The peak age of presentation is 60 years. The neoplastic clone of cells induces excess osteoclastic activity, which results in osteoporosis, osteolytic lesions, pathological fractures and hypercalcaemia. Bone pain is the most common presenting symptom. Progressive marrow infiltration results in anaemia, infections and bleeding. Renal failure has multiple causes: deposition of light chains in the tubules, hypercalcaemia, hyperuricaemia and amyloid deposition in the kidneys. Paraproteins may form aggregates in the blood, which greatly increase the viscosity, leading to blurred vision, gangrene and bleeding.

Investigations

The diagnosis is made by demonstrating the following:

- Plasma cell infiltration on bone marrow aspirate or trephine biopsy
- Osteolytic bone lesions (often in the skull) on skeletal survey
- Monoclonal ('M') bands on serum protein electrophoresis, or Bence-Jones protein in the urine.

Other essential investigations are as follows:

- Blood count, which may show anaemia, thrombocytopenia and leukopenia. The ESR is almost always high.
- Serum biochemistry may show evidence of renal failure and hypercalcaemia. The alkaline phosphatase is usually normal.

Management

Combination chemotherapy with alkylating agents (melphalan or cyclophosphamide) given in conjunction with prednisolone has improved the median survival of patients with myeloma from 7 months to 2 years. Selected patients are treated with high-dose melphalan supported by autologous BMT or PBPC. Adjuvant interferon therapy following chemotherapy has been shown to prolong remission. Localized bone pain can be helped by radiotherapy, and pathological fractures prevented by pinning of lytic bone lesions. Renal failure (page 301) and hypercalcaemia (page 246) may be corrected by adequate hydration alone. Hyperviscosity is treated by plasmapheresis together with systemic therapy.

Prognosis

The median survival with treatment is about 2 years.

Waldenström's macroglobulinaemia

As in myeloma the neoplastic B cells secrete a monoclonal immunoglobulin. However, unlike myeloma, but similar to lymphoma, the tumour infiltrates the lymphoid tissues, including bone marrow, spleen and lymph nodes.

Clinical features

The most common features are malaise, weight loss, lymph node enlargement and symptoms of hyperviscosity.

Investigations

- Blood count may show a normal or low Hb and WCC, although the ESR is almost always high.
- Protein electrophoresis shows an IgM paraprotein.
- Bone marrow aspirate shows infiltration with lymphoplasmacytoid cells.

Management

Treatment is with alkylating agents or doxorubicin-containing regimens. Hyperviscosity is treated with plasmapheresis.

Monoclonal gammopathy of undetermined significance

This is usually seen in older patients, where a raised level of paraprotein (usually IgA) is found in the blood, but without other features of myeloma. Patients are often asymptomatic and no treatment is required. Regular follow-up is usually indicated in case they later develop lymphoma or myeloma.

Rheumatology

5

Musculoskeletal problems are common and account for about one in six GP consultations. Most of these are non-articular problems (see below). Osteoarthritis and rheumatoid arthritis are more commonly seen in hospital clinics. Pain is the most common presenting symptom of joint disease and may be localized to a single joint or affect many joints.

Arthralgia is the term used to describe joint pains when the joint appears normal on examination. *Arthritis* is the term used when there is objective evidence of joint inflammation (swelling, deformity or an effusion). In a patient presenting with joint pains, the history and examination must assess the distribution of joints affected (symmetrical?, axial or peripheral?), the presence of morning stiffness (common in inflammatory arthropathies), aggravating and relieving factors, past medical history and family history. Table 5.1 lists the likely causes of joint pains based on the age and sex of the patient and the presence of associated features.

Pain in or around a single joint may arise from the joint itself (articular problem) or from structures surrounding the joint (periarticular problem). Enthesitis (inflammation at the site of attachment of ligaments, tendons and joint capsules), bursitis and tendinitis are all causes of periarticular pain. Pain arising from the joint may be the result of a mechanical problem (e.g. torn meniscus) or an inflammatory problem. The causes of a large joint monoarthritis include osteoarthritis, gout, pseudogout, trauma and septic arthritis. The key investigation is synovial fluid aspiration with Gram stain and culture, and analysis for crystals (in gout and pseudogout). Less common causes are rheumatoid arthritis, the spondyloarthropathies, tuberculous infection and haemarthrosis (e.g. in haemophilia).

Table 5.1 Differential diagnosis of polyarticular disease in adults in the UK

Age	Predominantly males	Predominantly females
Young	Reiter's syndrome Reactive arthritis Ankylosing spondylitis	Systemic lupus erythematosus Rheumatoid arthritis Sjögren's syndrome
	Psoriatic arthropathy Enteropathic arthropathy	
Middle age	Gout	Rheumatoid arthritis Sjögren's syndrome Generalized osteoarthritis
Elderly		Polymyalgia rheumatica Pseudogout
Uncommon arthropathies	Malignancy (hypertrophic pulmonary osteoarthropathy), Lyme disease, rheumatic fever, Henoch–Schönlein purpura, Behçet's syndrome	

ARTHRITIS

Osteoarthritis

Osteoarthritis is a condition characterized by cartilage loss with an accompanying periarticular bone response, and is the commonest form of arthritis. Radiological changes of osteoarthritis may be seen in about 10% of the population as a whole, and in 50% of those aged over 60, although only a proportion of these have symptoms.

Epidemiology

Osteoarthritis (OA) occurs throughout the world, although it is uncommon in the black population. It is twice as common in women as in men, and there is a marked familial tendency.

Pathology and pathogenesis

Osteoarthritis is the result of active, sometimes inflammatory but potentially reparative processes, rather than the inevitable result of trauma and ageing. It is characterized by a progressive destruction and loss of articular cartilage. The exposed subchondral bone becomes sclerotic, with increased vascularity and cyst formation. Attempts at repair produce cartilaginous growths at the margins of the joint which later become calcified (osteophytes).

There are several mechanisms that have been suggested for the pathogenesis. These include the production of metalloproteinases, such as stromelysin and collagenase, which degrade collagen, and proteoglycans, the production of inflammatory mediators such as a interleukin-1 and tumour necrosis factor-α, and genetic factors.

Most osteoarthritis is primary. Secondary osteoarthritis occurs in joints that have been damaged in some way (e.g. intra-articular fractures, avascular necrosis) or are congenitally abnormal (e.g. slipped femoral epiphysis).

Clinical features

Although OA is not always symptomatic the main symptom is pain, which is made worse by movement and relieved by rest. Stiffness occurs after sitting down and for a short period (<1/2 h) on waking in the morning. The joints most commonly involved are the distal interphalangeal joints (DIPJ) and first carpometacarpal joint of the hands, first metatarsophalangeal joint of the foot and the weight-bearing joints – vertebrae, hips and knees. On examination there is deformity and bony enlargement of the joints, limited joint movement and muscle wasting of surrounding muscle groups. There may occasionally be a joint effusion. Heberden's nodes are bony swellings at the distal interphalangeal joints. Bouchard's nodes are similar but occur at the proximal interphalangeal joint.

Differential diagnosis

Osteoarthritis is differentiated from rheumatoid arthritis by the pattern of joint involvement (Figure 5.1) and the absence of the systemic features that occur in rheumatoid arthritis. Pyrophosphate arthropathy (page 231) affects a similar age group as osteoarthritis but the wrists are usually involved. Chronic tophaceous gout (page 228) and psoriatic arthritis affecting the DIPJ (page 214) may mimic osteoarthritis.

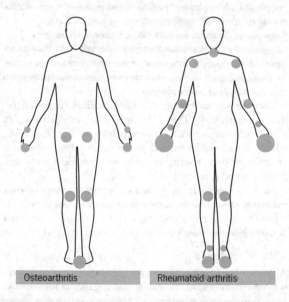

Osteoarthritis   Rheumatoid arthritis

Figure 5.1
The pattern of joint involvement in osteoarthritis compared with rheumatoid arthritis. Both conditions are usually bilateral and symmetrical in distribution.

Investigations

- Radiology. X-rays are only abnormal if the joint is damaged, and may show narrowing of the joint space (resulting from loss of cartilage), osteophytes, subchondral sclerosis and cyst formation.
- MRI demonstrates early cartilage changes.
- Other tests. The FBC and ESR are both normal. Rheumatoid factor is negative, but low-titre tests may occur incidentally in elderly people.

Management

Treatment should focus on the symptoms and disability, not the radiological appearances. There are three main types of treatment: physical measures, drugs and surgery. Obese patients should be encouraged to lose weight, particularly if weight-bearing joints are affected.

- Physical therapy. The application of heat to an affected joint may provide pain relief. Exercises maintain muscle power and improve the mobility of weight-bearing joints. Hydrotherapy may be helpful.
- Drugs. Paracetamol and non-steroidal anti-inflammatory drugs (NSAIDs) are used to control symptoms, and should ideally be used on an intermittent rather than a continuous basis. Intra-articular steroids can be used for inflammatory exacerbations, but systemic corticosteroid therapy is not used.
- Surgery. Replacement of the joint is indicated if pain and loss of function have failed to respond to drugs and physical therapy.

Rheumatoid arthritis

Rheumatoid arthritis (RA) is a chronic symmetrical polyarthritis of unknown cause. It is a systemic disorder associated with extra-articular involvement, e.g. the lungs and many other organs.

Epidemiology

Rheumatoid arthritis affects 1–3% of the population worldwide, with a peak prevalence between the ages of 30 and 50 years. Women are affected three times more often than men. There is an increased incidence in those with a family history of rheumatoid arthritis and an association with HLA-DR4 in most ethnic groups.

Aetiology

The cause of rheumatoid arthritis is unknown. The most widely held view is that an interplay of genetic factors, sex hormones and an infectious agent initiates an autoimmune mechanism with inflammatory and destructive features.

Pathology

Rheumatoid arthritis is a disease of the synovium. There is infiltration by chronic inflammatory cells: lymphocytes, plasma cells and macrophages. The synovium then proliferates and grows out over the surface of cartilage, producing a tumour-like mass called 'pannus'. Pannus destroys the articular cartilage and subchondral bone, producing bony erosions.

Subcutaneous nodules (rheumatoid nodules) have a characteristic appearance with a central area of necrosis surrounded by macrophages and fibrous tissue. Similar lesions occur in the pleura, pericardium and lung.

Clinical features

The typical presentation is with an insidious onset of pain, stiffness and swelling in the small joints of the hands and feet, which is most marked on waking in the mornings. Early in the disease there is spindling of the fingers caused by swelling of the proximal but not the distal interphalangeal joints; the metacarpophalangeal joints and wrist joints are also swollen. As the disease progresses there is weakening of joint capsules, causing joint instability, subluxation (partial dislocation) and deformity. The characteristic deformities of the rheumatoid hand are shown in Figure 5.2. Most patients eventually have many joints involved, including the wrists, elbows, shoulders, cervical spine, knees, ankles and feet. The dorsal and lumbar spine are not involved. Joint effusions and wasting of muscles around the affected joints are early features. Later there is joint deformity, subluxation and instability.

Less common presentations are 'explosive' (sudden onset of widespread arthritis), palindromic (relapsing and

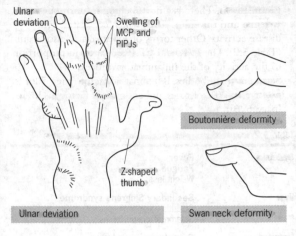

Figure 5.2
Characteristic hand deformities in rheumatoid arthritis. MCP, metacarpophalanges; PIPJs, proximal interphalangeal joints; (Adapted from Read et al (1992) Essential Medicine. Churchill Livingstone, Edinburgh.)

remitting monoarthritis of different large joints), or with a systemic illness with few joint symptoms initially.

Extra-articular manifestations

Periarticular features of rheumatoid arthritis include bursitis, tenosynovitis, muscle wasting and nodule formation. Rheumatoid nodules are found in about 20% of cases, usually on the ulnar surface of the forearm just below the elbow. Patients with nodules are usually seropositive (see later).

Other extra-articular disease manifestations are summarized in Table 5.2. The most common manifestations are highlighted; these may be present but cause few symptoms, e.g. a pericardial rub is often heard (up to 30%) but pericarditis is seldom a clinical problem. Atlantoaxial subluxation is commonly seen on a cervical radiograph, but much less commonly causes problems.

Investigations

The diagnosis is usually clinical, but appropriate investigations include:

207

- Blood count. There is a normochromic/normocytic anaemia and thrombocytosis which correlates with disease activity. Other forms of anaemia may also occur (Table 5.2). The ESR and CRP are raised in proportion to the activity of the inflammatory process.
- Serum autoantibodies. Rheumatoid factor (page 706) is positive in 70% of cases and antinuclear factor in 30% (page 696).

Table 5.2 Extra-articular manifestations of rheumatoid arthritis

Systemic	**Fever**
	Fatigue
	Weight loss
Eyes	**Secondary Sjögren's syndrome**
	Scleritis
	Scleromalacia perforans
Neurological	**Carpal tunnel syndrome**
	Atlantoaxial subluxation
	Cord compression
	Polyneuropathy, predominantly sensory
	Mononeuritis multiplex
Reticuloendothelial	**Lymphadenopathy**
	Felty's syndrome (rheumatoid arthritis, splenomegaly, neutropenia)
Blood	**Anaemia caused by**
	Chronic disease
	NSAID-induced gastrointestinal blood loss
	Haemolysis
	Hypersplenism
	Thrombocytosis
Pulmonary	**Pleural effusion**
	Diffuse fibrosing alveolitis
	Rheumatoid nodules
	Rheumatoid pneumoconiosis (Caplan's syndrome)
	Small airway disease
Heart	**Pericarditis**
	Pericardial effusion
Kidneys	Amyloidosis
	Analgesic nephropathy
Vasculitis	Leg ulcers
	Nailfold infarcts
	Gangrene of fingers and toes

The most common manifestations are in bold.

- Radiology. Radiographs of the affected joints may show joint narrowing, erosions at the joint margins, porosis of periarticular bone and cysts.
- Synovial fluid. Is sterile with a high neutrophil count in uncomplicated disease.

Differential diagnosis

In the patient with symmetrical peripheral arthritis, nodules and positive rheumatoid factor the diagnosis is straightforward. Rheumatoid must be distinguished from the symmetrical seronegative arthropathy occurring in psoriasis, and severe rheumatoid from 'arthritis mutilans' (page 214). In a young woman presenting with joint pains SLE must be considered, but characteristically the joints are normal on examination in this condition.

Management

Effective management of rheumatoid arthritis requires a multidisciplinary approach, with input from rheumatologists, orthopaedic surgeons (joint replacement, arthroplasty), occupational therapists (aids to reduce disability) and physiotherapists (teaching of exercise to improve muscle power and to maintain mobility to prevent flexion deformities).

NSAIDs are effective in relieving the joint pain and stiffness of rheumatoid arthritis, but they do not slow disease progression or alter inflammatory markers. Slow-release indomethacin taken at night may produce dramatic relief of symptoms on the following day. The main side effects are peptic ulceration, with the risk of bleeding and perforation, fluid retention and chronic tubulointerstitial nephritis.

Disease-modifying drugs should probably now be used early in the disease to prevent the irreversible effects of long-term inflammation of the joints. These drugs, which act mainly through inhibition of inflammatory cytokines, reduce inflammation and slow the development of joint erosions, though they may take up to 6 months to achieve maximum effect. The most effective drugs are methotrexate, penicillamine and azathioprine. Hydroxychloroquine, sulphasalazine and auranofin are a little less effective but safer. Methotrexate is now considered to be the drug of first choice for most patients, though all drugs can have serious side effects (Table 5.3) so careful monitoring with blood tests is necessary. The antimalarial drug hydroxychloroquine may produce corneal deposits (which disappear when treatment is stopped) and more rarely retinopathy, which may be permanent. Visual acuity must be checked and ophthalmoscopy performed 6 monthly.

Table 5.3 Side effects of drugs used in long-term suppressive therapy for rheumatoid arthritis. Rash is an additional side effect of most of the drugs listed

Drug	Side effects
Methotrexate	Neutropenia
	Liver fibrosis
Penicillamine	Thrombocytopenia
	Proteinuria
Azathioprine	Neutropenia
	Nausea and vomiting
Intramuscular gold (sodium aurothiomalate)	Thrombocytopenia
Oral gold (auranofin)	Diarrhoea
Hydroxychloroquine	Retinopathy
Sulphasalazine	Nausea
	Male infertility (reversible)

Corticosteroids suppress disease activity but the dose required is often large, with the considerable risk of long-term toxicity (osteoporosis, diabetes mellitus, hypertension and myopathy). They are seldom used except in the elderly patient with explosive rheumatoid arthritis or in patients with severe extra-articular manifestations. Local injection of a troublesome joint (see below) with a long-acting corticosteroid improves pain, synovitis and effusion. Repeated injections into an individual joint are possible, but this is usually limited to four a year because too-frequent injections may accelerate joint damage.

In patients presenting with disproportionate involvement of a single joint, septic arthritis (page 215) must be considered and excluded before the symptoms are attributed to a disease flare-up.

Prognosis

The prognosis is variable. After 10 years 10% of patients will be severely crippled and 25% will have minimal, if any, symptoms. Other patients lie between these two extremes.

THE SERONEGATIVE SPONDARTHRITIDES

This title describes a group of conditions affecting the spine and peripheral joints which cluster in families and are linked to certain type I HLA antigens (Table 5.4). The joint involvement is more limited than that seen in RA and its distribution is different. The synovitis itself is difficult to distinguish from that of RA histologically, but there is no production of rheumatoid factors, hence 'seronegative'. All are associated with an increased frequency of sacroiliitis and an increased frequency of HLA-B27 or structurally associated class I antigens which cross-react with HLA-B27. The explanation for the association with HLA-B27 is unknown.

Table 5.4 Seronegative spondarthritides

Ankylosing spondylitis (AS)
Psoriatic arthritis
Reactive arthritis
   Sexually acquired (Reiter's disease)
   Post-dysenteric reactive arthritis
Ulcerative colitis/Crohn's (enteropathic) arthritis

Ankylosing spondylitis

This is an inflammatory disorder of the back affecting mainly young adults. Although the disease affects women as commonly as men, men are usually affected more severely.

Clinical features

The typical patient with ankylosing spondylitis is a young man (late teens, early 20) who presents with increasing pain and morning stiffness in the lower back. There is a progressive loss of spinal movement. Inspection of the spine reveals two characteristic abnormalities:

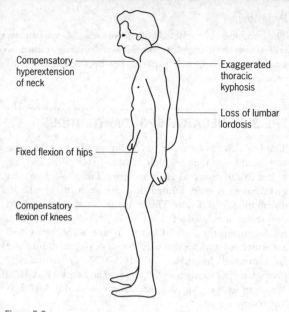

Compensatory hyperextension of neck

Exaggerated thoracic kyphosis

Loss of lumbar lordosis

Fixed flexion of hips

Compensatory flexion of knees

Figure 5.3
Ankylosing spondylitis – the typical posture in advanced cases. (Adapted from Calin (1994) Seronegative spondylarthritides. Medicine International 22: 148.)

- Loss of lumbar lordosis and increased kyphosis (Figure 5.3)
- Variable limitation of spinal flexion and a reduction in chest expansion.

Other features include Achilles tendinitis and planter fasciitis (enthesitis) and tenderness around the pelvis and chest wall.

Non-articular features are iritis (in 25%) and, rarely, aortic incompetence, cardiac conduction defects and apical lung fibrosis.

Investigations

- Blood count. The ESR and CRP are often raised.
- Radiology. Radiographs may be normal or show erosion and sclerosis of the margins of the sacroiliac joints,

proceeding to ankylosis (immobility and consolidation of the joint). In the spinal column, squaring of the vertebrae (caused by erosion of the corners) and progressive calcification of the interspinous ligaments produce the 'bamboo spine'.

Management

- Regular exercises (twice daily) are essential to maintain posture and mobility.
- Drugs. Slow-release NSAIDs taken at night are particularly effective in relieving night pain and morning stiffness. Sulphasalazine or methotrexate may help the peripheral arthritis but there is little evidence that they control the spinal disease.

Prognosis

Most patients are able to lead a normal active life and remain at work. In severe cases the spine becomes completely fused and brittle, with a risk of fracture (on minimal trauma) and cord compression. The fixed kyphosis of the cervical and thoracic spine may impair ventilation.

Reiter's syndrome

Reiter's syndrome consists of the triad of a seronegative reactive arthritis, non-specific urethritis and conjunctivitis. Two types are recognized:

- Following a gastrointestinal infection with *Shigella*, *Salmonella*, *Yersinia* or *Campylobacter* (enteric)
- Following non-specific urethritis.

Clinical features

Arthritis The typical case is a young man who presents with an acute arthritis shortly (within 4 weeks) after an enteric or venereal infection, which may have been mild or asymptomatic. The joints of the lower limbs are particularly affected in an asymmetrical pattern; the knees, ankles and feet are the most common sites.

Urethritis is associated with a sterile urethral discharge and dysuria.

Conjunctivitis occurs in one-third of patients and is usually mild and bilateral.

Occasional additional features are iritis, enthesiopathy (planter fasciitis, Achilles tendinitis), circinate balanitis (superficial ulceration around the penile meatus) and keratoderma blenorrhagica, an intense scaling of the soles of the feet resembling pustular psoriasis.

Investigations

The diagnosis is clinical. The ESR is raised in the acute stage. Aspirated synovial fluid is sterile, with a high neutrophil count.

Management

Treatment is with NSAIDs together with local joint aspiration and injection of corticosteroid. In chronic cases sulphasalazine or azathioprine may be necessary.

Prognosis

The acute arthritis resolves within a few months. However, 50% of patients develop recurrent arthritis, iritis or ankylosing spondylitis.

Reactive arthritis

The full triad of Reiter's syndrome is rare, but a large joint arthritis following enteric or venereal infection is common and is the most common cause of arthritis in young men.

Psoriatic arthritis

This is a seronegative arthritis occurring in 5–8% of patients with psoriasis, particularly in those with nail disease (page 629).

Clinical features

There are several types:

- *Asymmetrical involvement* of the small joints of the hand, including the distal interphalangeal joints
- *Symmetrical polyarthritis* resembling rheumatoid arthritis
- *Arthritis mutilans*, a severe form with destruction of the small bones in the hands and feet
- *Ankylosing spondylitis* occurs with increased frequency in patients with psoriasis.

Investigations

- Blood count. Routine blood tests are unhelpful in the diagnosis. The ESR is often normal.
- Radiology. Radiographs may show erosions and periarticular osteoporosis in the terminal interphalangeal joints.

Treatment

This is with analgesia and NSAIDs. Local synovitis responds to intra-articular corticosteroid injections. In more severe cases methotrexate or cyclosporin may be used, as they control both the arthritis and the skin lesions.

Enteropathic arthritis

Enteropathic arthritis is a large joint mono- or asymmetrical oligoarthritis occurring in 10–15% of patients with ulcerative colitis and Crohn's disease. It parallels the activity of the inflammatory bowel disease and consequently improves as bowel symptoms improve. Ankylosing spondylitis occurs in 5% of patients with inflammatory bowel disease but is not related to disease activity.

INFECTIVE ARTHRITIS

Joint infection is uncommon but is important because it can lead to considerable joint destruction. Infection of the joints may be caused by the following:

- Bacteria (see below)
- Viruses: rubella, mumps and hepatitis B virus infections are associated with a mild self-limiting arthritis. HIV infection is associated with an intermittent arthritis
- Spirochaetes and fungi (rare).

Septic arthritis

Septic arthritis results from infection of the joint with pyogenic organisms, most commonly *Staphylococcus aureus*. The organism reaches the joint through the bloodstream from a distant site of infection, from local spread of adjacent osteomyelitis, or through direct injury or trauma.

Clinical features

Classically there is a hot painful red joint, often the knee, which has developed acutely. There may be fever and evidence of infection elsewhere. Fever and systemic reactions may be absent in those with rheumatoid arthritis or in patients taking corticosteroids.

Investigations

- Joint aspiration is the single most important diagnostic procedure. The synovial fluid is usually purulent, with $>50\,000 \times 10^6/l$ white blood cells, predominantly neutrophils. Gram staining may show the presence of organisms, which may be confirmed by culture.
- Blood cultures may be positive.
- Radiology. Radiographs play little part in the diagnosis because these only become abnormal when joint destruction has occurred.

Management

Treatment should be started immediately because joint damage can occur rapidly. The joint should be rested and immobilized. Appropriate antibiotics should be given parenterally for the first 2 weeks, followed by oral antibiotics for the following 4 weeks. Treatment depends on the organism concerned, but a suitable 'blind' regimen would be flucloxacillin 1–2 g 6 hourly intravenously, together with oral fusidic acid 500 mg 8 hourly. Adequate joint drainage, usually with needle aspiration, is also required as long as the effusion is detectable.

Tuberculous arthritis

Approximately 1% of patients with TB have skeletal involvement, which is usually caused by haematogenous spread from pulmonary or renal disease.

Clinical features

Spinal involvement is particularly common (50%) but the knee, hip, sacroiliac and other joints may be involved. There is an insidious onset of pain, swelling and dysfunction, often associated with general symptoms of malaise, anorexia and night sweats.

Diagnosis

Culture of the synovial fluid may give the diagnosis. Occasionally, synovial biopsy is required.

Treatment

Treatment is as for tuberculosis elsewhere (see page 420), in addition to joint rest and immobilization.

Meningococcal arthritis

Meningococcal arthritis usually occurs as part of a meningococcal septicaemia and results from the deposition of circulating immune complexes containing meningococcal antigens. It is a migratory polyarthritis, not associated with joint destruction. Treatment is with penicillin.

Gonococcal arthritis

Gonococcal arthritis occurs secondary to genital or oral infection (often asymptomatic) and presents with a mild inflammatory polyarthritis. Concomitant skin involvement is common (maculopapular pustules). It affects particularly young women and homosexual men. The organism can usually be cultured from the bloodstream, and from the joints in 25% of cases. Treatment is with penicillin.

Salmonella arthritis

Salmonella arthritis presents as a mild polyarthritis and occurs with types of salmonellae that invade the bloodstream rather than staying within the gastrointestinal tract. Gastrointestinal symptoms may therefore be minor or absent. Treatment is with amoxycillin.

CONNECTIVE TISSUE DISEASE

The term 'connective tissue disease' is used for three diseases:

- Systemic lupus erythematosus (SLE)
- Systemic sclerosis (scleroderma)
- Polymyositis and dermatomyositis.

Their relationship is illustrated in Figure 5.4.

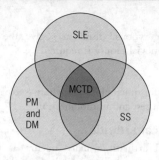

Figure 5.4
The family of connective tissue diseases. MCTD, mixed connective tissue disorders; PM, DM, poly- and dermatomyositis; SLE, systemic lupus erythematosus; SS, systemic sclerosis.

These diseases have a number of features in common, including arthritis, immune complex deposition and vasculitis. Features of all three occur in mixed connective tissue disease.

Systemic lupus erythematosus

SLE is the most common of the connective tissue disorders and is characterized by the presence of serum antibodies against nuclear components. It is a multisystem disease and has a varied clinical presentation.

Epidemiology

SLE is mainly a disease of young women, with a peak age of onset between 20 and 40 years. It affects about 0.1% of the population but is much more common in Africans.

Aetiology

The cause of the disease is unknown but is probably multifactorial. Factors that are thought to play a role include the following:

- *Genetic factors*: there is a 70% concordance for SLE between identical twins and an increased incidence of HLA-B8 and -DR3
- *Immunological factors*: antinuclear antibodies are present which are thought to result from polyclonal activation of B cells by an antigenic stimulus, possible viral antigens. This may be associated with impaired T-cell regulation and deficiencies in complement. Most of the

visceral lesions are mediated by vascular immune complex (DNA-anti-DNA) deposition
- *Drugs*: hydralazine and procainamide may cause a mild lupus-like syndrome, which often resolves after the drug is withdrawn
- *Infection*: viral infections may be responsible
- *Hormonal factors*: the high incidence in women suggests that female hormones may modify the immune response.

Clinical features

These are illustrated in Figure 5.5. A migratory asymmetrical arthralgia is one of the most common

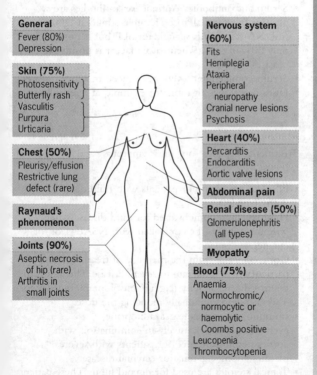

General
Fever (80%)
Depression

Skin (75%)
Photosensitivity
Butterfly rash
Vasculitis
Purpura
Urticaria

Chest (50%)
Pleurisy/effusion
Restrictive lung defect (rare)

Raynaud's phenomenon

Joints (90%)
Aseptic necrosis of hip (rare)
Arthritis in small joints

Nervous system (60%)
Fits
Hemiplegia
Ataxia
Peripheral neuropathy
Cranial nerve lesions
Psychosis

Heart (40%)
Percarditis
Endocarditis
Aortic valve lesions

Abdominal pain

Renal disease (50%)
Glomerulonephritis (all types)

Myopathy

Blood (75%)
Anaemia
  Normochromic/ normocytic or haemolytic
  Coombs positive
Leucopenia
Thrombocytopenia

Figure 5.5
Clinical features of SLE.

presenting features. Synovitis and joint effusions are uncommon and joint destruction is very rare. Non-specific features such as fever, malaise and depression may dominate the clinical picture.

Discoid lupus is often a benign variant of the disease, in which skin involvement may be the only feature. There is a characteristic facial rash with erythematous plaques which progress to scarring and pigmentation. Sunlight is an exacerbating factor in most patients.

Investigations

- Blood count usually shows a normochromic/normocytic anaemia, often with neutropenia and thrombocytopenia. The ESR is raised but the CRP is usually normal.
- Serum autoantibodies. Antinuclear antibodies are positive in almost all cases. Double-stranded DNA (dsDNA) binding is specific for SLE but is positive in only 50% of cases. Rheumatoid factor is positive in 50% of cases.
- Serum complement levels are reduced in active disease.
- Histological investigation, for example of a renal biopsy, shows a vasculitis.

Management

Treatment depends on the symptoms and severity of disease.

- NSAIDs are useful for patients with mild disease and with arthralgia.
- Hydroxychloroquine is used for mild disease when symptoms cannot be controlled with NSAIDs, or for cutaneous disease.
- Corticosteroids from the mainstay of treatment, particularly in moderate to severe disease. The aim is to control disease activity (e.g. prednisolone 30 mg/day for 4 weeks) before gradually reducing the dose.
- Immunosuppressives (e.g. azathioprine, cyclophosphamide), usually in combination with corticosteroids, are used for patients with severe manifestations, e.g. renal or cerebral disease.
- Topical steroids are used for discoid lupus. These patients should also avoid excessive sunlight.

Prognosis

The disease is characterized by relapses and remissions even in severe disease. The 10-year survival is about 90%. Infection has replaced renal failure as the most common cause of death in SLE.

Antiphospholipid syndrome

This syndrome is characterized by the presence of antoantibodies to β_2 glycoprotein I, a phospholipid binding protein. The antibodies are thought to play a role in thrombosis by an effect on platelet membranes, endothelial cells and clotting compounds such as prothrombin, protein C and protein S (page 177). It was first described in patients with SLE, but it has become clear that it is much more common than SLE and most patients (often young women) with the syndrome do not have SLE.

Clinical features

The major clinical features are the result of thrombosis:

- *In arteries*: stroke, transient ischaemic attacks, myocardial infection
- *In veins*: deep vein thrombosis, Budd–Chiari syndrome
- In the placenta: recurrent abortions.

Other features include valvular heart disease, migraine, epilepsy and thrombocytopenia.

Investigations

Anticardiolipin antibodies are diagnostic.

Management

Small doses of aspirin are used in mild cases; warfarin is used in more severe cases.

Systemic sclerosis

Systemic sclerosis (scleroderma) is a chronic multisystem disease which predominantly affects the skin and is usually accompanied by Raynaud's phenomenon (page 389). It is three to five times more common in women than men, and presents before the age of 50 years.

Aetiology

The cause of systemic sclerosis is unknown, although many abnormalities in both cellular and humoral immunity have been documented. There is an increase in dermal collagen and a decrease in elastic tissue which leads to the typical thickening and immobility.

Clinical features

Limited cutaneous scleroderma This starts initially with Raynaud's phenomenon, often prior to the development of cutaneous manifestations. The skin changes that dominate this disease are usually limited to the hands, face and feet. Typically the skin is thickened, bound down to underlying structures, and the fingers taper (sclerodactyly). There is often a characteristic facial appearance, with beaking of the nose, a fixed expression, radial furrowing of the lips and limitation of mouth movements. There may be telangiectasia and palpable subcutaneous nodules of calcium deposition in the fingers (calcinosis).

The CREST syndrome (Calcinosis, Raynaud's phenomenon, oEsophageal involvement, Sclerodactyly, Telangiectasia) and morphoea (dermal fibrosis producing plaques of thickened skin) are variants of systemic sclerosis which carry a better prognosis.

Diffuse cutaneous scleroderma The skin changes develop more rapidly after the development of Raynaud's phenomenon and there is early involvement of other organs (Table 5.5).

Investigations

- Blood count shows a normochromic/normocytic anaemia and the ESR may be raised.
- Serum autoantibodies. Antinuclear antibodies are often positive. Specific types are antinucleolar and anti-Scl 70 (page 701). Anticentomere antibodies occur in the CREST syndrome.
- Radiology. A radiograph of the hands may show deposits of calcium around the fingers, and there may be erosion and resorption of the tufts of the distal phalanges.
- Oesophageal manometry demonstrates failure of peristalsis in the distal oesophagus, with reduced oesophageal sphincter pressure.

Management

Management is symptomatic. There is no specific treatment.

Table 5.5 Major clinical features of scleroderma

Organ	Clinical manifestation	Involved in (%)
Skin	Thickened skin, sclerodactyly, telangiectasia, calcinosis	90
Vascular	Raynaud's phenomenon	80
Oesophagus	Impaired peristalsis causing reflux with eventual stricture formation	80
Lungs	Fibrosis, pulmonary hypertension	45
Heart	Myocardial fibrosis with arrhythmias and conduction defects	40
Kidney	Obliterative endarteritis of renal vessels with renal failure and malignant hypertension	35
Eyes	Sjögren's syndrome	
Joints/muscle	Joint deformity, myopathy, myositis	20–25

Control of hypertension is important when the kidneys are involved.

Prognosis

The 10-year cumulative survival is approximately 65%. Lung disease is now the major cause of death (previously accelerated hypertension and renal failure).

Polymyositis and dermatomyositis

Polymyositis is a rare muscle disorder of unknown aetiology in which there is inflammation and necrosis of muscle fibres. When accompanied by a rash it is called dermatomyositis.

Clinical features

Peak ages of onset are in childhood and in the fifth and sixth decades. Muscle weakness affecting the proximal muscles of the shoulder and pelvic girdle is the chief symptom. Patients have difficulty squatting, going upstairs, rising from a chair and raising their hands above the head. This may be accompanied by pain, tenderness and muscle wasting. The skin changes of dermatomyositis are characteristic: a heliotrope (purple) periorbital skin rash, a photosensitive scaling rash on the face, and erythematous plaques over the dorsal aspects of the fingers and knuckles. Other features include arthralgia or arthritis, dysphagia resulting from oesophageal muscle involvement, and

Raynaud's phenomenon. Dermatomyositis is associated with an increased incidence of underlying malignancy, particularly in the older age groups.

Investigations

- ESR is usually elevated.
- Muscle enzymes (aldolase or creatine phosphokinase) are elevated in the serum.
- Anti-Jo-1 antibodies are positive.
- Electromyography (EMG) shows characteristic changes.
- Muscle biopsy shows inflammation and necrosis of muscle cells.
- MRI may show characteristic changes.

Management

Oral prednisolone (40–60 mg/day, reducing to a lower maintenance dose) is the treatment of choice. Sometimes immunosuppressive therapy with azathioprine or methotrexate is required.

Prognosis

Fifty per cent of affected children die within 2 years. In adults the prognosis is better, except in association with malignancy.

Mixed connective tissue disease

This rare disorder combines features of more than one of the connective tissue diseases. Cerebral and renal disease are unusual and the prognosis is good. High titres of antibodies to extractable nuclear antigens (page 701) such as ribonucleoprotein (RNP) are commonly found.

Sjögren's syndrome

Sjögren's syndrome is a chronic autoimmune disorder predominantly affecting middle-aged women. It is characterized by immunologically mediated destruction of epithelial exocrine glands.

Clinical features

The main features are dry eyes (keratoconjunctivitis sicca) and dry mouth (xerostomia). It occurs as an isolated disorder (primary Sjögren's syndrome), also known as the sicca syndrome, or more often in association with another autoimmune disease (secondary Sjögren's syndrome), which is rheumatoid arthritis in 50% of cases. Other features of primary Sjögren's syndrome are arthritis, Raynaud's phenomenon and interstitial nephritis. Six per cent develop lymphomas.

Investigations

- Antinuclear antibodies are found in 60–70% of patients. Anti-Ro and anti-La antibodies are present in 70% of patients with primary Sjögren's syndrome.
- Labial gland biopsy shows characteristic changes of lymphocyte infiltration and destruction of acinar tissue.
- A positive Schirmer test confirms defective tear production. (Schirmer test: a standard strip of filter paper is placed on the inside of the lower eyelid; wetting of less than 10 mm in 5 min is positive.)

Management

Treatment is aimed at symptomatic relief using artificial tears.

Vasculitis

Vasculitis is inflammation of the blood vessel walls and may be associated with SLE, rheumatoid arthritis, polymyositis and some allergic drug reactions. The term 'systemic vasculitides' describes a group of multisystem disorders in which vasculitis is the principal feature. These disorders are all rare except for giant cell (temporal) arteritis. Classification of the systemic vasculitides is based on the size of the vessels affected (Table 5.6).

Polymyalgia and temporal arteritis

Polymyalgia and temporal arteritis are clinical syndromes affecting elderly people that form part of the spectrum of giant cell arteritis.

Clinical features

Polymyalgia is characterized by an abrupt onset of stiffness and intense pain in the proximal muscles of the shoulder and pelvic girdle. Significant objective weakness is

Table 5.6 Classification of vasculitis

Large-vessel vasculitis (aorta and its major branches)
Giant-cell arteritis
Takayasu's arteritis (affects young women, causing coronary and CNS ischaemia)

Medium-sized-vessel vasculitis (main visceral vessels, e.g. renal, coronary)
Classic polyarteritis nodosum
Kawasaki's disease (affects young children)

Small-vessel vasculitis (small arteries, arterioles, venules and capillaries)
ANCA associated
    Microscopic polyangiitis
    Wegener's granulomatosis (page 425)
    Churg–Strauss syndrome
Immune complex
    Henoch–Schönlein purpura
    Cutaneous leucocytoclastic angiitis
    Essential cryoglobulinaemia

ANCA, antineutrophil cytoplasmic antibodies (page 695).

uncommon. There may be constitutional symptoms, with malaise, fever, weight loss and anorexia. Arteritic involvement by inflammation is most frequently noticed in the superficial temporal arteries and causes localized headache, temporal artery tenderness and loss of pulsation (page 608). Giant cell arteritis affecting the vertebrobasilar, and sometimes the carotid, circulation may result in stroke.

Investigations

The diagnosis is usually based on clinical findings.

- Blood count usually shows a very high ESR (around 100 mm/h) and a normochromic/normocytic anaemia.
- Temporal artery biopsy may be performed if arteritis is suspected.

Management

Treatment of polymyalgia rheumatica and temporal arteritis is with corticosteroids. The usual starting dose is 15 mg/day for polymyalgia and 60 mg/day for temporal arteritis. The dose is gradually reduced by weekly decrements of 5 mg. Once 10 mg is reached a reduction of 1 mg every 2–4 weeks is usually sufficient. The dose is titrated against symptoms and the ESR. Patients may relapse when treatment is stopped.

Polyarteritis nodosa (classic polyarteritis nodosa)

Polyarteritis nodosa (PAN) predominantly affects middle-aged men. Hepatitis B surface antigen is detected in some patients and may be involved in the pathogenesis. There is a necrotizing arteritis associated with microaneurysm formation, thrombosis and infarction. Clinical features include fever, malaise, weight loss, mononeuritis multiplex, abdominal pain (resulting from visceral infarcts), renal impairment and hypertension. Diagnosis is made on histological investigations and angiography (often of renal vessels showing microaneurysms).

Microscopic polyangiitis

A necrotizing focal segmental glomerulonephritis causes haematuria, proteinuria and sometimes progressive renal failure. Other features include arthralgia and purpuric rashes. Diagnosis is by renal biopsy and measurement of serum perinuclear antineutrophil cytoplasmic antibodies (pANCA) (present in 70%; see page 695).

Churg–Strauss syndrome

This is characterized by a triad of asthma, eosinophilia and a systemic vasculitis. The treatments for Churg–Strauss syndrome, PAN and microscopic polyangiitis are similar, using prednisolone, azathioprine and cyclophosphamide.

Henoch–Schönlein purpura

This condition is most commonly seen in children and presents as a purpuric rash, mainly on the legs and buttocks. The rash is caused by a vasculitis with intradermal bleeding. Abdominal pain, arthritis, haematuria and nephritis also occur. It is characterized by vascular deposition of IgA-dominant immune complexes, and the onset is often preceded by an acute upper respiratory tract infection. Recovery is usually spontaneous.

Arthritis in children

There are three main types: juvenile chronic arthritis, juvenile rheumatoid arthritis and juvenile ankylosing spondylitis.

CRYSTAL DEPOSITION DISEASES

Two main types of crystal account for the majority of crystal-induced arthritis: sodium urate and calcium pyrophosphate. Neutrophils ingest the crystals and initiate a proinflammatory reaction. Crystals may be found in asymptomatic joints.

Gout

Gout is an abnormality of uric acid metabolism resulting in the deposition of sodium urate crystals in:

- Joints, causing arthritis
- Soft tissue, causing tophi and tenosynovitis
- Urinary tract, causing urate stones and renal failure.

Epidemiology

The prevalence of gout is about 0.2% in Europeans. The disease is 10 times more common in men, rarely occurs before puberty and is more prevalent in the upper social classes. One-third have a positive family history.

Pathogenesis

The biochemical abnormality is hyperuricaemia resulting from overproduction or renal underexcretion of uric acid. Urate is derived from the breakdown of purines (adenine and guanine in DNA and RNA), which are synthesized in the body or ingested (a minor component). In idiopathic (primary) gout, the most common form, impaired renal excretion is the most common cause of hyperuricaemia. The causes of hyperuricaemia are shown in Table 5.7.

Clinical features

The typical patient is an obese middle-aged man who presents with acute gout, characterized by the sudden onset of severe pain and swelling, most frequently in the metatarsophalangeal joint of the big toe. The joint becomes red, hot, swollen and exquisitely tender. The attack may be precipitated by a surgical operation, dietary or alcoholic excess, starvation or drugs, particularly thiazide diuretics. With persisting hyperuricaemia there is recurrent acute arthritis affecting more joints, associated with the

Table 5.7 Causes of hyperuricaemia

Impaired excretion of uric acid	Increased production of uric acid
Idiopathic (primary) gout	Idiopathic (primary) gout
Chronic renal disease (clinical gout unusual)	Increased turnover of purines
Drug therapy, e.g. thiazide diuretics, low-dose aspirin	Myeloproliferative disorders, e.g. polycythaemia vera
Hypertension	Lymphoproliferative disorders, e.g. leukaemia
Lead toxicity	Others, e.g. carcinoma, severe psoriasis
Alcohol	Increased de novo purine synthesis (very rare)
Glucose-6-phosphatase deficiency	HGPRT deficiency (Lesch–Nyhan syndrome)
	PPS overactivity

HGPRT, hypoxanthine-guanine phosphoribosyltransferase; PPS, phosphoribosyl-pyrophosphate synthetase.

permanent deposition of urate in and around joints (chronic tophaceous gout). Tophaceous urate deposits may also occur in cartilage, particularly the pinna of the ear. Acute attacks must be diffentiated from other causes of monoarthritis, particularly septic arthritis.

Investigations

- Synovial fluid examination reveals long needle-shaped crystals which are negatively birefringent under polarized light.
- Serum uric acid should be measured and is usually raised, but may be normal in acute gout. However, the diagnosis is excluded if the serum uric acid is in the lower half of the normal range. Conversely, asymptomatic hyperuricaemia is common.
- Serum urea and creatinine for signs of renal impairment.

Management

Acute attacks are treated with anti-inflammatory drugs:

- NSAIDs, e.g. naproxen, diclofenac, are the treatment of choice.
- Intra-articular corticosteroid injection after aspiration of effusion.
- Other treatments: intramuscular ACTH is very effective for difficult cases. Oral colchicine may be useful if NSAIDs are contraindicated, e.g. active peptic ulceration.

Long-term therapy is considered when the acute attack subsides. Obese patients should lose weight, alcohol consumption should be reduced, and drugs such as thiazides and salicylates should be withdrawn. Drugs used to reduce serum uric acid include:

- Allopurinol, which inhibits xanthine oxidase (an enzyme in the purine breakdown pathway) and is the drug of choice, but may precipitate an acute attack; thus it should be used initially in conjunction with an NSAID.
- Probenecid, a uricosuric agent, may be used in those allergic to allopurinol.

Pyrophosphate arthropathy (pseudogout)

This condition is associated with the deposition of calcium pyrophosphate dihydrate in articular cartilage and periarticular tissue. The acute attacks of synovitis that occur in 25% of patients are known as pseudogout. The aetiology is unknown and it occurs most commonly in elderly women. It may occur secondary to other diseases, including primary hyperparathyroidism, haemochromatosis, hypothyroidism and gout.

Clinical features

The clinical picture is similar to primary osteoarthritis, with acute attacks most commonly involving the knee. There is often polyarticular involvement or involvement of unusual joints such as the wrist, and the patient may be pyrexial.

Investigations

- Blood count may show a raised white cell count.
- Synovial fluid examination reveals small brick–shaped pyrophosphate crystals which are positively birefringent under polarized light (compare uric acid).
- Radiograph of the knee may show linear calcification parallel to the articular surfaces (chondrocalcinosis).
- Serum calcium is normal.

Management

Rest with joint aspiration and NSAIDs forms the mainstay of treatment. Injection of local corticosteroids may also be useful.

Unusual arthropathies

BACK PAIN

Lumbar back pain

Lumbar back pain is an extremely common symptom experienced by most people at some time in their lives. Mechanical back pain is a common cause in young people. It starts suddenly, is often unilateral, and may be helped by rest. It may arise from the facet joints, spinal ligaments or muscle. The history, physical examination and simple investigations will also often identify the minority of patients with a more sinister cause of back pain (Table 5.8).

Table 5.8 Causes of lumbar back pain

		Relevant points in the history and examination
Mechanical	Prolapsed intervertebral disc Osteoarthritis Fractures Spondylolisthesis Spinal stenosis	Often sudden onset Pain worse in the evening Morning stiffness is absent Exercise aggravates pain
Inflammatory	Ankylosing spondylitis Infection (see below)	Gradual onset Pain worse in the morning Morning stiffness is present Exercise relieves pain
Serious cause	Metastatic carcinoma Myeloma Tuberculosis osteomyelitis Bacterial osteomyelitis Cord or cauda equina compression	Constant pain without relief Systemically unwell: fever, weight loss Localized bone tenderness Bilateral signs in the legs Neurological deficit involving more than one root level
Others	Osteomalacia, Paget's disease, referred pain from pelvic/abdominal disease	

The age of the patient is important in deciding the aetiology of back pain because certain causes are more common in particular age groups. These are illustrated in Table 5.9.

Investigations

A detailed history and physical examination (see Table 5.8) will lead to the diagnosis in many cases. The key points are age, speed of onset, the presence of motor or sensory symptoms, involvement of the bladder or bowel, and the presence of stiffness and the effect of exercise. Young adults

Table 5.9 Disorders most commonly found in specific age groups

15–30 years	30–50 years	50 years and over
Mechanical	Mechanical	Degenerative joint disease
Prolapsed intervertebral disease	Degenerative joint disease	Osteoporosis
Ankylosing spondylitis	Prolapsed intervertebral disease	Paget's disease
Spondylolisthesis	Malignancy	Malignancy
Fractures (all ages)		Myeloma
Infective lesions (all ages)		

with a history suggestive of mechanical back pain and with no physical signs do not need further investigation.

- Blood count is usually normal. The ESR may be raised with inflammatory back pain and tumours.
- Serum biochemistry. A raised calcium and alkaline phosphatase suggest metastases. Typically with myeloma the calcium is raised, with a normal alkaline phosphatase. A raised alkaline phosphatase with a normal calcium occurs with metabolic bone disease. Prostate specific antigen should be measured if secondary prostatic disease is suspected.
- Radiology. Radiographs may be useful for excluding serious disease, although they may be misleading, e.g. degenerative disease is virtually always present in older people.
- Technetium bone scan will show increased uptake with infection or malignancy.
- MRI is useful when neurological symptoms and signs are present. It is useful for the detection of disc and cord lesions, and has largely taken over from CT and myelography.

Management

The treatment depends on the cause. Mechanical back pain is managed with analgesia, brief rest and physiotherapy. Exercise programmes reduce long-term problems.

....

INTERVERTEBRAL DISC DISEASE

Acute disc disease

Acute disc disease is a syndrome in which there is prolapse of the intervertebral disc resulting in acute back pain (lumbago), with or without radiation of the pain to areas supplied by the sciatic nerve (sciatica). It is a disease of younger people (20–40 years) because the disc degenerates with age and in elderly people is no longer capable of prolapse. In older patients sciatica is more likely to be the result of compression of the nerve root by osteophytes in the lateral recess of the spinal canal.

Clinical features

There is a sudden onset of severe back pain, often following a strenuous activity. The pain is often clearly related to position and is aggravated by movement. Muscle spasm leads to a sideways tilt when standing. The radiation of the pain and the clinical findings depend on the disc affected (Table 5.10), the lowest three discs being those most commonly affected.

Investigations

Investigations are of very limited value in acute disc disease and radiographs are often normal. MRI or myelography are usually reserved for patients in whom surgery is being considered (see later).

Management

Treatment is aimed at the relief of symptoms and has little effect on the duration of the disease. In the acute stage treatment consists of bed rest on a firm mattress, analgesia, and occasionally epidural corticosteroid injection in severe disease. Surgery is only considered for severe or increasing neurological impairment, e.g. foot drop or bladder symptoms. Physiotherapy plays an important role in the recovery phase, helping to correct posture and restore movement.

Chronic disc disease

This common syndrome is characterized by the presence of chronic lower back pain associated with 'degenerative'

Table 5.10 Symptoms and signs of common root compression syndromes produced by lumbar disc prolapse

Root lesion	Pain	Sensory loss	Motor weakness	Reflex lost	Other signs
S1	From buttock down back of thigh and leg to ankle and foot	Sole of foot and posterior calf	Plantar flexion of ankle and toes	Ankle jerk	Diminished straight leg raising
L5	From buttock to lateral aspect of leg and dorsum of foot	Dorsum of foot and anterolateral aspect of lower leg	Dorsiflexion of foot and toes	None	As above
L4	Lateral aspect of thigh to medial side of calf	Medial aspect of calf and shin	Dorsiflexion and inversion of ankle; extension of knee	Knee jerk	Positive femoral stretch test

changes in the lower lumbar discs and apophyseal joints. Pain is usually of the mechanical type (see above). Sciatic radiation may occur and there may be a history of acute disc prolapse. Usually the pain is long-standing and the prospects for cure are limited. However, measures that have been found useful include NSAIDs, physiotherapy and weight reduction. Surgery can be considered when pain arises from a single identifiable level which has failed to respond to conservative measures. Fusion at this level, with decompression of the affected nerve roots, can be successful.

Mechanical problems

Spondylolisthesis

Spondylolisthesis is characterized by a slipping forward of one vertebra on another, most commonly at L4/L5. It arises because of a defect in the pars interarticularis of the vertebra, and may be either congenital or acquired (e.g. trauma). The condition is associated with mechanical pain which worsens throughout the day. The pain may radiate to one or other leg and there may be signs of nerve root irritation. Small spondylolistheses, often associated with degenerative disease of the lumbar spine, may be treated conservatively with simple analgesics. A large spondylolisthesis causing severe symptoms should be treated with spinal fusion.

Spinal stenosis

Narrowing of the lower spinal canal compresses the cauda equina, resulting in back and buttock pain typically coming on after a period of walking and easing with rest. Accordingly it is sometimes called spinal claudication. Causes include disc prolapse, degenerative osteophyte formation, tumour and congenital narrowing of the spinal canal. CT and MRI will demonstrate cord compression and treatment is by surgical decompression.

Neck pain

Pain in the neck may be caused by rheumatoid arthritis, ankylosing spondylitis or fibrositis (chronic muscle pain in young women with no underlying cause; large psychological overlay in some patients). In addition, disc disease, both acute and chronic, the latter in association with osteoarthritis, may occur in the neck as well as in the lumbar spine. The three lowest cervical discs are most often affected, and there is pain and stiffness of the neck with or without root pain radiating to the arm. Chronic cervical disc disease is known as cervical spondylosis.

BONE DISEASE

Bone normally consists of 70% mineral and 30% organic matrix (mostly type 1 collagen fibres). The mineral component consists mostly of a complex crystalline salt of calcium and phosphate called hydroxyapatite. Although major skeletal growth occurs in childhood, adult bone is continuously being remodelled, with bone formation and resorption. Two major cell types are involved in bone remodelling:

- Osteoblasts produce type 1 collagen and growth factors, and also regulate osteoclast activity.
- Osteoclasts produce lysosomal enzymes which degrade collagen matrix.

Control of calcium and bone metabolism

Vitamin D and parathyroid hormone (PTH) are the major factors that control plasma calcium concentration and bone turnover. Bone metabolism is also controlled by calcitonin, glucocorticoids, sex hormones, growth hormone and thyroid hormone.

Vitamin D

The metabolism and actions of vitamin D are shown in Figure 5.6.

Parathyroid hormone (PTH)

PTH levels rise as serum ionized calcium falls. The effects are several, all serving to increase plasma calcium and decrease plasma phosphate:

- Increased osteoclastic resorption of bone
- Increased intestinal absorption of calcium
- Increased synthesis of $1,25\text{-}(OH)_2D_3$
- Increased tubular reabsorption of calcium
- Increased renal excretion of phosphate.

Osteomalacia

Inadequate mineralization of the osteoid framework, leading to soft bones, produces rickets during bone growth and osteomalacia following epiphyseal closure.

Aetiology

- Deficiency of vitamin D as a result of a combination of poor diet and inadequate sunlight. This is seen in immobile elderly people and in female Asian immigrants
- Malabsorption, e.g. coeliac disease and small bowel resection
- Renal disease leading to inadequate conversion of $25\text{-}(OH)D_3$ to $1,25\text{-}(OH)_2D_3$ (Figure 5.6)

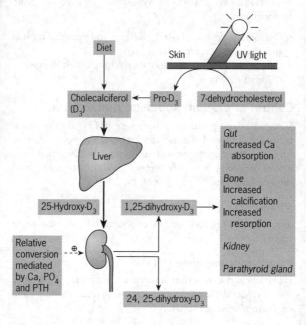

Figure 5.6
The metabolism and actions of vitamin D. Cholecalciferol is predominantly formed from photoactivation of 7-dehydrocholesterol in the skin. In the liver, cholecalciferol is converted to 25-hydroxycholecalciferol, which is then converted to the much more active form, 1,25-dihydroxycholecalciferol, in the kidney. PTH, parathyroid hormone.

- Other causes include liver failure, renal phosphate loss and anticonvulsant therapy (caused by increased vitamin D inactivation).

Clinical features

In the adult osteomalacia produces muscle and bone pain and fractures. In addition, a proximal myopathy leads to a 'waddling' gait and difficulty in rising from a chair.

Investigations

- Serum biochemistry shows a low phosphate, low or low–normal calcium and increased alkaline phosphatase.
- Radiology. Radiographs are characteristic, showing defective mineralization and Looser's zones (low-density bands extending from the cortex inwards in the shafts of the long bones).
- Bone biopsy is the definitive investigation and shows increased non-mineralized bone. However, this procedure is uncomfortable and rarely necessary.

Management

The treatment is with oral vitamin D; the dose and formulation depends on the cause (Table 5.11). Treatment is monitored by measurement of serum alkaline phosphatase and calcium.

Table 5.11 Treatment of osteomalacia

Vitamin D deficiency	Vitamin D_2 10 µg (400 U) daily
Malabsorption	Vitamin D_2 1–2.5 mg (40 000–100 000 U) daily
Renal failure	1α-Hydroxycholecalciferol (alfacalcidol or 1α (OH)D_3) or 1,25-dihydroxycholecalciferol (calcitriol or 1,25 (OH)$_2D_3$)

Osteoporosis

Osteoporosis means thin bone and the term implies a reduction in bone mass, including all components of bone, not just calcium. The bone is fragile, with an increased risk of fracture.

Aetiology

Bone resorption is part of the normal ageing process, occurring more in women than in men, largely as a result of postmenopausal oestrogen deficiency. The risk factors for osteoporosis are:

- Increasing age
- Female sex
- Early menopause
- Oophorectomy
- Slender habitus
- Smoking
- Lack of exercise
- Family history
- Excess alcohol.

Classification

There are two types of osteoporosis:

- Type 1 (postmenopausal) is the result of oestrogen deficiency. Trabecular bone loss leads to vertebral fractures between the ages of 50 and 75 years.
- Type 2 (senile) affects the over-70s. Reduced intake of calcium and vitamin D leads to increased parathyroid hormone activity. This results in cortical bone resorption and hip fractures.

Osteoporosis may also occur secondary to endocrine disease (Cushing's disease, thyrotoxicosis and hypogonadism), drugs (corticosteroids, heparin) and systemic disease (e.g. rheumatoid arthritis and chronic renal failure).

Clinical features

Symptoms of osteoporosis are the result of fractures, which typically occur at three sites: the thoracic and lumbar vertebrae, neck of the femur and the distal radius (Colles' fracture). Vertebral fractures may lead to kyphosis and height loss.

Investigations

- Serum biochemistry. Calcium, phosphate and alkaline phosphatase are normal.
- Radiology. Radiographs will demonstrate fractures and may show reduced bone density (osteopenia).

- Bone densitometry. Dual-energy X-ray absorptiometry (DEXA) scanning is of increasing importance in screening people at risk and in monitoring the effects of treatment.
- Bone biopsy is occasionally needed.

Management

Prevention is better than treatment of established disease. This is an area of change, and indications and treatment protocols may alter as more studies are completed.

- Oestrogen therapy as hormone replacement therapy (HRT) should be considered for women at high risk (see list on page 240) to reduce bone loss during the postmenopausal years. Oestrogens are combined with progestogens in women with an intact uterus because oestrogens alone increase the risk of developing endometrial cancer.
- Calcium intake should be maintained and regular exercise may retard bone loss.
- Bisphosphonates, which inhibit bone resorption, are often given to older patients, i.e. postmenopausal women. Oral alendronate is given with calcium supplements.
- Smoking accelerates bone loss and patients should be advised to stop.
- Corticosteroid induced osteoporosis. Corticosteroids produce a net loss of bone through a number of mechanisms which result in a greater rate of bone resorption than bone loss. Prolonged use (>6 months) of prednisolone in doses over 7.5 mg per day is associated with increased risk of osteoporosis, and may occur in high risk patients (postmenopausal women) at lower doses. Patients on long-term corticosteroid treatment who have significant osteoporosis on DEXA scanning should be treated, usually with HRT or bisphosphonates. Patients without significant loss of bone mineral density should have a repeat scan in one year and those found to have bone loss of >4% per year should also be treated.

Paget's disease

Paget's disease is characterized by excessive osteoclastic bone resorption followed by disordered osteoblastic activity, leading to abundant new bone formation which is structurally abnormal and weak.

Aetiology

Osteoclasts contain viral inclusion bodies, suggesting a possible 'slow viral' aetiology.

Epidemiology

The incidence increases with age; it is rare in the under 40s and affects up to 10% of adults by the age of 90.

Clinical features

The most common sites are the femur, pelvis, tibia, skull and lumbosacral spine, although any bone can be involved. Most cases are asymptomatic, but features include the following:

* *Bone pain*
* *Apparent joint pain* when the involved bone is close to a joint
* *Deformities:* enlargement of the skull, bowing of the tibia
* *Complications:*
  - nerve compression (deafness, paraparesis)
  - fractures
  - rarely cardiac failure, osteogenic sarcoma.

Investigations

The diagnosis is often clinical but is supported by:

* Serum biochemistry, which shows a raised alkaline phosphatase concentration (reflects level of bone formation), often >1000 U/l, with a normal calcium and phosphate.
* X-rays showing characteristic changes, most often in the pelvis, skull or spine. There is localized bony enlargement and distortion, sclerotic changes (increased density) and osteolytic areas (loss of bone and reduced density).
* Radionuclide bone scans showing increased uptake of bone-seeking radionuclides, which is due to increased bone formation. The appearances on bone scans and plain X-rays may be difficult to distinguish from metastatic carcinoma, especially sclerotic secondaries seen with breast and prostate cancer.

- Urinary hydroxyproline is usually increased and reflects the level of bone resorption.

Treatment

When asymptomatic, Paget's disease requires no treatment. Pain, which is the usual indication for treatment, may respond to simple analgesics and NSAIDs. With more specific treatment, disease activity is monitored by symptoms and the measurement of serum alkaline phosphatase.

- Bisphosphonates inhibit bone resorption by decreasing osteoclastic activity. Oral alendronate should be first-choice therapy. Etidronate has also been used but carries the risk of osteomalacia when used at high doses.
- Calcitonin (salmon or porcine) administered intramuscularly or subcutaneously inhibits osteoclast activity and decreases bone resorption. It is extremely expensive, with troublesome side effects (nausea, flushing and the development of neutralizing antibodies). Calcitonin nasal spray has fewer side effects but large doses are needed to decrease bone turnover.

CALCIUM AND THE PARATHYROIDS

Total plasma calcium is normally 2.2–2.6 mmol/l. Usually only 40% of total plasma calcium is ionized and physiologically relevant; the remainder is bound to albumin and thus unavailable to the tissues. Routine analytical methods measure total plasma calcium and this must be corrected for the serum albumin concentration: add or subtract 0.02 mmol/l for every g/l by which the simultaneous albumin lies below or above 40 g/l. For critical measurements samples should be taken in the fasting state without the use of an occluding cuff, which may increase the local plasma protein concentration.

Hypocalcaemia and hypoparathyroidism

Aetiology

The causes of hypocalcaemia are listed in Table 5.12. Renal failure is the most common cause of hypocalcaemia, which results from the inadequate production of active vitamin D

Table 5.12 Causes of hypocalcaemia

Increased serum phosphate levels
   Chronic renal failure
   Phosphate therapy

Hypoparathyroidism
   Post-thyroidectomy and parathyroidectomy (usually transient)
   Congenital deficiency (DiGeorge's syndrome)
   Idiopathic hypoparathyroidism (autoimmune)
   Severe hypomagnesaemia (inhibits PTH release)

Vitamin D deficiency
   Osteomalacia
   Resistance

End-organ resistance to PTH
   Pseudohypoparathyroidism

Drugs
   Calcitonin
   Bisphosphonates

Miscellaneous
   Acute pancreatitis
   Citrated blood in massive transfusion

Indicates common cause of hypocalcaemia

and renal phosphate retention, leading to microprecipitation of calcium phosphate in the tissues. Mild transient hypocalcaemia often occurs after parathyroidectomy, and a few patients develop long-standing hypoparathyroidism.

Clinical features

Hypocalcaemia causes increased excitability of nerves. There is numbness around the mouth and in the extremities, followed by cramps, tetany (carpopedal spasm: opposition of the thumb, extension of the interphalangeal and flexion of the metacarpophalangeal joints), convulsions and death if untreated. Two important physical signs are Chvostek's sign (tapping over the facial nerve in the region of the parotid gland causes twitching of the facial muscles) and Trousseau's sign (carpopedal spasm induced by inflation of the sphygmomanometer cuff to a level above systolic blood pressure). With prolonged hypocalcaemia there may be cataract formation and rarely papilloedema.

Tetany may also develop in the presence of alkalosis, and potassium and magnesium deficiency as well as in hypocalcaemia. Hyperventilation alters the protein binding of calcium such that the ionized fraction is decreased, and may therefore cause hypocalcaemic tetany even with a normal plasma total calcium.

Investigations

The clinical picture is usually diagnostic and is confirmed by a low corrected serum calcium. Additional tests identify the cause.

- Serum urea and creatinine for renal disease
- Serum parathyroid hormone levels
- Serum parathyroid antibodies – present in autoimmune disease
- Serum 25-hydroxy vitamin D level.

Management

- Acute (e.g. with tetany): 10 ml of 10% calcium gluconate intravenously and repeated as necessary as an infusion over 4 hours.
- Maintenance therapy is with alfacalcidol (1_α-OH D_3).

Hyperparathyroidism and hypercalcaemia

Mild asymptomatic hypercalcaemia occurs in about one in 1000 of the population, especially elderly women, and is usually the result of primary hyperparathyroidism.

Aetiology

Most cases are the result of primary hyperparathyroidism or malignancy (Table 5.13). Tumour-related hypercalcaemia is caused by the secretion of a peptide with PTH-like activity, or by direct invasion of bone and production of local factors that mobilize calcium. Ectopic PTH secretion by tumours is very rare.

Hyperparathyroidism may be primary, secondary or tertiary.

Primary hyperparathyoidism is usually caused by a single adenoma, occasionally hyperplasia, and rarely carcinoma.

Secondary hyperparathyroidism is a physiological response to hypocalcaemia (e.g. in renal failure or vitamin D deficiency). Calcium is low or low–normal.

Tertiary hyperparathyroidism is the development of apparently autonomous parathyroid hyperplasia after long-

Table 5.13 Causes of hypercalcaemia

Excess PTH
  Primary hyperparathyroidism (commonest cause)*
  Tertiary hyperparathyroidism
  Ectopic PTH (very rare)

Excess action of vitamin D
  Self-administered vitamin D*
  Sarcoidosis

Excess calcium intake
  'Milk-alkali' syndrome

Malignant disease (second commonest cause)*
  Multiple myeloma   Prostate
  Breast cancer   Renal cell
  Bronchus   Lymphoma
  Thyroid

Other endocrine disease
  Thyrotoxicosis
  Addison's disease

Drugs
  Thiazides

Miscellaneous
  Long-term immobility

* Conditions causing severe hypercalcaemia (>3.5 mmol/l)

standing secondary hyperparathyroidism, most often in renal disease. Plasma calcium and PTH are both raised. Treatment is parathyroidectomy.

Clinical features

Mild hypercalcaemia is often asymptomatic and discovered on biochemical screening. Symptoms are general malaise and depression, bone pain, abdominal pain, nausea and constipation. Calcium deposition in the renal tubules causes polyuria and nocturia. Renal calculi and renal failure may develop. With very high levels there is dehydration, confusion, clouding of consciousness and a risk of cardiac arrest.

Investigations

- Serum biochemistry. Corrected calcium is raised; low phosphate, low bicarbonate and raised chloride support primary hyperparathyroidism.

- Serum PTH levels. Detectable levels during hypercalcaemia are inappropriate and imply hyperparathyroidism.
- Radiology. Subperiosteal erosions in the phalanges are seen in hyperparathyroidism.
- Hydrocortisone suppression test is less often used with modern PTH assays; plasma calcium in hyperparathyroidism and some malignancies are resistant to suppression by steroids. Suppression is seen in most other causes of hypercalcaemia.
- Other investigations. Protein electrophoresis for myeloma, thyroid function tests and investigations (e.g. MRI, selective venous sampling) to localize parathyroid adenomas before surgery.

Management

This involves lowering of the calcium levels to near normal and treatment of the underlying cause. Severe

---

! Emergency

- **Rehydrate with intravenous fluid (0.9% saline)**
  4–6 litres of intravenous saline over 24 h and then 3–4 litres for several days thereafter
  Amount and rate depends on clinical assessment and measurement of serum urea and electrolytes

- **After minimum of 2 litres of intravenous fluids give biphosphonate infusion**
  Pamidronate disodium 15–60 mg as an intravenous infusion in 0.5 litre 0.9% saline over 2 h

- **Measure**
  Serum urea and electrolytes at least daily
  Do not measure serum calcium for a least 48 h after initiation of treatment, normalization may take 3–5 days

- **Prednisolone (30–60 mg daily)**
  May be useful in some cases (myeloma, sarcoidosis and vitamin D excess) but in most cases ineffective

- **Prevent recurrence**
  Treat underlying cause if possible
  With untreatable malignancy consider maintenance treatment with bisphosphonates

Emergency Box 5.1
The treatment of acute hypercalcaemia

hypercalcaemia (>3.5 mmol/l) is a medical emergency which must be treated aggressively whatever the underlying cause (Emergency Box 5.1). Treatment is based on the corrected calcium value.

Treatment of primary hyperparathyroidism

The treatment of a symptomatic parathyroid adenoma is surgical removal. Conservative therapy may be indicated in asymptomatic patients with mildly raised calcium levels (2.65–3 mmol/l). In those with parathyroid hyperplasia all four glands are removed.

Water and electrolytes

6

BODY FLUID COMPARTMENTS

A 75 kg man contains approximately 45 litres of water (i.e. about 50–60% of total body weight is water) and 3000 mmol of osmotically active sodium (Table 6.1). Maintenance of the total amount depends on the balance between intake and loss. Water and electrolytes are taken in as food and water, and lost in urine, sweat and faeces (Table 6.2). In addition, about 500 ml water are lost daily in expired air.

Table 6.1 Normal adult total body content and serum electrolyte concentrations

Cation	Total body content (mmol)	Extracellular/ intracellular distribution	Serum concentration (mmol/l)	Dietary intake/day (mmol)
Sodium	3000	95% extracellular	136–144	140
Potassium	4000	98% intracellular	3.6–5.0	80–150
Magnesium	1000	1% extracellular	0.7–1.1	12–14

Table 6.2 The normal daily water and sodium balance in a 75 kg man

	Input		Output	
Water (ml)				
Drink	1500	Urine	1500	
Food	800	Insensible loss	800	
Metabolism	200	(skin, lungs)		
		Faeces	200	
Total	2500		2500	
Sodium (mmol)				
Food and drink	140	Urine	140	
		Sweat	Negligible	
		Faeces	Negligible	

Body water is distributed between three major compartments:

* The intracellular fluid (28 litres, about 35% of lean body weight)
* The interstitial fluid that bathes the cells (9.4 litres, about 12%)
* Plasma (4.6 litres, about 4–5%).

Water moves freely between compartments and the distribution is determined by the osmotic equilibrium between them. Osmolality is determined by the concentration of osmotically active particles. Thus 1 mole of sodium chloride dissolved in 1 kg of water has an osmolality of 2 mmol/kg, as sodium chloride freely dissociates into two particles, the sodium ion and the chloride ion. One mole of urea (which does not dissociate) in 1 kg of water has an osmolality of 1 mmol/kg. Sodium is the major extracellular ion and therefore the main determinant of plasma osmolality. The plasma osmolality can be calculated from the plasma concentrations of sodium, urea and glucose, as follows:

Calculated plasma osmolality (mmol)
= $(2 \times [Na+]) + [urea] + [glucose]$.

The factor of 2 applied to sodium concentration allows for associated anions. The other extracellular solutes, e.g. calcium, potassium and magnesium, and their associated anions exist in very low concentrations and contribute so little to osmolality that they can be ignored when calculating the osmolality. The normal plasma osmolality is 285–300 mmol/kg.

The *calculated* osmolality is the same as the osmolality *measured* by the laboratory, unless there is an unmeasured, osmotically active substance present. For instance, plasma alcohol or ethylene glycol concentration (substances sometimes taken in cases of poisoning) can be estimated by subtracting the calculated from the measured osmolality.

Distribution of extracellular fluid

The distribution of extracellular water between vascular and extravascular (interstitial space) is determined by the equilibrium between hydrostatic pressure (i.e. capillary

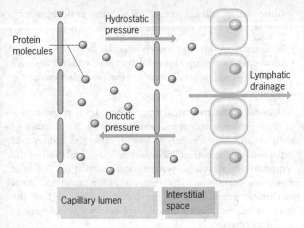

Figure 6.1
Distribution of water between the vascular and extravascular (interstitial) spaces. This is determined by the equilibrium between hydrostatic pressure, which tends to force fluid out of the capillaries, and oncotic pressure, which acts to retain fluid within the vessel. The net flow of fluid outwards is balanced by 'suction' of fluid into the lymphatics, which returns it to the bloodstream. Similar principles govern the volume of the peritoneal and pleural spaces.

pressure), which tends to force fluid out of the capillaries, and oncotic pressure (i.e. osmotic pressure exerted by plasma proteins), which acts to retain fluid within the vessel. The net flow of fluid outwards is balanced by 'suction' of fluid into the lymphatics which returns it to the bloodstream (Figure 6.1).

Oedema is defined as an increase in interstitial fluid and results from:

- Increased hydrostatic pressure, e.g. sodium and water retention in cardiac failure
- Reduced oncotic pressure, e.g. as a result of nephrotic syndrome and hypoalbuminaemia
- Obstruction to lymphatic flow.

Regulation of extracellular volume

Extracellular volume is controlled by the total body content of sodium. Control of body sodium is exerted by tight control over renal excretion. This is achieved by activation of 'volume' receptors (which respond to extracellular volume rather than changes in sodium concentration). There are two types of volume receptors:

- Extrarenal: in the large vessels near the heart
- Intrarenal: in the afferent renal arteriole, which controls the renin–angiotensin system via the juxtaglomerular apparatus.

A decreased effective circulating volume leads to activation of these volume receptors, which leads to an increase in sodium (and hence water) reabsorption by the kidney and expansion of the extracellular volume via stimulation of the sympathetic nervous system and activation of the renin–angiotensin system (page 512). In contrast, atrial natriuretic peptide (ANP), produced by the atria of the heart in response to an increase in blood volume, increases sodium excretion.

Regulation of body water content

Body water is controlled mainly by changes in the plasma osmolality. An increased plasma osmolality, sensed by osmoreceptors in the hypothalamus, causes thirst and the release of antidiuretic hormone (ADH, vasopressin) from the posterior pituitary, which increases water reabsorption from the renal collecting ducts. In addition, non-osmotic stimuli may cause the release of ADH even if serum osmolality is normal or low. These include hypovolaemia, stress (surgery and trauma) and nausea.

ABNORMALITIES OF EXTRACELLULAR VOLUME

Increased extracellular volume

Extracellular volume expansion is the result of increased sodium (and hence water) reabsorption or impaired excretion by the kidney.

Aetiology

- *Cardiac failure* caused by impaired perfusion (therefore effective hypovolaemia) of the volume receptors.
- *Hypoalbuminaemia* Loss of plasma oncotic pressure leads to loss of water from the vascular to the interstitial space, and therefore activation of intravascular volume receptors.

- *Cirrhosis* This is through a complex mechanism, but there is vasodilatation and hence underperfusion of the volume receptors. There may also be hypoalbuminaemia.
- *Sodium retention* This may be as a result of renal impairment, where there is a reduction in renal capacity to excrete sodium, or due to drugs such as mineralocorticoids or NSAIDs.

Clinical features

These depend on the distribution of extracellular water, e.g. with hypoalbuminaemia caused by loss of plasma oncotic pressure there is predominantly interstitial volume overload. Cardiac failure leads to expansion of both compartments.

- *Interstitial volume overload* – ankle oedema, pulmonary oedema, pleural effusion and ascites.
- *Intravascular volume overload* – raised jugular venous pressure, cardiomegaly, and a raised arterial pressure in some cases.

This must be differentiated from local causes of oedema (e.g. ankle oedema as a result of venous damage following thrombosis) which do not reflect a disturbance in the control of extracellular volume.

Management

The underlying cause must be treated. The cornerstone of treatment is diuretics, which increase sodium and water excretion in the kidney. There are a number of different classes of diuretic, of which the most potent are the loop diuretics, e.g. frusemide (Table 6.3).

Decreased extracellular volume

This may be the result of loss of sodium and water, plasma or blood.

Aetiology

Volume depletion occurs in haemorrhage, plasma loss in extensive burns, or loss of salt and water from the kidneys, gastrointestinal tract or skin (Table 6.4).

Clinical features

Symptoms include thirst, nausea and postural dizziness. Interstitial fluid loss leads to loss of skin elasticity ('turgor').

Table 6.3 The main classes of diuretics in clinical use

Class	Example	Mechanism of action	Relative potency
Loop diuretics	Frusemide	Reduce Na^+ and Cl^- reabsorption in ascending limb of loop of Henle	++++
Thiazides	Bendrofluazide	Reduce sodium reabsorption in distal convoluted tubule	++
Potassium-sparing diuretics	Spironolactone	Aldosterone antagonist	+
	Amiloride	Prevents potassium exchange for sodium in distal tubule	

Table 6.4 Causes of extracellular volume depletion

Haemorrhage
External
Concealed, e.g. leaking aortic aneurysm

Burns

Gastrointestinal losses
Vomiting, diarrhoea, ileostomy losses

Renal losses
Diuretic use, impaired tubular sodium conservation, e.g. reflux nephropathy, papillary necrosis

Loss of circulating volume causes peripheral vasoconstriction and tachycardia, a low jugular venous pressure and postural hypotension. Severe depletion of circulating volume causes hypotension, which may impair cerebral perfusion, resulting in confusion and eventual coma.

Investigations

The diagnosis is usually made clinically. A central venous line allows the measurement of central venous pressure which helps in assessing the response to treatment. Plasma urea may be raised because of increased urea reabsorption and, later, prerenal failure (when the creatinine rises as well). This is, however, very non-specific. Urinary sodium is low (<20 mmol/l) if the kidneys are working normally, which can be misleading if the cause of the volume depletion involves the kidneys (e.g. diuretics or intrinsic renal disease).

Management

The overriding aims of treatment are to replace what is missing:

- Haemorrhage involves the loss of whole blood. The rational treatment of acute haemorrhage is therefore whole blood, or a combination of red cells and a plasma substitute.
- Loss of plasma, as in burns or severe peritonitis, should be treated with human plasma or a plasma substitute (see page 442).
- Loss of sodium and water, as in vomiting, diarrhoea or excessive renal losses, should be treated with replacement of water and electrolytes. This is best done

orally if possible, with an increased intake of water and salt. Glucose–electrolyte solutions are often used to restore fluid balance in patients with diarrhoeal diseases. This is based on the fact that the presence of glucose stimulates intestinal absorption of salt and water (page 22).

- In the acute situation if there have been large losses of sodium and water patients are usually treated with intravenous physiological saline (Tables 6.5 and 6.6) and replacement is assessed clinically and by measurement of serum electrolytes.
- Loss of water alone, e.g. diabetes insipidus, only causes extracellular volume depletion in severe cases because the loss is spread evenly over all the compartments of body water. The correct treatment is to give water. If

Table 6.5 Intravenous fluids in general use*

	Na+	K+	HCO₃⁻	Cl⁻ mmol/l
Normal plasma constituents	142	4.5	26	103
Sodium chloride 0.9% (isotonic physiological saline)	150	–	–	150
Glucose 5%	–	–	–	–
Sodium chloride (0.18%) + glucose 4% (1/5 physiological saline)	30	–	–	30

* Accounting for 95% of the fluids used in clinical practice.

Table 6.6 Guidelines for intravenous fluid administration in maintenance and replacement of losses

For maintenance fluid balance
Each day 2500 ml fluid containing about 140 mmol sodium and 60 mmol potassium are required to maintain balance in a 75 kg man. A good regimen is 2 litres 5% dextrose and 1 litre physiological saline every 24 h

For hypovolaemic patients
An estimate of the losses is made (e.g. in hospital patients from a review of the input/output charts) and these must be given in addition to the normal daily requirements

intravenous treatment is required, water is given as 5% dextrose (pure water is not given because it would cause osmotic lysis of blood cells).

....

DISORDERS OF SODIUM REGULATION

As discussed above, sodium content is regulated by volume receptors, with water content adjusted to maintain a normal osmolality and a normal plasma sodium concentration. Disturbances of sodium concentration are usually caused by disturbances of water balance, rather than an increase or decrease in total body sodium.

Hyponatraemia

Hyponatraemia (serum sodium <135 mmol/l) may be the result of the following:

- Relative water excess (dilutional hyponatremia); this is the most common cause
- Salt loss in excess of water, e.g. diarrhoea and renal diseases as described above
- Pseudohyponatraemia, in which hyperlipidaemia or hyperproteinaemia results in a spuriously low measured sodium concentration. The sodium is confined to the aqueous phase but its concentration is expressed in terms of the total volume of plasma (i.e. water plus lipid). In this situation plasma osmolality is normal and therefore treatment of 'hyponatraemia' is unnecessary.
- True hyponatraemia must be differentiated from artefactual 'hyponatraemia' caused by taking blood from the drip arm into which a fluid of low sodium is being infused.

Once preliminary evaluation reveals that the hyponatraemia reflects hypo-osmolality (i.e. it is not pseudohyponatraemia or artefactual), assessment of the extracellular volume (page 253) allows patients to be classified as hypovolaemic, normovolaemic or hypervolaemic. (Figure 6.2).

Hyponatraemia resulting from salt loss (hypovolaemic hyponatraemia)

These patients have a deficit of both total body sodium and water, with the sodium deficit exceeding the water deficit.

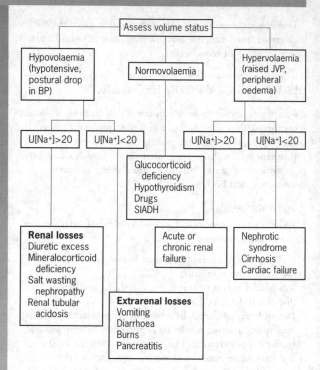

U[Na⁺] = Urinary sodium concentration in mmol/l
SIADH = Syndrome of inappropriate ADH secretion

Figure 6.2
Diagnosis of hyponatraemia.

Measurement of urinary sodium will help to differentiate between renal and extrarenal sources of fluid loss (Figure 6.2). For example, vomiting and diarrhoea are associated with avid sodium retention as the kidney responds to volume contraction by conserving NaCl.

Diuretics are the most common cause of hypovolaemic hyponatraemia with a high urinary [Na⁺].

Clinical features

These are usually a result of the hypovolaemia and extracellular volume depletion (page 253). Symptoms directly related to the hyponatraemia are rare, as the loss of both sodium and water limits osmotic shifts in the brain.

Management

Restoration of extracellular volume with crystalloids or colloids interrupts non-osmotic release of ADH and normalizes serum sodium.

Hyponatraemia resulting from water excess (dilutional hyponatraemia)

An excess of body water relative to sodium is differentiated from hyponatraemia caused by sodium loss, because there are none of the clinical features of extracellular volume depletion. This is the most common mechanism of hyponatraemia seen in hospital patients.

Aetiology

Hyponatraemia is often seen in patients with severe cardiac failure, hepatic cirrhosis or the nephrotic syndrome, in which there is an inability of the kidney to excrete 'free water'. This is compounded by the use of diuretics. There is evidence of volume overload and the patient is usually oedematous. Where there is no evidence of extracellular volume overload, causes include the syndrome of inappropriate ADH secretion (SIADH), Addison's disease and hypothyroidism.

Clinical features

Symptoms rarely occur until the serum sodium is less than 120 mmol/l. They result from the movement of water into the brain cells in response to the fall in extracellular osmolality, and include headache, confusion, convulsions and coma.

Investigation

Hyponatraemia in association with cardiac failure, cirrhosis or nephrotic syndrome is usually clinically obvious and no further investigation is necessary. If there is no evidence of volume overload the most probable cause is SIADH or diuretic therapy (page 508).

Management

The underlying cause must be corrected where possible. Most cases (those without symptoms) are simply managed by water restriction (to 1000 ml or even 500 ml/day) with a review of diuretic treatment. Management of SIADH syndrome is described on page 508. Patients with hyponatraemia developing acutely, in less than 48 hours (often a hospital patient on intravenous dextrose), are at the greatest risk of developing cerebral oedema and should be treated more urgently (see Emergency Box 6.1).

 Emergency

Treat the underlying cause

Restrict water intake to 500–1000 ml/day

With acute symptomatic hyponatraemia:
- Infuse 3% NaCl at a rate of 1–2 ml/kg/h
- Aim to raise serum sodium by 2 mmol/l/h until symptoms resolve
- Give frusemide 40–80 mg i.v. to enhance free water excretion
- If there are severe neurological symptoms (seizures, obtundation), NaCl can be infused at 4–6 ml/kg/h
- Subsequent correction should be very slow so that the total increase in serum sodium is less than 8 mmol/l in 24 h
- A rapid rise in extracellular osmolality, particularly if there is 'overshoot' to high serum sodium and osmolality, may result in severe shrinking of brain cells and the syndrome of 'central pontine myelinolysis', which can be fatal

Emergency Box 6.1
Management of hyponatraemia resulting from water excess

Hypernatraemia

Hypernatraemia (serum sodium >145 mmol/l) is almost always the result of reduced water intake or water loss in excess of sodium. More rarely it is caused by excessive administration of sodium.

Aetiology

Insufficient fluid intake is most often found in elderly people, neonates or unconscious patients when access to water is denied or confusion or coma eliminates the normal response to thirst. The situation is exacerbated by increased losses of fluid, e.g. sweating, diarrhoea.

Water loss relative to sodium occurs in pituitary diabetes insipidus, nephrogenic diabetes insipidus, osmotic diuresis and water loss from the lungs or skin.

Clinical features

Symptoms are non-specific and include nausea, vomiting, fever and confusion.

Investigations

Simultaneous urine and plasma osmolality and sodium should be measured.

The passage of urine with an osmolality lower than that of plasma in this situation is clearly abnormal and indicates diabetes insipidus (page 509). If urine osmolality is high this suggests an osmotic diuresis or excessive extrarenal water loss (e.g. heat stroke).

Management

Treatment is that of the underlying cause and replacement of water, either orally if possible or intravenously with 5% dextrose. The aim is to correct over 48 hours, as over-rapid correction may lead to cerebral oedema. In severe hypernatraemia (>170 mmol/l), 0.9% saline (150 mmol/l) should be used to avoid too rapid a drop in serum sodium. In addition, if there is clinical evidence of volume depletion this implies that there is a sodium deficit as well as a water deficit, and intravenous 0.9% saline should be used.

DISORDERS OF POTASSIUM REGULATION

Dietary intake of potassium varies between 80 and 150 mmol daily. Potassium is predominantly an intracellular ion, only 2% of total body potassium being extracellular. Serum levels are mainly controlled by renal excretion under the influence of aldosterone in the renal tubules. Levels are also influenced by extrarenal losses (e.g. gastrointestinal) and uptake of K^+ into cells. Alkalosis associated with a fall in intracellular H^+ concentration results in a net flux of potassium into cells, with a fall in plasma potassium; acidosis has the reverse effect.

Hypokalaemia

This is a serum potassium concentration of <3.5 mmol/l.

Aetiology

The most common causes of hypokalaemia (Table 6.7) are diuretic treatment and hyperaldosteronism.

Table 6.7 Causes of hypokalaemia

Increased renal excretion (spot urinary K+ >20 mmol/l)	Diuretics, e.g. thiazides, loop diuretics
	Solute diuresis, e.g. glycosuria
	Hypomagnasaemia
	Increased aldosterone secretion
	Liver failure
	Heart failure
	Nephrotic syndrome
	Cushing's syndrome
	Conn's syndrome
	Exogenous mineralocorticoid
	Corticosteroids
	Carbenoxolone
	Liquorice
	Renal tubular acidosis:
	types 1 and 2
	Renal tubular damage
Gastrointestinal losses	Vomiting, diarrhoea, villous adenoma, fistulae, ileostomies
Severe dietary deficiency	
Redistribution into cells	Alkalosis, β-agonists, insulin

Clinical features

Hypokalaemia is usually asymptomatic, although muscle weakness may occur if severe. There is an increased risk of cardiac arrhythmias, particularly in patients with cardiac disease. Hypokalaemia also predisposes to digoxin toxicity.

Management

The underlying cause should be identified and treated where possible. Usually withdrawal of purgatives, assessment of diuretic treatment, and replacement with oral potassium supplements is all that is required. Serum magnesium concentrations should be normalized, as hypomagnasaemia makes hypokalaemia difficult or impossible to correct. Indications for the intravenous infusion of potassium include hypokalaemic diabetic ketoacidosis and severe hypokalaemia (<2.5 mmol/l), which may be associated with cardiac arrhythmias. This should be performed slowly, and replacement at rates of greater than 20 mmol/h should only be done with ECG monitoring and hourly measurement of serum potassium.

Hyperkalaemia

This is defined as a serum potassium concentration of >5.0 mmol/l. True hyperkalaemia must be differentiated from artefactual hyperkalaemia, which results from lysis of red cells during vigorous phlebotomy.

Aetiology

The most common causes (Table 6.8) are renal impairment and drug interference with potassium excretion.

Table 6.8 Causes of hyperkalaemia

Excessive intake

Impaired renal excretion
Renal failure
Potassium-sparing diuretics (amiloride)

Hypoaldosteronism
Addison's disease
Hyporeninaemic hypoaldosteronism
Angiotensin-converting enzyme (ACE) inhibitors

Release from cells
Acidosis
Crush injury
Suxamethonium

Clinical features

Hyperkalaemia usually produces few symptoms or signs until it is high enough to cause cardiac arrest. It is often associated with metabolic acidosis causing Kussmaul's respiration.

Management

A serum potassium of more than 7 mmol/l is a medical emergency (Emergency Box 6.2) and may be associated with typical ECG changes (Figure 6.3).

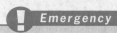

Emergency

1. **Protect myocardium from hyperkalaemia (if ECG changes present)**
   10 ml of 10% calcium gluconate bolus i.v. over 2–3 min with ECG monitoring
   Repeat as necessary
   Nb: Does not alter serum K+

2. **Drive K+ potassium into cells**
   Soluble insulin 10 units + 50 ml 50% dextrose intravenously over 15–30 min and/or correction of severe acidosis with $NaHCO_{3=}$ (1.26%)
   Effects last 1–2 h; repeated doses may be necessary

3. **Deplete body K+**
   Calcium or sodium resonium orally (15 g three times daily with laxatives) or rectally (30 g)
   Treat the cause
   Haemodialysis or peritoneal dialysis

4. **Monitor**
   Blood glucose (finger-prick Stix testing) hourly during and after insulin/dextrose infusion
   Serum potassium 2–4-hourly acutely, and daily thereafter

Emergency Box 6.2

DISORDERS OF MAGNESIUM REGULATION

Disturbance of magnesium balance is uncommon and usually associated with more obvious fluid and electrolyte disturbance. Like potassium, magnesium is mainly an intracellular cation and balance is maintained mainly via the kidney.

Hypomagnesaemia
Aetiology

A low serum magnesium is most often caused by loss of magnesium from the gut or kidney. Gastrointestinal causes include diarrhoea, malabsorption, extensive bowel resection and intestinal fistulae. Excessive renal loss of magnesium occurs with diuretics, alcohol abuse, and with an osmotic diuresis such as glycosuria in diabetes mellitus.

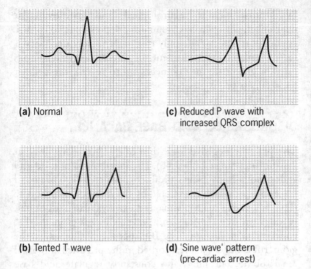

(a) Normal

(c) Reduced P wave with increased QRS complex

(b) Tented T wave

(d) 'Sine wave' pattern (pre-cardiac arrest)

Figure 6.3
Progressive ECG changes with increasing hyperkalaemia.

Clinical features

Hypomagnesaemia increases renal excretion of potassium, inhibits secretion of parathyroid hormone and leads to PTH resistance. Many of the symptoms of hypomagnesaemia are therefore due to hypokalaemia (page 262) and hypocalcaemia (page 244).

Management

The underlying cause must be corrected where possible and oral supplements given (magnesium chloride 5–20 mmol daily). Symptomatic severe magnesium deficiency should be treated by intravenous infusion (50 mmol of MgCl in 1 litre of 5% dextrose over 12–24 h), plus a loading dose (4 mmol over 10 min) if there are seizures or ventricular arrhythmias.

Hypermagnesaemia

Hypermagnesaemia is rare and then is usually iatrogenic, occurring in patients with renal failure who have been given magnesium-containing laxatives or antacids.

Symptoms include neurological and cardiovascular depression, with narcosis, respiratory depression and cardiac conduction defects. The only treatment usually necessary is to stop magnesium treatment. In severe cases intravenous calcium gluconate may be necessary to reverse the cellular toxic effects of magnesium.

DISORDERS OF ACID–BASE BALANCE

The pH (the negative logarithm of $[H^+]$) is maintained at 7.4 (normal range 7.35–7.45). The metabolism of food and endogenous body tissues produces about 70–100 mmol of H^+ each day, which is excreted by the kidneys. Bicarbonate (HCO_3^-) is the main plasma and extracellular fluid buffer. It mops up free H^+ ions and prevents increases in the H^+ concentration (Figure 6.4). Bicarbonate is filtered at the glomerulus but is then reabsorbed in the proximal and distal renal tubule. The lungs also constantly regulate acid–base balance through the excretion of CO_2. Between production and excretion of H^+ ions there is an extremely effective buffering system maintaining a constant H^+ ion concentration inside and outside the cell. Buffers include haemoglobin proteins, bicarbonate and phosphate.

Acid–base disturbances may be caused by:

- Abnormal carbon dioxide removal in the lungs ('respiratory' acidosis and alkalosis)
- Abnormalities in the regulation of bicarbonate and other buffers in the blood ('metabolic' acidosis and alkalosis).

Both may, and usually do, coexist. For instance, metabolic acidosis causes hyperventilation (via medullary chemo-receptors), leading to increased removal of CO_2 in the lungs and partial compensation for the acidosis. Conversely,

$$\text{carbonic anhydrase}$$

$$H^+ + HCO_3^- \rightleftharpoons H_2CO_3 \rightleftharpoons H_2O + CO_2$$

Figure 6.4
The carbonic anhydrase reaction.

respiratory acidosis is accompanied by renal bicarbonate retention, which could be mistaken for primary metabolic alkalosis.

Measurement of pH, PCO_2 and $[HCO_3^-]$ will reveal which type of disturbance is present (Table 6.9). These measurements are made on an arterial blood sample (page 638) using an automated blood gas analyser.

Table 6.9 Changes in arterial blood gases

	pH	P_aCO_2	HCO_3^-
Respiratory acidosis	Normal or reduced	Increased ++	Increased
Respiratory alkalosis	Normal or increased	Reduced ++	Reduced
Metabolic acidosis	Normal or reduced	Reduced	Reduced ++
Metabolic alkalosis	Normal or increased	Increased	Increased ++

The pH may be at the limits of the normal range if the acidosis or alkalosis is compensated, e.g. respiratory compensation (hyperventilation) of a metabolic acidosis. The clue to the abnormality from the blood gases will be the abnormal P_aCO_2 and HCO_3^-

Respiratory acidosis

This is usually associated with ventilatory failure, with retention of carbon dioxide (page 450). Treatment is of the underlying cause.

Respiratory alkalosis

Hyperventilation results in increased removal of carbon dioxide, resulting in a fall in P_aCO_2 and $[H^+]$.

Metabolic acidosis

This is the result of the accumulation of any acid other than carbonic acid. The most common cause is lactic acidosis following shock or cardiac arrest.

Clinical features

These include hyperventilation, hypotension caused by arteriolar vasodilatation and the negative inotropic effect of acidosis, and cerebral dysfunction associated with confusion and fits.

Differential diagnosis (the anion gap)

The first step is to identify whether the acidosis is the result of retention of HCl or of another acid. This is achieved by measurement of the anion gap. The main electrolytes measured in plasma are sodium, potassium, chloride and bicarbonate. The sum of the cations, sodium and potassium, normally exceeds that of chloride and bicarbonate by 6–12 mmol/l. This anion gap is usually made up of negatively charged proteins, phosphate and organic acids. If the anion gap is normal in the presence of acidosis, it can be concluded that HCl is being retained or $NaHCO_3$ is being lost. The causes of a normal anion gap acidosis are given in Table 6.10.

Table 6.10 Causes of metabolic acidosis with a normal anion gap

Increased gastrointestinal HCO_3 loss
Diarrhoea
Ileostomy
Ureterosigmoidostomy

Increased HCO_3^- renal loss
Acetazolamide ingestion
Proximal (type 2) renal tubular acidosis
Hyperparathyroidism
Tubular damage, e.g. drugs, heavy metals

Decreased renal H+ excretion
Distal (type 1) renal tubular acidosis
Type 4 renal tubular acidosis

Increased HCl production
Ammonium chloride ingestion
Increased catabolism of lysine, arginine

If the anion gap is increased (i.e. >12 mmol/l), the acidosis is the result of an exogenous acid, e.g. salicylates or one of the acids normally present in small unmeasured quantities, such as lactate. Causes of a high anion gap acidosis are given in Table 6.11.

Lactic acidosis

Increased production of lactic acid occurs when cellular respiration is abnormal, resulting from either lack of oxygen (type A) or a metabolic abnormality (type B). The most common form in clinical practice is type A lactic acidosis, occurring in septicaemic or cardiogenic shock.

Table 6.11 Causes of a high anion gap metabolic acidosis

Renal failure (sulphate, phosphate)

Ketoacidosis
Diabetes
Starvation
Alcohol poisoning

Lactic acidosis
Type A
    Methanol
    Ethylene glycol
    Strenuous exercise
    Shock
    Severe hypoxia

Type B
    Metformin accumulation
    Leukaemia, lymphoma
    Poisoning, ethanol, paracetamol
    Acute liver failure

Drug poisoning
Salicylates

Diabetic ketoacidosis

This is a high anion gap acidosis caused by the accumulation of organic acids, acetoacetic acid and hydroxybutyric acid (see page 526).

Renal tubular acidosis

Renal tubular acidosis may occur in the absence of renal failure and is a normal anion gap acidosis. There is failure of the kidney to acidify the urine adequately. This group of disorders is uncommon and only rarely a cause of significant clinical disease.

Type 4 renal tubular acidosis This is the most common of these disorders and is also known as hyporeninaemic hypoaldosteronism. Typical features are acidosis and hyperkalaemia occurring in the setting of mild chronic renal failure, usually caused by tubulointerstitial disease or diabetes. Plasma aldosterone and renin are low and do not respond to stimulation. Treatment is with fludrocortisone, diuretics, sodium bicarbonate and ion exchange resins for the reduction of serum potassium.

Proximal (type 2) renal tubular acidosis This is failure to absorb bicarbonate in the proximal tubule. Typical features are hypokalaemia, and inability to produce an acid urine in spite of systemic acidosis and the appearance of bicarbonate in the urine. This disorder normally occurs as part of a generalized tubular defect, together with other features such as glycosuria and amino aciduria. Treatment is with oral sodium bicarbonate.

Distal (type 1) renal tubular acidosis There is failure of H^+ excretion in the distal tubule. Typical features include hypokalaemia and an inability to produce an acid urine in spite of systemic acidosis. Causes include autoimmune diseases, SLE and nephrocalcinosis. Presentation is often with renal stones as a result of hypercalciuria, low urinary citrate (citrate inhibits calcium phosphate precipitation) and alkaline urine (favours precipitation of calcium phosphate). Treatment is with sodium bicarbonate.

Uraemic acidosis

Reduction of the capacity to secrete H^+ and NH_4^+, in addition to bicarbonate wasting, contributes to the acidosis of chronic renal failure. Acidosis occurs particularly when there is tubular damage, such as reflux and chronic obstructive nephropathy. It is associated with hypercalciuria and renal osteodystrophy because H^+ ions are buffered by bone in exchange for calcium. Treatment is with calcium or sodium bicarbonate, although acidosis in end-stage renal failure is only usually fully corrected by adequate dialysis.

Metabolic alkalosis

This is much less common than acidosis and is often associated with potassium or volume depletion. The main causes are persistent vomiting, diuretic therapy or hyperaldosteronism. Vomiting causes alkalosis both by causing volume depletion and through loss of gastric acid.

Clinical features

Cerebral dysfunction is an early feature of alkalosis. Respiration may be depressed.

Management

This includes fluid replacement, if necessary, with replacement of sodium, potassium and chloride. The bicarbonate excess will correct itself.

Renal disease

···

7

PRESENTING FEATURES OF RENAL DISEASE

The most common diseases of the kidney and urinary tract are benign prostatic hypertrophy in men and urinary tract infection (UTI) in women. The symptoms suggesting renal tract disease are frequency of micturition, dysuria, haematuria, urinary retention and alteration of urine volume (either polyuria or oliguria). In addition there may be pain situated anywhere along the renal tract, from loin to groin. Non-specific symptoms may be the presenting features, e.g. lethargy, anorexia and pruritus, which occur in chronic renal failure.

Renal disease may be asymptomatic and discovered by the incidental finding of hypertension, a raised serum urea, or proteinuria and haematuria on stix testing.

Urine stix testing (page 650)

Commercial reagent stix detect the presence of protein, glucose, ketones, bilirubin, urobilinogen and blood in the urine. They also measure urine pH, which is useful in the investigation and management of renal tubular acidosis (page 269). Each test is based on a colour change in a strip of absorbent cellulose impregnated with the appropriate reagent. The stix is dipped briefly into a fresh specimen of urine collected in a clean container and the colour changes compared with the manufacturer's colour charts on the reagent strip container. The degree of colour change is a semiquantitative assessment of the amount of substance present. Haematuria or proteinuria suggest renal tract disease. Dipsticks are also available for testing for bacteriuria (page 284).

Proteinuria

The glomerular ultrafiltrate normally contains a small amount of protein, most of which is absorbed in the proximal renal tubule and only small amounts (up to 200 mg/24 h) appear in the urine. Most reagent stix can detect a protein concentration of 150 mg/l or more in the urine. Pyrexia, exercise and adoption of the upright posture may all produce a mild increase in urinary protein output. 'Postural proteinuria' is the term used when proteinuria occurs in the upright posture but not when supine. It may be diagnosed by testing for protein in several early morning urine samples passed after overnight recumbency, and then testing several samples after being up and about. The condition is usually benign and the amount of protein excreted small.

Persistent proteinuria (Figure 7.1) detected on stix testing requires full investigation. The first step is to quantify protein excretion by a 24-hour urine collection. Proteinuria greater than 2 g/24 h is usually the result of glomerular disease (page 275) and greater than 3–5 g/24 h may result in the nephrotic syndrome (page 280).

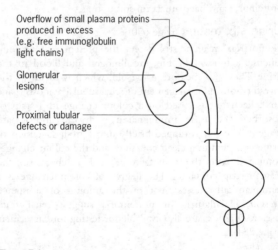

Overflow of small plasma proteins produced in excess (e.g. free immunoglobulin light chains)

Glomerular lesions

Proximal tubular defects or damage

Figure 7.1
Sources of urinary protein. (Adapted from Mallick (1991) Presenting features of renal disease. Medicine International 85: 3512.)

Proteinuria caused by failure of proximal tubular reabsorption is uncommon and is seldom an isolated defect: there are usually multiple proximal tubular defects causing glycosuria, aminoaciduria, phosphaturia and renal tubular acidosis (Fanconi's syndrome). Bence-Jones proteins (immunoglobulin light chains in patients with myeloma) are not detected by stix and are identified by immunoelectrophoresis of urine.

Haematuria

Haematuria may arise from any site in the kidney or urinary tract (Figure 7.2) and may be macroscopic, with bloody urine, or microscopic and found only on stix testing. A positive stix test must always be followed by careful microscopy of fresh urine to confirm the presence of red cells, to look for red cell casts and to exclude

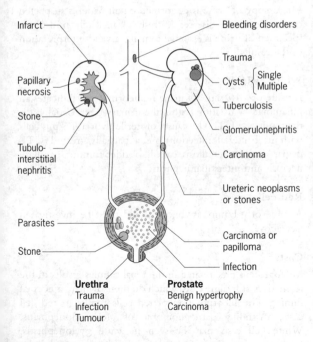

Figure 7.2
Sites and causes of bleeding from the urinary tract.

haemoglobinuria, which is uncommon but also results in a positive test. The presence of red cell casts on urine microscopy indicates bleeding of glomerular origin (see later). In the absence of red cell casts, further investigations, such as urine cytology, intravenous urography and cystoscopy, are required to define the site of bleeding.

With macroscopic haematuria the source of bleeding may be suggested by a careful history. Haematuria that is only apparent at the start of micturition is usually associated with urethral disease. Haematuria that occurs at the end of micturition suggests bleeding from the prostate or bladder base, whereas blood seen as an even discoloration throughout the urine suggests bleeding from a source in the bladder or above.

Urine microscopy

Microscopy of urine is performed on all patients suspected of having renal disease. A fresh clean-catch midstream specimen of urine is essential to make a valid interpretation of the results.

White cells

A value of >10/mm³ of urine is abnormal and indicates an inflammatory reaction within the urinary tract. Usually it is the result of a UTI. The causes of sterile pyuria (i.e. pus cells without bacterial infection) are a partially treated UTI, urinary tract tuberculosis, calculi, bladder tumour, papillary necrosis and interstitial nephritis.

Red cells

A value of >1/mm³ is abnormal and must be investigated (see above).

Casts

Mucoprotein precipitated in the renal tubules results in the formation of hyaline casts, which on their own are a normal finding. The incorporation of red cells results in red cell casts, a finding pathognomonic of glomerulonephritis. White cell casts may be seen in acute pyelonephritis. Granular casts result from the disintegration of cellular debris and indicate renal disease.

Bacteria

A bacterial count over 100 000 organisms per ml of urine in a fresh midstream specimen is a reliable indicator of a UTI (page 284).

··

GLOMERULONEPHRITIS

Normal glomerular structure

A renal glomerulus (there are about 1 million glomeruli in each kidney) consists of a capillary plexus invaginating the blind end of the proximal renal tubule (Figure 7.3). The glomerular capillaries are lined by a fenestrated endothelium which rests on the glomerular basement membrane (GBM). External to the GBM are the visceral epithelial cells (podocytes). These cells only make contact with the GBM by finger-like projections, called foot processes, which are separated from one another by 'slit pores' (Figure 7.3). This unique structure of the glomerular membrane accounts for its tremendous permeability, allowing 125–200 ml of glomerular filtrate to be formed every minute (this is the glomerular filtration rate, or GFR). The composition of the glomerular filtrate is similar to plasma but contains only small amounts of protein (all of low molecular weight), most of which is reabsorbed in the proximal tubule. The water and electrolyte composition of the glomerular filtrate is normally substantially altered by tubular reabsorption and secretion until it reaches the renal pelvis as urine.

Glomerulonephritis is a general term for a group of disorders in which there is bilateral, symmetrical immunologically mediated injury to the glomerulus. Two chief pathogenic mechanisms are recognized:

- Deposition or in situ formation of immune complexes (most human glomerulonephritides). Circulating antigen –antibody complexes are deposited in the kidney, or complexes are formed locally when antigen becomes trapped in the glomerulus. The antigen may be exogenous, e.g. β-haemolytic streptococci, or endogenous, e.g. DNA in systemic lupus erythematosus.

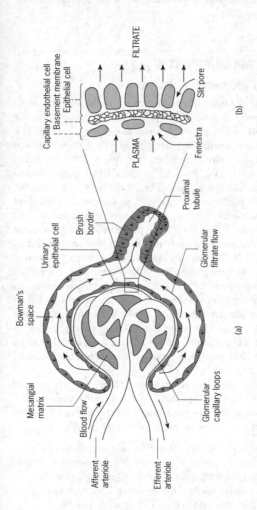

Figure 7.3
(a) Diagrammatic representation of the normal glomerulus. **(b)** Components of the glomerular membrane. (Adapted from Read et al (1993) Essential Medicine. Churchill Livingstone, Edinburgh; Guyton (1987) Human Physiology and Mechanisms of Disease, 4th edn. WB Saunders, London.)

- Deposition of antiglomerular basement membrane antibody (anti–GBM, <5% of glomerulonephritides). Anti–GBM antibody reacts with an antigen in the GBM, producing glomerular damage. The antibody may also react with alveolar capillary basement membrane and can cause both lung haemorrhage and glomerulonephritis (Goodpasture's syndrome).

In some glomerulonephritides, e.g. associated with Wegener's granulomatosis and microscopic polyarteritis, there is no evidence of immune complex deposition. Injury is mediated by a vasculitis causing a focal segmental necrotizing glomerulonephritis with haematuria, proteinuria and deteriorating renal function.

Pathogenesis

Deposition of immune complexes in the glomerulus leads to an inflammatory response which triggers secondary mechanisms of glomerular injury. These include complement activation, fibrin deposition, platelet aggregation and activation of kinin systems. The histological response to immune complex deposition is very variable.

Glomerulonephritis is classified on the basis of light microscopic appearances supplemented by information gained from immunohistochemical techniques and electron microscopy (EM). The main forms of histopathologically identified glomerulonephritis and the clinical features most often associated with each are listed in Table 7.1. The terms 'focal' and 'diffuse' refer to the kidney as a whole, and 'segmental' and 'global' refer to the glomeruli. Thus in focal segmental glomerulonephritis only some glomeruli are affected and only a part of the glomerulus.

Aetiology

In most patients with immune complex-mediated glomerulonephritis the cause is unknown, i.e. the nature of the antigen is not determined. In a minority of cases antigens derived from viruses, bacteria, parasites, drugs and from the host may be involved (Table 7.2)

Clinical features

Glomerulonephritis presents in one of four ways:

Table 7.1 Categories of glomerulonephritis (GN) and associated clinical condition*

Histological type	Light microscopic appearances	Most common clinical presentation
Proliferative glomerulonephritis		
Diffuse	Endothelial and mesangial cell proliferation	Acute nephritic syndrome
Focal segmental	As above but changes are focal	Haematuria, proteinuria
With crescent formation (rapidly progressive GN)	Crescent formation (aggregates of macrophages and epithelial cells in Bowman's space)	Acute renal failure
Mesangiocapillary (mesangioproliferative)	Thickening of GBM, mesangial cell proliferation	Haematuria, proteinuria, nephritic and nephrotic syndrome
IgA nephropathy	Mesangial cell proliferation	Haematuria in young men
Membranous GN	Thickening of GBM	Nephrotic syndrome in adults
Minimal change nephropathy	Normal (fusion of epithelial cell foot processes on EM)	Nephrotic syndrome in children
Focal glomerulosclerosis	Segmental scarring of glomerull	Proteinuria or nephrotic syndrome

* There is not a complete correlation between the histopathological types and the clinical features. GBM, glomerular basement membrane.

Table 7.2 Some causes of immune complex-mediated glomerulonephritis

Infections
Lancefield group A β-haemolytic streptococci
Streptococcus viridans (infective endocarditis)
Mumps virus
Hepatitis B and C virus
Tropical infections: schistosomiasis, *Plasmodium malariae*, filariasis

Systemic disease
Systemic lupus erythematosus (SLE)

Malignant tumours

Drugs, e.g. penicillamine

- Asymptomatic proteinuria/haematuria (page 272)
- Acute nephritic syndrome
- Nephrotic syndrome
- Renal failure, acute and chronic (page 298).

Acute nephritic syndrome

Diffuse proliferative glomerulonephritis underlies many of the cases of acute nephritic syndrome in adults and children. The prototype exogenous pattern is poststreptococcal glomerulonephritis, whereas that produced by an endogenous antigen is lupus nephritis, seen in SLE. The typical case of poststreptococcal glomerulonephritis develops in a child 1–3 weeks after a streptococcal infection (pharyngitis or cellulitis) with a Lancefield group A β-haemolytic streptococcus. The bacterial antigen becomes trapped in the glomerulus, leading to an acute diffuse proliferative glomerulonephritis.

Clinical features

The syndrome comprises:

- Haematuria (macroscopic or microscopic)
- Proteinuria (usually <2 g/day)
- Hypertension caused by salt and water retention
- Oedema (periorbital, leg or sacral)
- Oliguria
- Uraemia.

Investigations

A thorough history and examination are essential to assess the severity of the illness and to determine any associated underlying conditions. The investigations to consider in nephritic syndrome are listed in Table 7.3. If the clinical diagnosis of a nephritic illness is clear-cut, e.g. in poststreptococcal glomerulonephritis, renal ultrasonography and renal biopsy are usually unnecessary.

Management

Poststreptococcal glomerulonephritis usually has a good prognosis and supportive measures are often all that is required until spontaneous recovery takes place. Hypertension is treated with salt restriction, loop diuretics and vasodilators. Fluid balance is monitored by daily weighing and daily recording of fluid input and output. In oliguric patients with evidence of fluid overload (e.g. oedema, pulmonary congestion and severe hypertension) fluid restriction is necessary. Life-threatening complications such as hypertensive encephalopathy (see page 304), pulmonary oedema and severe uraemia (see page 304) are treated in the usual ways.

In glomerulonephritis complicating SLE or the systemic vasculitides (see below), immunosuppression with prednisolone, cyclophosphamide or azathioprine improves renal function.

Nephrotic syndrome

Nephrotic syndrome consists of heavy proteinuria (>3–5 g/24 h), hypoalbuminaemia and oedema. Structural damage to the glomerular basement membrane leads to loss of electrostatic and physical barriers which normally prevents the passage of large molecular weight proteins into the glomerular filtrate. Increased protein loss, in addition to increased catabolism of protein in the kidney, leads to hypoalbuminaemia. The pathogenesis of oedema in the nephrotic syndrome is poorly understood. The classic explanation is that intravascular hypovolaemia (hypoalbuminaemia reduces plasma oncotic pressure, salt and water move into extravascular compartment) results in activation of the renin–angiotensin–aldosterone system, which promotes sodium and water reabsorption in the

Table 7.3 Investigations indicated in glomerular disease

Investigations	Significance
Baseline measurements	
Measurement of creatinine clearance	To determine current status, monitor progress and response to treatment
24-hour urinary protein excretion	
Serum urea and electrolytes	
Serum albumin	
Diagnostically useful tests	
Urine microscopy	Red cell casts indicate glomerulonephritis
Culture (swab from throat or infected skin }	Diagnosis of recent streptococcal infection
Serum antistreptolysin-O titre	
Blood glucose	Diagnosis of diabetes mellitus
Antinuclear and anti-DNA antibodies	Positive in SLE
ANCA (page 695)	Positive in Wegener's granulomatosis
ANCA (page 696)	Positive in microscopic polyarteritis
Antiglomerular basement membrane antibody	Goodpasture's disease
Hepatitis B surface antigen	Negative result excludes HBV infection
Chest radiograph	Cavities in Wegener's granulomatosis, malignancy?
Renal biopsy	Indicated in some adults with nephrotic or nephritic syndrome

distal nephron. However, it seems probable that there is also a primary intrarenal defect in sodium excretion.

Aetiology

All types of glomerulonephritis can cause the nephrotic syndrome, although in Europe and the USA membranous disease is the most common cause in adults and minimal change glomerulonephritis in children. Membranous glomerulonephritis is usually idiopathic but may occur in association with drugs, neoplasms or infections (see Table 7.2).

Minimal change glomerulonephritis occurs most commonly in boys under 5 years of age. It accounts for 90% of cases of nephrotic syndrome in children and 20–25% in adults; however, it is rare in black African populations. The pathogenesis of this condition is not known; immune complexes are absent on immunofluorescence but the increase in glomerular permeability is thought to be immunologically mediated in some way.

Amyloid (page 546) involving the kidneys and diabetes mellitus (page 533) are also important causes of the nephrotic syndrome but, unlike minimal change and membranous glomerulonephritis, the mechanism is not immune mediated.

Other renal diseases, e.g. polycystic kidneys, chronic pyelonephritis, may cause proteinuria, but are rarely severe enough to cause the nephrotic syndrome.

Clinical features

Oedema of the ankles, genitals and abdomen is the principal finding. The face (periorbital oedema) and arms may also be involved in severe cases.

Differential diagnoses

Nephrotic syndrome must be differentiated from other causes of oedema and hypoalbuminaemia. In congestive cardiac failure (page 341) there is oedema and a raised jugular venous pressure (JVP). In nephrotic syndrome the JVP is normal or low unless there is concomitant renal failure and oliguria. Hypoalbuminaemia and oedema occur in cirrhosis, but there are usually signs of chronic liver disease on examination (page 112).

Investigations

The diagnosis is established by demonstrating:

- Heavy proteinuria (>3–5 g daily in adults)
- Hypoalbuminaemia (<30 g/l).

Hyperlipidaemia is common in the nephrotic syndrome and is the result of increased hepatic synthesis of cholesterol and triglycerides, which accompanies hepatic albumin synthesis. Further investigations to be considered are listed in Table 7.3.

In the UK most cases of childhood nephrotic syndrome are caused by minimal change glomerulonephritis, and therefore treatment is usually started with corticosteroids without recourse to a renal biopsy. In adults a renal biopsy is performed unless the diagnosis is clear-cut, e.g. nephrotic syndrome in a patient with long-standing diabetes mellitus must be advanced diabetic glomerulopathy. If a drug is implicated, e.g. penicillamine, the correct management is to stop the drug.

Management

General Oedema is treated with bed rest, dietary salt restriction and diuretic therapy. Intravenous diuretics and occasionally intravenous salt-poor albumin may be required to initiate a diuresis which, once established, can usually be maintained with oral diuretics alone. If diuresis is too vigorous it may precipitate circulatory collapse and acute renal failure.

Specific treatment Minimal change disease is almost always steroid responsive in children, although less commonly in adults. High-dose prednisolone therapy (40–60 mg daily) should be given over a period of 8 weeks and then reduced slowly. Of patients who enter remission 30–50% will have a relapse within 3 years, and this is treated with a further course of steroids. In patients with frequent relapses and in steroid-unresponsive patients, immunosuppressive therapy with cyclophosphamide or cylcosporin may be used.

The benefits of immunosuppressive therapy in membranous glomerulonephritis remain contentious. In other types of glomerulonephritis remission may occur if the underlying disease can be treated, e.g. in patients with

SLE treatment with steroids or cyclophosphamide may induce long-term remission.

Complications

- *Venous thrombosis* Hypovolaemia and a hypercoagulable state predispose to thrombus formation in both renal (seen on ultrasonography) and peripheral veins. Prolonged bed rest should be avoided but, if necessary, patients should receive prophylactic anticoagulation with subcutaneous heparin (page 185). Renal vein thrombosis presents with renal pain, haematuria and a deterioration in renal function.
- *Sepsis* Loss of immunoglobulin in the urine increases the susceptibility to infection which is an important cause of death in these patients.
- *Acute renal failure* is rarely the result of progression of the underlying renal disease. However, acute renal failure may occur as a result of hypovolaemia, particularly after diuretic therapy or with renal vein thrombosis.

URINARY TRACT INFECTION

Urinary tract infection is common in women, with about 35% having symptoms of a UTI at some time in their lives. It is relatively uncommon in children and in men, when it usually indicates underlying disease.

Pathogenesis

Infection of the urinary tract is most often via the ascending transurethral route, and this is facilitated by sexual intercourse and urethral catheterization. Women are more susceptible to infection because the short urethra and its proximity to the anus facilitates the transfer of bowel organisms to the bladder. Infection is most often caused by bacteria from the patient's own bowel flora (Table 7.4), but in 20–30% of young women it is caused by skin organisms: *Staphylococcus saprophyticus* or *Staph. epidermidis*.

Abnormalities that encourage bladder infection (*cystitis*) include:

- Urinary obstruction or stasis
- Previous damage to the bladder epithelium

Table 7.4 Organisms causing urinary tract infection in domiciliary practice

Organism	Approximate frequency (%)
Escherichia coli and other coliforms	68+
Proteus mirabilis	12
*Klebsiella aerogenes**	4
Enterococci*	6
Staphylococcus saprophyticus or *Staph. epidermidis*†	10

* More common in hospital practice.
† More common in women.

- Bladder stones
- Poor bladder emptying.

Ascending infection of the ureters results in renal parenchymal infection (*acute pyelonephritis*). This is facilitated by vesicoureteric reflux and dilated hypotonic ureters. *Chronic pyelonephritis* (also called atrophic pyelonephritis or reflux nephropathy) arises from childhood UTIs in combination with vesicoureteric reflux, leading to progressive renal scarring. It presents as hypertension or chronic renal failure in childhood and adult life.

Clinical features

The most common symptoms of lower urinary tract infection are frequency of micturition, dysuria (painful voiding), suprapubic pain, and tenderness, haematuria and smelly urine.

In acute pyelonephritis there may also be loin pain and tenderness, with fever and systemic upset. However, localization of infection on the basis of symptoms alone is unreliable.

In elderly people the symptoms may be atypical, with incontinence, nocturia or just a vague change in wellbeing.

Investigations

- Dipstick tests can be used to detect the presence of nitrites (produced by reduction of urinary nitrates by bacteria) and elastase produced by neutrophils. Dipstick tests positive for both nitrite and elastase are highly predictive of acute infection.

- Urine microscopy and culture. The diagnosis depends on finding more than 100 000 of the same organism per ml of urine in a clean-catch midstream urine specimen (MSU). Lower counts or mixed growths are of uncertain significance and the test should be repeated. If in doubt, urine must be obtained by suprapubic bladder aspiration, where any growth of a uropathogenic organism is evidence of infection.
- Excretion urography (page 701) is performed to look for physiological and anatomical abnormalities of the urinary tract which may predispose to UTI. It is indicated in women with repeated infections and after a single infection in children and men.

Management

A 3–5-day course of oral amoxycillin, nitrofurantion or trimethoprim is usually effective. A high fluid intake should be encouraged during treatment and for some weeks afterwards. In women with relapsing infection, low-dose prophylactic antibiotics may be required for a period of 6–12 months. Patients with acute pyelonephritis may be acutely ill and usually require initial treatment with parenteral antibiotics, such as intravenous cefuroxime, ciprofloxacin or an aminoglycoside (e.g. gentamicin). In patients with an indwelling catheter treatment is indicated in the presence of symptoms.

Complications

In fit patients with normal urinary tracts UTIs rarely result in serious kidney damage. In patients with abnormal urinary tracts (e.g. stones) or systemic disease involving the kidney (e.g. diabetes mellitus), the complications are renal papillary necrosis (page 296) and the development of a renal or perinephric abscess with the risk of Gram-negative septicaemia. Abscesses can be seen on ultrasonography and usually require surgical drainage as well as antibiotic therapy.

Urinary tract infection in pregnancy

Approximately 6% of pregnant women have significant bacteriuria in pregnancy; if untreated, 20% of these will develop acute pyelonephritis. Early detection and treatment of bacteriuria is thus indicated.

Abacteriuric frequency or dysuria ('urethral syndrome')

The urethral syndrome occurs in women and presents with dysuria and frequency but in the absence of bacteriuria. It may be associated with vaginitis in postmenopausal women, irritant chemicals (e.g. soaps) and sexual intercourse.

Tuberculosis of the urinary tract

Tuberculosis (TB) of the urinary tract may present with all the symptoms of a UTI, i.e. dysuria, frequency or haematuria, and should be considered particularly in the Asian immigrant population of the UK. Classically, there is sterile pyuria (page 274). Diagnosis depends on culture of mycobacteria from early morning urine samples. Treatment is as for pulmonary tuberculosis (page 420).

....

TUBULOINTERSTITIAL NEPHRITIS

Interstitial inflammation with tubular damage is a regular feature of bacterial pyelonephritis but, contrary to former belief, it rarely, if ever, leads to chronic renal damage in the absence of reflux, obstruction or other complicating factors. The importance of other factors, particularly drugs, in the causation of this disorder has now been realized.

Acute tubulointerstitial nephritis

Acute tubulointerstitial nephritis is most often the result of a hypersensitivity reaction to drugs (Table 7.5), most commonly drugs of the penicillin family and non-steroidal anti-inflammatory drugs (NSAIDs).

Table 7.5 Common causes of acute tubulointerstitial nephritis

Penicillins
NSAIDs
Sulphonamides
Allopurinol
Cephalosporins
Rifampicin
Diuretics – frusemide, thiazides
Cimetidine
Phenytoin

Patients present with acute renal failure and the features of a hypersensitivity reaction: fever, arthralgia, skin rashes and blood eosinophilia. Renal biopsy shows an intense interstitial cellular infiltrate, predominantly eosinophils, and variable tubular necrosis. Management involves withdrawal of the offending drug and treatment of acute renal failure (page 304). High-dose prednisolone therapy is often used, although its value has not been proven. The prognosis is generally good; patients should avoid further exposure to the offending drug.

Chronic tubulointerstitial nephritis

The most common cause of chronic tubulointerstitial nephritis is prolonged consumption of large amounts of analgesic drugs, particularly NSAIDs and drugs containing phenacetin (now withdrawn) ('analgesic nephropathy'). Some causes are shown in Table 7.6.

Table 7.6 Causes of chronic tubulointerstitial nephritis

Chronic pyelonephritis
NSAIDs
Diabetes mellitus
Sickle-cell disease
Sjögren's syndrome
Hyperuricaemic nephropathy

Presentation is usually with polyuria, proteinuria (usually <1 g/day) or uraemia. Polyuria and nocturia are the result of tubular damage in the medullary area of the kidney, leading to defects in the renal concentrating ability. Necrosis of the papillae, which may subsequently slough off and be passed in the urine, sometimes causes ureteric colic or acute ureteral obstruction. Management is largely supportive. In cases of analgesic nephropathy the drug should be stopped and replaced if necessary with paracetamol or dihydrocodeine.

HYPERTENSION AND THE KIDNEY

Hypertension may be the cause or the result of renal disease, and it may be difficult to differentiate between the two on clinical grounds. Investigations, as described on page 386, should be performed on all patients, although intravenous urography (IVU) is usually unnecessary.

Essential hypertension

Hypertension leads to characteristic histological changes in the renal vessels and intrarenal vasculature over time. These include intimal thickening with reduplication of the elastic lamina, reduction in kidney size, and an increase in the proportion of sclerotic.glomeruli. The changes are usually accompanied by some deterioration in renal function.

Accelerated or malignant phase hypertension is marked by the development of fibrinoid necrosis in afferent glomerular arterioles and fibrin deposition in arteriolar walls. A rapid rise in blood pressure may trigger these arteriolar lesions, and a vicious circle is then established whereby fibrin deposition leads to renal damage, increased renin release and a further increase in blood pressure.

Treatment of hypertension is described on page 387. The outlook is good if treatment is started before renal impairment has occurred.

Renal hypertension

Bilateral renal disease

Hypertension commonly complicates bilateral renal disease, such as chronic glomerulonephritis, bilateral reflux nephropathy or analgesic nephropathy. Two main mechanisms are responsible:

- Activation of the renin–angiotensin–aldosterone system
- Retention of salt and water, leading to an increase in blood volume and hence blood pressure.

Good control of blood pressure is important to prevent further deterioration in renal function, with angiotensin-converting enzyme (ACE) inhibitors normally being the drugs of choice.

Unilateral renal disease

Hypertension may arise as a result of unilateral renal artery stenosis (caused by fibromuscular hyperplasia in young women, atheroma in elderly people) or unilateral reflux nephropathy. The mechanism of hypertension is illustrated in Figure 7.4.

Screening for unilateral renal disease

- *Rapid sequence excretion urography* is widely employed. Injected contrast medium is filtered more slowly and concentrated to a greater extent within the nephron on the side of the stenosis.
- *Radionucleotide studies* using technetium-labelled diethylenetriaminepentaacetic acid ([99 mTC]DTPA). With significant renal artery stenosis, a fall in uptake of isotope on the affected side follows administration of an ACE inhibitor, such as captopril.
- *Renal arteriography* remains the gold standard for the diagnosis of renal artery disease, though the technique is invasive and requires cannulation of the femoral artery.

Management

Most patients do well with hypotensive therapy without the need for surgery. ACE inhibitors are avoided because they can lead to acute renal failure in the presence of renal artery stenosis. Surgical options for renal artery stenosis include

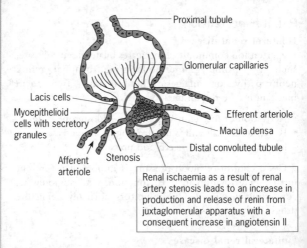

Proximal tubule
Glomerular capillaries
Lacis cells
Myoepithelioid cells with secretory granules
Efferent arteriole
Macula densa
Distal convoluted tubule
Afferent arteriole
Stenosis

Renal ischaemia as a result of renal artery stenosis leads to an increase in production and release of renin from juxtaglomerular apparatus with a consequent increase in angiotensin II

Figure 7.4
The mechanism of hypertension in unilateral renal artery stenosis. (Adapted from Davidson (1991) Principles and Practice of Medicine. Churchill Livingstone, Edinburgh.)

transluminal angioplasty to dilate the stenotic region, reconstructive vascular surgery and nephrectomy. With good patient selection more than 50% are cured or improved by intervention. In unilateral reflux nephropathy nephrectomy is advocated, particularly if the abnormal kidney is making an insignificant contribution to overall excretion function.

RENAL STONE DISEASE

In the UK approximately 2% of the population will experience renal stone disease at some time in their life. There is a male:female ratio of 2:1.

Aetiology

Calcium-containing stones are the most common (Table 7.7).

Table 7.7 Types and frequency of renal stones

Type	Approximate frequency (%)
Calcium-containing	80
Calcium oxalate (65%)	
Calcium phosphate (15%)	
Magnesium ammonium phosphate	10–15
Uric acid	3–5
Cystine	1–2

Calcium stones More than half of all patients with calcium oxalate stones have idiopathic hypercalciuria. People with this condition both absorb from the gut and excrete in the urine a higher fraction of dietary calcium than normal people. Serum calcium levels are normal. Less common causes of hypercalciuria are:

- Hypercalcaemia (page 245): most patients with hypercalcaemia who form stones have primary hyperparathyroidism
- Excessive dietary intake of calcium
- Excessive resorption of calcium from the skeleton, as occurs with prolonged immobilization or weightlessness.

Increased oxalate excretion favours the formation of calcium oxalate, even if calcium excretion is normal:

- Primary hyperoxaluria is a rare autosomal recessive enzyme deficiency leading to increased oxalate production and corresponding oxalate excretion. There is widespread calcium oxalate crystal deposition in the kidneys, and later in other tissues (myocardium, tissues and bone). Renal failure typically develops in the late teens or early 20s. More frequent causes of mild hyperoxaluria are dietary or enteric hyperoxaluria.
- Dietary hyperoxaluria from excessive ingestion of high oxalate-containing foods (e.g. spinach, rhubarb and tea), or from dietary calcium restriction with compensatory increased absorption of oxalate.
- Enteric hyperoxaluria: small bowel disease, e.g. Crohn's disease or resection, is associated with increased absorption of oxalate from the colon. Dehydration secondary to fluid loss from the gut also plays a part in stone formation.

Primary renal disease may lead to calcium stone formation. Medullary sponge kidney is associated with hypercalciuria and a tendency to develop stones (page 295). The alkaline urine seen in the renal tubular acidoses favours the precipitation of calcium phosphate.

Infection–induced stones Urinary tract infection with organisms that produce urease (*Proteus*, *Klebsiella* and *Pseudomonas* spp.) is associated with stones containing ammonium, magnesium and calcium. Urease hydrolyses urea to ammonia and thus raises the urine pH. An alkaline urine and high ammonia concentration favour stone formation. These stones are often large and fill the pelvicalyceal system, producing the typical radio-opaque staghorn calculus.

Uric acid stones Uric acid stones are sometimes associated with hyperuricaemia with or without clinical gout (page 228). Patients with ileostomies are also at risk of developing urate stones, as loss of bicarbonate from gastrointestinal secretions results in the production of an acid urine (uric acid is more soluble in an alkaline than an acid medium).

Cystine stones These may occur with cystinuria, an autosomal recessive condition affecting cystine and dibasic amino acid transport (lysine, ornithine and arginine) in the epithelial cells of renal tubules and the gastrointestinal tract. The excessive urinary excretion of cystine, which is the least soluble of the naturally occurring amino acids, leads to the formation of crystals and calculi.

Clinical features (Table 7.8)

Most people with urinary tract calculi are asymptomatic; pain is the most common symptom. Large staghorn renal calculi may cause loin pain. *Ureteric stones* cause renal colic, a severe intermittent pain lasting for hours. The pain is felt anywhere between the loin and the groin, and may radiate into the scrotum or labium or into the tip of the penis. Nausea and vomiting are common. Microscopic haematuria is almost always present. The patient will be pyrexial only if there is a UTI associated with the stone. *Bladder stones* present with urinary frequency and haematuria. *Urethral stones* may cause bladder outflow obstruction, resulting in anuria and painful bladder distension.

Table 7.8 Clinical features of urinary tract calculi

Asymptomatic
Pain
Haematuria
Urinary tract infection
Urinary tract obstruction

Investigations

In a patient presenting with renal colic the clinical diagnosis is confirmed by plain abdominal radiograph (KUB: kidney, ureters and bladder) and emergency intravenous urography. Ninety per cent of renal stones are radio-opaque and calcification may be seen in the line of the renal tract. Intravenous urography (IVU) shows a delayed nephrogram on the side of the stone.

A detailed history may reveal possible aetiological factors for stone formation, e.g. vitamin D consumption, gouty arthritis, recurrent UTIs, intestinal resection. The subsequent work-up for a renal calculus is indicated in Table 7.9.

Table 7.9 Investigations in a patient with urinary calculi

First line	Second line in recurrent stone formers

Urine
  Chemical analysis of any stone passed
  MSU for culture and sensitivity
	Two 24 h urine collections for calcium, oxalate and uric acid output

Blood
  Serum urea and electrolytes
  Serum calcium
  Serum uric acid
  Serum bicarbonate
	Random urine for cystine screening

Radiography
  Plain film
  Excretion urography	

Management

Initial treatment In the case of renal colic, a strong analgesic (e.g. an opiate or an NSAID) should be given to relieve the pain. Most ureteric stones that are 5 mm or less in diameter will pass spontaneously. Indications for surgical intervention include persistent pain, infection above the site of obstruction, and failure of the stone to pass down the ureter. The options for stone removal include the following:

- Percutaneous nephrolithotomy for stones in the renal pelvis and calyces
- Extracorporeal shock wave lithotripsy for renal stones
- Cystoscopic removal of ureteric and bladder stones
- Open surgery for very large stones.

Prevention of recurrence Further therapy depends on the type of stone and any underlying condition identified during screening investigations. For prevention of all stones, whatever the cause, it is important to maintain a high intake of fluid (to produce a urine volume of 2–2.5 l/day), particularly during the summer months. When no metabolic or renal abnormality has been identified ('idiopathic stone formers') adequate hydration is the mainstay of treatment.

- Idiopathic hypercalciuria. Reduction of dietary intake of calcium by avoiding milk, cheese and white bread is recommended, though its value has been questioned. A water softener may be helpful for patients who live in hard water areas. If hypercalciuria persists a thiazide diuretic, e.g. bendrofluazide, will reduce urinary calcium excretion.
- Mixed infective stones. Recurrent stones should be prevented by maintenance of a high fluid intake and measures to stop bacteriuria. This will require long-term follow-up and may demand the use of long-term, low-dose, prophylactic antibiotics.
- Uric acid stones are prevented by the long-term use of the xanthine oxidase inhibitor, allopurinol, which allows the excretion of the soluble precursor compound, hypoxanthine, in preference to uric acid. Oral sodium bicarbonate supplements to maintain an alkaline urine, and hence increased solubility of uric acid, is an alternative approach in those patients unable to tolerate allopurinol.
- Cystine stones. Patients may be unable to tolerate the very high fluid intake (5 litres of water in 24 hours) needed to maintain solubility of cystine in the urine. An alternative is D-penicillamine, which chelates cystine, forming a more soluble complex.

Nephrocalcinosis (Table 7.10)

The term 'nephrocalcinosis' means diffuse renal parenchymal calcification that is detectable radiologically. The condition is typically painless. Hypertension and renal impairment commonly occur. The treatment is of the underlying cause.

Table 7.10 Common causes of nephrocalcinosis

Mainly medullary
Hypercalcaemia
Renal tubular acidosis
Primary hyperoxaluria
Medullary sponge kidney
Tuberculosis

Mainly cortical (rare)
Renal cortical necrosis

URINARY TRACT OBSTRUCTION

The urinary tract may be obstructed at any point along its length between the kidney and the urethral meatus. This results in dilatation of the tract above the obstruction. Dilatation of the renal pelvis is known as *hydronephrosis*.

Aetiology

The causes of obstruction may be classified into four groups, listed in Table 7.11. In adults the most common causes are prostatic obstruction, gynaecological cancer and calculi.

Table 7.11 Causes of urinary tract obstruction

Within the lumen
Calculi
Blood clots
Sloughed renal papillae (diabetes, NSAIDs, sickle cell disease or trait)
Tumour

Within the wall
Stricture: ureteric or urethral
Neuropathic bladder
Pelviureteric junction obstruction (functional disturbance in peristalsis of collecting system)
Obstructive megaureter (defective peristalsis at lower end of ureter)

Pressure from outside
Prostatic hypertrophy/tumour
Pelvic tumours
Phimosis
Retroperitoneal fibrosis

Clinical features

- *Upper urinary tract obstruction* results in a dull ache in the flank or back which may be provoked by an increase in urine volume, e.g. high fluid intake or diuretics. Complete anuria is strongly suggestive of complete bilateral obstruction or complete obstruction of a single functioning kidney. Partial obstruction causes polyuria as a result of tubular damage and impairment of concentrating mechanisms.
- *Bladder outlet obstruction* results in hesitancy, poor stream, terminal dribbling and a sense of incomplete emptying.

Retention with overflow is characterized by the frequent passage of small quantities of urine. Infection commonly occurs and may precipitate acute retention of urine.

Depending on the site of obstruction an enlarged bladder or hydronephrotic kidney may be felt on examination. Pelvic and rectal examination is essential in determining the cause of obstruction.

Investigations

Imaging studies are performed to identify the site and nature of the obstruction and, together with serum biochemistry, to assess function of the affected kidney.

- Ultrasonography and excretion urography are the initial investigations. Ultrasonography confirms the diagnosis of obstruction and may show hydronephrosis. Excretion urography identifies the site of obstruction and shows a characteristic appearance (a delayed nephrogram, which eventually becomes denser than the non-obstructed side).
- Radionuclide studies (page 705) contribute to the management of obstruction by quantifying the degree of obstruction and function of the kidney. In general, absence of uptake of the radiopharmaceutical indicates renal damage that is sufficiently severe to render correction of the obstruction unprofitable.
- Subsequent investigations may include CT, retrograde and anterograde uretography, cystoscopy and pressure–flow studies during bladder filling and voiding. Anterograde uretography is particularly useful in both the diagnosis and therapy of patients with urinary obstruction. A fine catheter is introduced into the renal pelvis under ultrasound guidance. This allows the introduction of dye to determine the site and cause of obstruction; in addition, urine may be temporarily drained from an obstructed system while definitive treatment is planned.

Management

Surgery is the usual treatment for persistent urinary tract obstruction. Elimination of the obstruction may be associated with a massive postoperative diuresis, resulting partly from a solute diuresis from salt and urea retained during obstruction and partly from the renal concentrating defect. In some cases definitive relief of obstruction is not possible and urinary diversion may be required. This may be simply an indwelling urethral catheter, a stent placed across the obstructing lesion, or the formation of an ileal conduit.

RENAL FAILURE

The term 'renal failure' means failure of renal excretory function as a result of the depression of the glomerular filtration rate (GFR). This is accompanied to a variable extent by failure of erythropoietin production, vitamin D hydroxylation, regulation of acid–base balance, and regulation of salt and water balance and blood pressure.

- *Acute renal failure* (ARF) is a sudden and rapid decline in renal function which lasts days to weeks. It is usually reversible or self-limiting.
- *Chronic renal failure* (CRF) develops over months or years. It is usually not reversible but treatment may slow progression.

Acute renal failure

There is no universally accepted definition of acute renal failure (ARF), but commonly used definitions include an increase in the serum creatinine of more than 44 µmol/l or more than 50% over the baseline value.

Aetiology

ARF may be:

- Prerenal
- Renal
- Postrenal.

It may also result from a combination of these factors, e.g. in postsurgical ARF fluid depletion (prerenal), systemic infection and nephrotoxic drugs (renal) may all play a role. ARF may also complicate chronic renal failure ('*acute-on-chronic*').

Prerenal Failure of perfusion of the kidneys with blood occurs in prerenal failure. The kidney is able to maintain glomerular filtration close to normal in spite of wide variations in the renal perfusion pressure and volume status – so-called 'autoregulation'. Maintenance of a normal GFR in the face of decreased systemic pressure depends on the intrarenal production of prostaglandins and angiotensin II. With severe or prolonged hypovolaemia there is eventually a drop in glomerular filtration, termed 'prerenal failure'. Drugs that impair renal autoregulation, such as angiotensin-converting enzyme (ACE) inhibitors and non-steroidal anti-inflammatory drugs, increase the risk of prerenal failure in hypovolaemia. ACE inhibitors may also cause renal failure (ischaemic nephropathy) in patients with atherosclerotic renal artery stenosis (page 289), who may have evidence of atherosclerosis elsewhere, e.g ischaemic heart disease and peripheral vascular disease.

Prerenal failure is most commonly the result of hypovolaemia (Table 7.12), and is characterized in the early stages by lack of structural damage and rapid reversibility once normal renal perfusion has been restored. Hypovolaemia is identified from the clinical history and, on physical examination, by the presence of hypotension, a postural drop in blood pressure, a low jugular venous pressure (JVP) and reduced tissue turgor. Measurement of urinary electrolytes (Table 7.13) can help diffentiate

Table 7.12 Prerenal causes of acute renal failure

Hypovolaemia
Haemorrhage
Burns
Diarrhoea
Pancreatitis
Diabetic ketoacidosis
Diuretics
Sepsis

Decreased cardiac output
Myocardial infarction
Massive pulmonary embolism
Congestive cardiac failure

Severe liver failure (hepatorenal syndrome)

Renal artery obstruction

Table 7.13 Criteria for distinction between prerenal and intrinsic causes of renal dysfunction

	Prerenal	Intrinsic
Urine specific gravity	>1.020	<1.010
Urine osmolality (mOsmol/l)	>500	<350
Urine sodium (mmol/l)	<20	>40
Fractional excretion of sodium (Na^+)	<1%	>1%

$$\text{Fractional excretion of } Na^+ = \frac{[\text{Urine } Na^+/\text{Plasma Cr}]}{[\text{Plasma } Na^+/\text{Urine Cr}]} \times 100\%$$

where Cr is creatinine.

between prerenal ARF, in which the reabsorptive capacity of tubular cells and the concentrating ability of the kidney are preserved, and intrinsic renal failure, in which both these functions are impaired. However, the urinary indices do not completely segregate the two conditions and they are no substitute for a proper clinical assessment.

If, on the basis of the history and clinical examination, prerenal (hypovolaemia) failure is diagnosed or strongly suspected, the effect of volume repletion on renal function must be tested. Volume repletion should be with an appropriate fluid: blood in the case of posthaemorrhagic shock and physiological saline if fluid depletion is caused by vomiting, diarrhoea or polyuria. In some cases, e.g. with a very sick patient, volume replacement is guided by measurement of the central venous pressure. With pure prerenal failure, urine output should increase with volume replacement. If hypovolaemia is corrected (i.e. the JVP or CVP is normal) and urine output does not increase, the kidneys may respond to a strong diuretic stimulus (e.g. frusemide 120 mg i.v. over 10 minutes, which may be repeated once if there is no response). If urine output does not increase with these measures, then the patient has progressed to acute tubular necrosis (ATN) and the management is that of established intrinsic renal failure (see later).

Postrenal Postrenal ARF occurs when both urinary outflow tracts are obstructed or when one tract is obstructed in a patient with a single functional kidney (page 296). It is usually quickly reversed if the obstruction is relieved. All patients with ARF must be examined for evidence of obstruction (enlarged palpable kidneys or bladder, large prostate on rectal examination, pelvic masses on vaginal examination in women) and undergo renal ultrasonography to look for hydronephrosis and dilated ureters. Bladder outflow obstruction is ruled out by flushing of an existing catheter or insertion of a urethral catheter which should then be removed unless a large volume of urine is obtained. Treatment of obstruction is usually by a temporary measure, e.g. urethral/suprapubic catheterization or percutaneous nephrostomy until definitive treatment of the obstructing lesion can be undertaken.

Intrinsic renal failure Intrinsic renal diseases that result in ARF are categorized according to the primary site of injury: tubules, interstitium, renal vessels or glomerulus (Table 7.14). Injury to the tubules is most often ischaemic or toxic in origin. Prerenal ARF and ischaemic tubular necrosis represent a continuum, with the former leading to the latter when blood flow is sufficiently compromised to result in the death of tubular cells. In established renal failure the kidney loses its ability to concentrate the urine and conserve sodium. This may, in addition to clinical

Table 7.14 Causes of intrinsic renal failure

Acute tubular necrosis*
Ischaemia
Exogenous nephrotoxins: gentamicin, cephaloridine, intravenous contrast agents
Endogenous nephrotoxins: Bence-Jones protein, uric acid, myoglobin

Acute interstitial nephritis
Drug hypersensitivity
Infections

Large renal vessels
Renal artery thrombosis
Renal vein thrombosis

Small renal vessels
Vasculitis
Malignant hypertension
Haemolytic uraemic syndrome/thrombotic thrombocytopenic purpura

Acute glomerulonephritis

* Accounts for about 90% of intrinsic ARF.

examination, be useful in differentiating renal from prerenal failure where the kidney is able to concentrate the urine and conserve sodium (see Table 7.13).

Clinical features of established ARF

The early stages of renal failure are often completely asymptomatic. Symptoms are common when the plasma urea concentration is over 40 mmol/l, but many patients develop uraemic symptoms at lower levels of plasma urea. It is not the accumulation of urea itself that causes symptoms, but a combination of many different metabolic abnormalities.

- *Alteration of urine volume* Oliguria (urinary output <400 ml/day) usually occurs with acute renal failure, but there may be polyuria with the passage of large quantities of dilute urine.
- *Neurological* Weakness, fatigue and lassitude occur. Mental confusion, seizures and coma may also occur with severe uraemia, but this is less commonly seen since the introduction of effective renal replacement therapy.
- *Skin* Symptoms include pallor, pruritus, pigmentation and bruising.
- *Cardiopulmonary* Breathlessness occurs from a combination of anaemia and pulmonary oedema secondary to volume overload. There may be deep sighing respiration (Kussmaul's respiration) resulting from systemic metabolic acidosis. Pericarditis occurs with severe untreated uraemia and may be complicated by a pericardial effusion and tamponade.
- *Gastrointestinal* Nausea, anorexia and vomiting are common.
- *Haematological* Anaemia is most commonly seen in chronic renal failure but may occur in ARF. Impaired platelet function causes bruising and exacerbates gastrointestinal bleeding.

Investigation of the uraemic emergency

The purpose of investigation is:

- To differentiate acute from chronic renal failure (see page 308)

– To document the degree of renal impairment and obtain baseline values so that the response to treatment can be monitored. This is accomplished by measurement of serum urea and electrolytes, and a 24-hour creatinine clearance
– To establish whether ARF is prerenal, renal or postrenal, and to determine the underlying cause so that specific treatment (e.g. intensive immunosuppression in Wegener's granulomatosis) may be instituted as early as possible and thus prevent progression to irreversible renal failure.

- Blood count. Anaemia and a very high ESR may suggest myeloma or a vasculitis.
- Urine stix testing and microscopy. Glomerulonephritis is suggested by haematuria and proteinuria on urine stix testing and by the presence of red cell casts on urine microscopy (page 271).
- Urinary electrolytes. Measurement of urinary electrolytes (see Table 7.13) may help to exclude a significant prerenal element to ARF.
- Radiology. Every patient should undergo renal ultrasonography (for renal size and to exclude obstruction). CT is useful for the diagnosis of retroperitoneal fibrosis and some other causes of urinary obstruction, and may also indicate cortical scarring.
- Histological investigations. Renal biopsy should be considered in every patient with unexplained renal failure and normal-sized kidneys.
- Optional investigations (depending on the case):
  - Serum protein electrophoresis
  - Immunological: serum autoantibodies, ANCAs (page 695) and complement
  - Infectious screen: antibodies to hepatitis B and C and HIV
  - Blood cultures.

Management

The principles of management of established ARF are summarized in Emergency Box 7.1. In all patients with intrinsic renal failure, hypovolaemia and obstruction must be excluded as contributing factors.

> ! **Emergency**

Emergency resuscitation
To prevent death from hyperkalaemia (page 264) or pulmonary oedema (page 348)

Establish the aetiology and treat the underlying cause
- History, including family history, systemic disease, use of nephrotoxic drugs
- Examination includes assessment of haemodynamic status, pelvic and rectal examination
- Investigations, including bladder catheterization or flush of existing catheter

Prevention of further renal damage
Avoid sepsis, hypovolaemia, nephrotoxic drugs, NSAIDs and ACE inhibitors

Management of established renal failure
- Early specialist referral
- Once fluid balance has been corrected the daily fluid intake should equal fluid lost on the previous day plus insensible losses (approximately 500 ml)
- Adequate nutrition – enteral route preferred over parenteral
- Nursing care, e.g. prevention of pressure sores
- Adjust doses of drugs which are excreted by the kidney
- Monitor daily: urine volume, serum biochemistry, body weight
- Frequent review regarding the need for dialysis

Careful fluid and electrolyte balance during recovery phase
The patient may pass large volumes of dilute urine until the kidney recovers its concentrating ability

Emergency Box 7.1
Principles of management of a patient with acute renal failure

Indications for dialysis include:

- Hyperkalaemia not controlled by conservative measures
- Severe metabolic acidosis
- Pulmonary oedema
- Progressive uraemia with encephalopathy or pericarditis.

Whether haemodialysis, haemofiltration or peritoneal dialysis is used depends on the facilities available and the clinical circumstances, e.g. haemodialysis requires anticoagulation and thus would be inappropriate in a patient with recent haemorrhage from peptic ulceration.

Prognosis

The prognosis depends on the underlying cause. The most common cause of death is sepsis. In those who survive, renal function usually begins to recover within 2–3 weeks. ARF is irreversible in a few patients, probably because of cortical necrosis which, unlike tubules, which regenerate, heals with the formation of scar tissue.

Chronic renal failure

Aetiology

The causes of chronic renal failure (CRF) are listed in Table 7.15. In European countries diabetes mellitus is the single most common cause of end-stage renal failure. Hypertensive nephropathy and glomerulonephritis are other common causes. Regardless of the underlying cause, fibrosis of the remaining tubules, glomeruli and small blood vessels results in progressive renal scarring and eventually end-stage renal failure.

Clinical features and investigations

Clinical features are summarized in Table 7.16. Investigations are similar to those in ARF (page 303).

Table 7.15 The causes of end-stage renal failure

Congenital and hereditary disease
Polycystic kidneys

Glomerular disease
Primary glomerular disease
Secondary glomerular disease, e.g. diabetes mellitus, amyloidosis, systemic lupus

Tubulointerstitial disease
Reflux nephropathy
Chronic pyelonephritis
Tuberculosis
Nephrocalcinosis
Interstitial nephritis, e.g. drugs, idiopathic

Vascular disease
Atherosclerotic renal artery stenosis
Hypertensive nephropathy
Vasculitis

Urinary tract obstruction

Other
HIV-associated nephropathy

Table 7.16 Symptoms and signs of chronic renal failure

Anaemia
Pallor, lethargy, breathlessness on exercise

Platelet abnormality
Epistaxis, bruising

Skin
Pigmentation
Pruritus

Gastrointestinal tract
Anorexia, nausea, vomiting, diarrhoea

Endocrine/gonads
Amenorrhoea, erectile impotence, infertility

Central nervous system
Confusion, coma, fits (in severe uraemia)

Cardiovascular system
Uraemic pericarditis, hypertension, peripheral vascular disease, heart failure

Renal
Nocturia, polyuria, salt and water retention causing oedema

Renal osteodystrophy
Osteomalacia, muscle weakness, bone pain, hyperparathyroidism, osteosclerosis

In addition there may be symptoms and signs resulting from the long-term complications of CRF.

Anaemia This is present in the great majority of patients with CRF. The pathogenesis is multifactorial:

- Decreased erythropoietin production by the diseased kidney
- Depressed bone marrow activity
- Shortened red cell survival
- Increased blood loss (from the gut, during haemodialysis and as a result of repeated sampling)
- Dietary deficiency of haematinics (iron and folate).

Bone disease The term 'renal osteodystrophy' embraces the various forms of bone disease that develop in CRF, i.e. osteomalacia, osteoporosis, secondary and tertiary hyperparathyroidism, and osteosclerosis. Renal phosphate retention and impaired production of 1,25-dihydroxyvitamin D (the active hormonal form of vitamin

D) lead to a fall in serum calcium concentration and hence to a compensatory increase in parathyroid hormone (PTH) secretion. A sustained excess of PTH results in skeletal decalcification with the classic radiological features described in Figure 7.5. Osteosclerosis (hardening of bone) may be a result of hyperparathyroidism. Alternate bands of sclerotic and porotic bone in the vertebra produce the characteristic 'rugger jersey spine' radiographic appearance.

Neurological A motor and sensory neuropathy may occur in uraemia. Most commonly the sensory neuropathy may manifest as peripheral paraesthesiae. Median nerve compression in the carpal tunnel is common and is usually caused by β_2-microglobulin-related amyloidosis (see later). Autonomic dysfunction may present as postural hypotension and disturbed gastrointestinal motility. Dialysis produces an improvement in neuropathy.

Cardiovascular disease The highest mortality in CRF is from cardiovascular disease, which is increased as a result of the presence of hypertension, abnormalities of lipid metabolism and vascular calcification. Renal disease also results in a form of cardiomyopathy with both systolic and diastolic dysfunction.

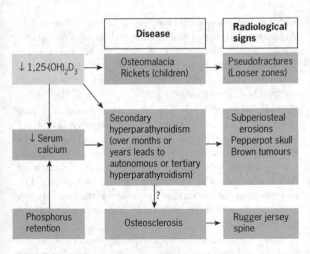

Figure 7.5
Pathogenesis and radiological features of renal osteodystrophy.

Other complications These include an increased risk of peptic ulceration, acute pancreatitis, hyperuricaemia, sexual dysfunction and, in children, failure to thrive.

Differentiating ARF from CRF

Distinction between ARF and CRF depends on the history, duration of symptoms and previous urinalysis or measurement of renal function. A normochromic anaemia, small kidneys on ultrasonography and the presence of renal osteodystrophy (see below) favour a chronic process.

Management

The underlying cause of renal disease should be treated aggressively wherever possible, e.g. tight metabolic control in diabetes.

Good blood pressure control may slow the decline in renal function. Of the antihypertensive agents, ACE inhibitors have particular protective effects on the glomeruli but must be used with caution in the presence of coexistent renal vascular disease. Low-protein diets, advocated on the basis that proteinuria accelerates renal scarring, are of uncertain value and patients are now usually advised to avoid high-protein diets.

Calcium and phosphate Hyperphosphataemia is treated by dietary restriction and oral calcium carbonate (a phosphate-binding agent). The serum calcium should be maintained in the normal range through the use of synthetic vitamin D analogues such as 1_α-cholecalciferol or the vitamin D metabolite 1,25-dihydroxyvitamin D_3 (1,25-$(OH)_2D_3$).

Anaemia Recombinant human erythropoietin is a very effective but expensive treatment for the anaemia of CRF and has largely replaced repeated blood transfusions. It is administered subcutaneously or intravenously three times weekly. Failure to respond may be the result of haematinic deficiency, bleeding, malignancy or infection. The disadvantages of treatment are that erythropoietin may accelerate hypertension and, rarely, lead to encephalopathy with convulsions.

Acidosis Systemic acidosis accompanies the decline in renal function and may contribute to increased serum potassium levels as well as dyspnoea and lethargy. Treatment is with

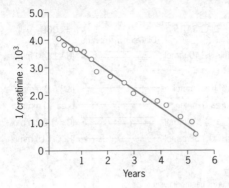

Figure 7.6
A reciprocal plot of serum creatinine against time. Such a slope is particular to an individual patient. It may be used to predict the time on onset of end-stage renal failure and thus prepare the patient for dialysis, e.g. the formation of an arteriovenous fistula.

oral sodium bicarbonate; the increased sodium load may exacerbate oedema and reduce blood pressure control.

Preparation for dialysis and transplantation In most patients with CRF there is a progressive loss of renal function, which proceeds at a constant rate for that patient (Figure 7.6). The graph of the reciprocal creatinine concentration plotted against time may be used to predict when the patient is likely to develop end-stage renal failure and thus require a form of renal replacement therapy. This may be haemodialysis, chronic ambulatory peritoneal dialysis or renal transplantation. Patients should be referred to a nephrologist by the time the serum creatinine reaches 350 μmol/l (250 μmol/l in diabetics), or earlier if the primary diagnosis is unknown.

··

RENAL REPLACEMENT THERAPY

Dialysis

'Uraemic toxins' can be efficiently removed from the blood by the process of diffusion across a semipermeable membrane towards the low concentrations present in dialysis fluid (Figure 7.7). The gradient is maintained by

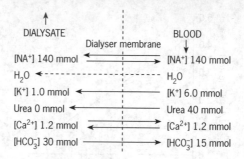

Figure 7.7
The principle of haemodialysis.

replacing used dialysis fluid with fresh solution. In haemodialysis, blood in an extracorporeal circulation is exposed to dialysis fluid separated by an artificial semipermeable membrane. In peritoneal dialysis the peritoneum is used as the semipermeable membrane and dialysis fluid is instilled into the peritoneal cavity.

Haemodialysis

Adequate dialysis requires a blood flow of at least 200 ml/min and the most reliable way of achieving this is by surgical construction of an arteriovenous fistula, usually in the forearm. This provides a permanent and easily accessible site for the insertion of needles. An adult of average size usually requires 4–5 hours of haemodialysis three times a week, which may be performed in hospital; in the UK some patients have self-supervised home haemodialysis. All patients are anticoagulated (usually with heparin) because contact of blood with foreign surfaces activates the clotting cascade. The most common acute complication of haemodialysis is hypotension, caused in part by excessive removal of extracellular fluid.

Haemofiltration

Haemofiltration is a form of haemodialysis (Figure 7.8) used most commonly in the treatment of ARF. The procedure employs a highly permeable membrane which allows large amounts of fluid and solute to be removed from

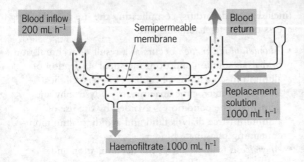

Figure 7.8
Principles of haemofiltration.

the patient which is then replaced by a solution with the desired biochemical composition. It is readily performed in intensive care units on very sick patients, as haemofiltration can be managed by ITU nursing staff rather than renal unit nurses.

Peritoneal dialysis

- *Continuous ambulatory peritoneal dialysis* (CAPD) requires the insertion of a permanent catheter (Tenkoff catheter) into the peritoneum via a subcutaneous tunnel. Up to 3 litres of dialysate are introduced and exchanged three to five times a day.
- *Intermittent peritoneal dialysis* Dialysate is introduced into the peritoneal cavity via a catheter and exchanged every 60–120 minutes, requiring the patient to remain in bed during treatment. It is mainly used in ARF.

Peritonitis is the most common serious complication of peritoneal dialysis. Infection with *Staph. epidermidis* accounts for 50% of cases. Treatment is with appropriate antibiotics, which are often given intraperitoneally.

Long-term complications of dialysis

Cardiovascular disease (as a result of atheroma) and sepsis are the leading causes of death in long-term dialysis patients. Causes of fatal sepsis include peritonitis complicating peritoneal dialysis and *Staph. aureus* infection (including endocarditis) complicating the use of indwelling access devices for haemodialysis.

- *Aluminium intoxication* occurs as a result of accumulation of dialysis solution and from intestinal absorption of aluminium-containing phosphate binders. Clinical features are microcytic anaemia, osteodystrophy and dementia. The condition is avoided by the use of aluminium-free dialysis fluid and avoiding aluminium-containing phosphate binders.
- *Amyloidosis* is the result of the accumulation and polymerization of β_2-microglobulin. This molecule (a component of HLA proteins on most cell membranes) is normally excreted by the kidneys, but is not removed by dialysis membranes. Deposition results in the carpal tunnel syndrome and joint pains, particularly of the shoulders.

Transplantation

Successful renal transplantation offers the potential for complete rehabilitation in end-stage renal failure. It allows freedom from dietary and fluid restriction, anaemia and infertility are corrected and the need for parathyroidectomy reduced. In the best centres graft survival is 80% at 10 years. Kidneys are obtained from cadavers or, less frequently, from healthy close relatives. The donor must be ABO compatible and good HLA matching increases the chances of successful transplantation. The donor kidney is placed in the iliac fossa and anastomosed to the iliac vessels of the recipient; the donor ureter is placed into the recipient's bladder. Graft rejection is reduced by giving long-term immunosuppressive treatment (unless the donor is an identical twin, i.e. genetically identical), which comprises corticosteroids, azathioprine and cyclosporin A, and sometimes tacrolimus. Antilymphocyte globulin is a potent immunosuppressive and is increasingly used in both the treatment and prevention of rejection. The complications of renal transplanation and immunosuppression include opportunistic infection (e.g. *Pneumocystis carinii*), hypertension, the development of tumours (skin malignancies and lymphomas) and, occasionally, recurrence of the renal disease (e.g. Goodpasture's syndrome).

CYSTIC RENAL DISEASE

Solitary and multiple renal cysts

Renal cysts are common, particularly with advancing age. They are usually asymptomatic and discovered incidentally on ultrasonography or excretion urography performed for some other reason. Occasionally they may cause pain and/or haematuria.

Adult polycystic disease

Adult polycystic disease (APCD) is an autosomal dominantly inherited condition in which multiple cysts develop throughout both kidneys. Cysts increase in size with advancing age and lead to renal enlargement and the progressive destruction of normal kidney tissue, with gradual loss of renal function. Most cases are due to a mutation in the *PKD-1* gene (short arm of chromosome 16), which encodes for a protein, polycystin, thought to be important in normal tubular development.

Clinical features

The disease presents at any age after the second decade. Presenting symptoms include the following:

- Acute loin pain and/or haematuria as a result of haemorrhage into a cyst
- Abdominal discomfort caused by renal enlargement
- Development of hypertension or symptoms of uraemia.

About 30% of patients will develop hepatic cysts, which are usually clinically insignificant. More rarely cysts develop in the pancreas, spleen, ovary and other organs. Berry aneurysms of the cerebral vessels are found in 8% of patients; these may result in subarachnoid haemorrhage.

Diagnosis

Clinical examination commonly reveals large irregular kidneys, hypertension and possibly hepatomegaly. A definitive diagnosis is established by ultrasonography.

Management

Treatment involves careful control of blood pressure and salt replacement if necessary. As the disease is always progressive, many patients will require renal replacement by dialysis and/or transplantation. Children and siblings of patients with the disease should be offered ultrasonographic screening. This is carried out in the second decade because diagnosis before this age is difficult and hypertension is rare in the very young.

Medullary sponge kidney

Medullary sponge kidney is an uncommon condition characterized by dilatation of the collecting ducts in the papillae with associated stasis of urine. In severe cases there are numerous cysts and the medullary area has a sponge-like appearance. In 20% of patients there is hypercalciuria or renal tubular acidosis (see page 270). The diagnosis is made by excretion urography. Most patients have intermittent colic, with the passage of small stones, or haematuria with well-preserved renal function.

TUMOURS OF THE KIDNEY AND GENITOURINARY TRACT

Renal cell carcinoma

Renal cell carcinomas (previously called hypernephroma or Grawitz's tumours) are the most common renal tumours in adults, presenting most commonly in the fifth decade, with a male:female ratio of 2:1. They arise from the proximal tubular epitheliums and may be solitary, multiple and occasionally bilateral.

Clinical features

Haematuria, loin pain and a mass in the flank are the most common presenting features. Other features include malaise, weight loss, fever and occasionally polycythaemia (page 166). Twenty-five per cent have metastases at presentation to bone, liver and the lung, where they are often solitary and large ('cannonball' metastases).

Investigations

Excretion urography will reveal a space-occupying lesion in the kidney.

Ultrasonography will demonstrate a solid lesion and can assess the patency of the renal vein and inferior vena cava.

MRI and CT are useful for tumour staging.

Management

Surgery forms the mainstay of treatment. Nephrectomy is carried out unless there is bilateral involvement or the contralateral kidney functions poorly. Medroxyprogesterone and α-interferon may be of value in controlling metastatic disease.

Prognosis

The 5-year survival rate is 60–70% when the tumour is confined to the renal parenchyma, but less than 5% in those with distant metastases.

Urothelial tumours

The calyces, renal pelvis, ureter, bladder and urethra are lined by transitional cell epithelium. Bladder tumours are the most common form of transitional cell malignancy. They occur most commonly after the age of 40 years and are four times more common in males. Predisposing factors include the following:

- Cigarette smoking
- Industrial chemicals, e.g. β-naphthylamine, benzidine
- Drugs, e.g. phenacetin, cyclophosphamide
- Chronic inflammation, e.g. schistosomiasis.

Clinical features

Painless haematuria is the most common symptom of bladder cancer, although pain may occur from clot retention. Transitional cell cancers of the kidney and ureters may cause haematuria and flank pain.

Investigations

- Cytology of the urine may show malignant cells.
- Excretion urography may show filling defects, but small tumours may not be seen.
- Cystoscopy if no evidence of upper urinary tract pathology has been found.

Management

Pelvic and ureteric tumours are treated with surgical resection. Treatment of bladder tumours depends on the stage, but options include local diathermy or cystoscopic resection, bladder resection, radiotherapy, and local and systemic chemotherapy.

DISEASES OF THE PROSTATE GLAND

Benign enlargement of the prostate gland

Benign prostatic enlargement is extremely common, occurring most commonly after the age of 60 years. There is hyperplasia of both glandular and connective tissue elements of the gland, although the aetiology of the condition remains unknown.

Clinical features

Frequency of micturition, nocturia, delay in initiation of micturition and postvoid dribbling are common symptoms. Acute urinary retention or retention with overflow incontinence may occur. An enlarged smooth prostate may be felt on rectal examination.

Investigations

Serum electrolytes and renal ultrasonography are performed to exclude renal damage resulting from obstruction. Serum prostate-specific antigen (PSA) is markedly raised in prostate cancer, which may present similarly (see below).

Management

Patients with mild or moderate symptoms may require no treatment or medical treatment only. Selective α_1-adrenoreceptor antagonists (prazosin, terazosin) relax smooth muscle in the bladder neck and prostate. 5_α-reductase inhibitors such as finasteride block the conversion of testosterone to dihydrotestosterone – the latter is thought to be responsible for the development of prostatic hypertrophy. α-Blockers provide better symptom relief than finasteride. Patients with severe symptoms or with dilatation of the upper urinary tract require surgery, most commonly with transurethral resection of the prostate (TURP).

Prostatic carcinoma

Prostatic adenocarcinoma is common, accounting for 7% of all cancers in men. Malignant change within the prostate is increasingly common with increasing age, being present in 80% of men aged 80 and over. In most cases these malignant foci remain dormant.

Clinical features

Most patients present with symptoms of bladder outflow obstruction identical to those of benign prostatic hypertrophy. Patients may also present with metastases, particularly to bone. In some cases malignancy is unsuspected until histological investigation is carried out on the resected specimen after prostatectomy. Rectal examination may reveal a hard irregular gland.

Investigation

Investigation is as for benign prostatic enlargement, with measurement of serum PSA. Supplemental tests include transrectal ultrasonography, which helps in tumour staging, and transrectal biopsy for histological confirmation.

Management

Microscopic tumour is sometimes managed by watchful waiting. Treatment of disease confined to the gland is radical prostatectomy or radiotherapy, both resulting in 80–90% 5-year survival. The treatment of metastatic disease depends on removing androgenic drive to the tumour. This is achieved by bilateral orchidectomy, synthetic luteinizing hormone-releasing hormone analogues, e.g. goserelin, or antiandrogens, e.g. cyproterone acetate.

Screening

Annual measurement of prostate-specific antigen in asymptomatic men results in earlier diagnosis of prostate cancer. Large scale trials are in progress to determine the potential benefits (i.e. increased survival) and drawbacks of screening (expense, side-effects of treatment, emotional impact of a positive result).

···

URINARY INCONTINENCE

Normal bladder physiology

As the bladder fills with urine two factors act to ensure continence until it is next emptied:

- Intravesical pressure remains low as a result of stretching of the bladder wall and the stability of the bladder muscle (detrusor), which does not contract involuntarily.

- The sphincter mechanisms of the bladder neck and urethral muscles.

At the onset of voiding the sphincters relax (mediated by decreased sympathetic activity) and the detrusor muscle contracts (mediated by increased parasympathetic activity). Overall control and coordination of micturition is by higher brain centres, which include the cerebral cortex and the pons.

Stress incontinence

Stress incontinence occurs as a result of sphincter weakness, which may be iatrogenic in men (post-prostactectomy) or the result of childbirth in women. There is a small leak of urine when intra-abdominal pressure rises, e.g. with coughing, laughing or standing up. In young women pelvic floor exercises may help. In postmenopausal women the contributing factor of urethral atrophy may be helped by oestrogen creams.

Urge incontinence

In urge incontinence there is a strong desire to void and the patient may be unable to hold his or her urine. The usual cause is detrusor instability, which occurs most often in women, and the aetiology is not known. Mild cases may respond to bladder retraining (gradually increasing the time interval between voids). More severe cases are treated with anticholinergic agents, which decrease detrusor excitability. Less commonly, urge incontinence is caused by bladder hypersensitivity from local pathology (e.g. UTI, bladder stones, tumours) and treatment is then of the underlying cause.

Overflow incontinence

Overflow incontinence is most often seen in men with prostatic hypertrophy causing outflow obstruction. There is leakage of small amounts of urine, and on abdominal examination the distended bladder is felt rising out of the pelvis. If the obstruction is not relieved then renal damage will develop.

Neurological causes

These are usually apparent from the history and examination, which reveal accompanying neurological deficits. Brain-stem damage, e.g. trauma, may lead to incoordination of detrusor muscle activity and sphincter relaxation, so that the two contract together during voiding. This results in a high-pressure system with the risk of obstructive uropathy. The aim of treatment is to reduce outflow pressure, either with α-adrenergic blockers or by sphincterotomy. Autonomic neuropathy, e.g. in diabetic individuals, decreases detrusor excitability and results in a distended atonic bladder with a large residual urine which is liable to infection. Permanent catheterization may be necessary.

In elderly people incontinence may be the result of a combination of factors: diuretic treatment, dementia (antisocial incontinence) and difficulty in getting to the toilet because of immobility.

COMMON PRESENTING SYMPTOMS OF HEART DISEASE

The common symptoms of heart disease are chest pain, breathlessness, palpitations and syncope.

Chest pain

Acute chest pain or discomfort is a common presenting symptom of cardiovascular disease and must be differentiated from non-cardiac causes. The site of pain, its character, radiation and associated symptoms will often point to the cause (Table 8.1).

Dyspnoea

Dyspnoea is an abnormal awareness of breathing. The causes are discussed on page 392. Left heart failure is the most

Table 8.1 Common causes of chest pain

Usually retrosternal	
Angina pectoris	Crushing pain on exercise, relieved by rest. May radiate to jaw or arms
Myocardial infarction	Similar in character to angina but more severe, occurs at rest, lasts longer
Pericarditis	Sharp pain aggravated by movement, respiration and changes in posture
Aortic dissection	Severe tearing chest pain which radiates to the back
Reflux oesophagitis	Pain may occur at night and when bending or lying down. Pain may radiate into the neck
Other sites	
Pulmonary infarct ⎫ Pneumonia ⎬ Pneumothorax ⎭	Typically pleuritic in nature, i.e. sharp, well localized pain aggravated by inspiration, coughing and movement
Costochondritis ⎫ ⎬ Fractured rib ⎭	Musculoskeletal pain is usually a sharp, well localized pain with a tender area on palpation

common cardiac cause of exertional dyspnoea, which may be accompanied by orthopnoea (breathlessness on lying flat).

Palpitations

A palpitation is an awareness of the heartbeat. The normal heartbeat is sensed when the patient is anxious, excited, exercising or lying on the left side. In other circumstances it usually indicates a cardiac arrhythmia, commonly ectopic beats or a paroxysmal tachycardia (page 327).

Syncope and dizziness

Syncope means a temporary impairment of consciousness as a result of cerebral ischaemia. There are many causes, but the most common is a simple faint. The cardiac causes of syncope are the result of either very fast (e.g. ventricular tachycardia) or very slow heart rates (e.g. complete heart block) which are unable to maintain an adequate cardiac output. Attacks occur suddenly and without warning. They last only 1 or 2 minutes, with complete recovery in seconds (compare with epilepsy, where complete recovery may be delayed for some hours). Obstruction to ventricular outflow also causes syncope (e.g. aortic stenosis, hypertrophic cardiomyopathy), which typically occurs on exercise when the requirements for increased cardiac output cannot be met.

Other symptoms

Tiredness, lethargy and exertional fatigue occur with cardiac failure and result from poor perfusion of brain and skeletal muscle. Heart failure also causes salt and water retention, leading to oedema, which in ambulant patients is most prominent over the ankles. In severe cases it may involve the genitalia and thighs.

The electrocardiogram

The electrocardiogram (ECG) is a recording from the body surface of the electrical activity of the heart. The standard ECG has 12 leads:

- Chest leads, V1–V6, which look at the heart in a *horizontal plane* (Figure 8.1)
- Limb leads, which look at the heart in a *vertical plane* (Figure 8.2). Limb leads are unipolar (AVR, AVL and AVF) or bipolar (I, II, III).

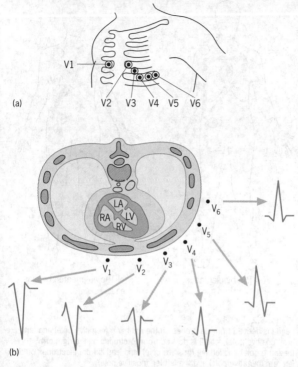

Figure 8.1
(a) The V leads are attached to the chest wall overlying the intercostal spaces as shown: V4 in the midclavicular line, V5 in the anterior axillary line, V6 in the midaxillary line. **(b)** Leads V1 and V2 look at the right ventricle, V3 and V4 at the interventricular septum, and V5 and V6 at the left ventricle. the normal QRS complex in each lead is shown.

The ECG machine is arranged so that when a depolarization wave spreads towards a lead the needle moves upwards, and when it spreads away from the lead the needle moves downwards.

ECG waveform and definitions (Figure 8.3)

The *heart rate*. At normal paper speed (25 mm/s in the UK) each 'big square' is 0.2 s. The heart rate (if the rhythm is

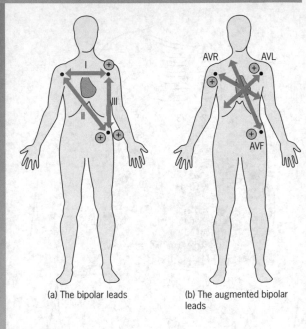

(a) The bipolar leads

(b) The augmented bipolar leads

Figure 8.2
Lead I is derived from electrodes on the right arm (negative pole) and left arm (positive pole), lead II is derived from electrodes on the right arm (negative pole) and left leg (positive pole), and lead III from electrodes on the left arm (negative pole) and the left leg (positive pole).

regular) is calculated by counting the number of big squares between consecutive R waves and dividing into 300.

The *P wave* is the first deflection and is caused by atrial depolarization. When abnormal it may be:

- Broad and notched (> 0.12 s) in left atrial enlargement ('P mitrale', e.g. mitral stenosis)
- Tall and peaked (> 2.5 mm) in right atrial enlargement ('P pulmonale', e.g. pulmonary hypertension)
- Replaced by flutter or fibrillation waves (page 332)
- Absent in sinoatrial block (page 328).

The *QRS complex* represents ventricular depolarization:

- A negative (downward) deflection preceding an R wave is called a Q wave. Normal Q waves are small and

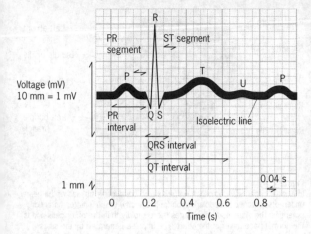

Figure 8.3
The waves and elaboration of the normal ECG. (Modified from Goldman (1976) Principles of Clinical Electrocardiography, 3rd edn. Longman, Los Altos.)

narrow; deep, wide Q waves (except in AVR and V1) indicate myocardial infarction (page 354).

- A deflection upwards is called an R wave whether or not it is preceded by a Q wave.
- A negative deflection following an R wave is termed an S wave.

Ventricular depolarization starts in the septum and spreads from left to right (Figure 8.4). Subsequently the main free walls of the ventricles are depolarized. Thus, in the right ventricular leads (V1 and V2) the first deflection is upwards (R wave) as the septal depolarization wave spreads towards those leads. The second deflection is downwards (S wave) as the bigger left ventricle (in which depolarization is spreading away) outweighs the effect of the right ventricle (see Figure 8.1). The opposite pattern is seen in the left ventricular leads (V5 and V6), with an initial downwards deflection (small Q wave reflecting septal depolarization) followed by a large R wave caused by left ventricular depolarization.

Left ventricular hypertrophy: the increased bulk of the left ventricular myocardium in left ventricular hypertrophy (e.g. with sytemic hypertension) increases the voltage induced

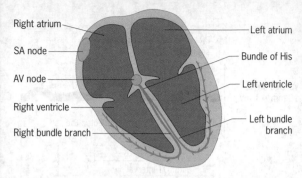

Right atrium

SA node

AV node

Right ventricle

Right bundle branch

Left atrium

Bundle of His

Left ventricle

Left bundle branch

Figure 8.4
In normal circumstances only the specialized conducting tissues of the heart
undergo spontaneous depolarization (automaticity) which initiates an action
potential. The sinus node discharges more rapidly than the other cells and is
the normal pacemaker of the heart. The impulse generated by the sinus
node spreads first through the atria, producing atrial systole, and then
through the atrioventricular node to the His–Purkinje system, producing
ventricular systole.

depolarization of the free wall of the left ventricle. This
gives rise to tall R waves (>25 mm) in the left ventricular
leads (V5,V6) and/or deep S waves (>30 mm) in the right
ventricular leads (V1,V2). The sum of the R wave in the left
ventricular leads and the S wave in the right ventricular
leads exceeds 40 mm. In addition to these changes there
may also be ST-segment depression and T wave flattening or
inversion in the left ventricular leads.

Right ventricular hypertrophy (e.g. in pulmonary
hypertension) causes tall R waves in the right ventricular
leads.

The QRS duration reflects the time that excitation takes
to spread through the ventricle. A wide QRS complex
(>0.10 s) occurs if conduction is delayed, e.g. with right or
left bundle-branch block, or if conduction is through
abnormal pathways, e.g. ventricular ectopic.

T waves result from ventricular repolarization. In general
the direction of the T wave is the same as that of the QRS
complex. Inverted T waves occur in many conditions and,
although usually abnormal, they are a non-specific finding.

The *PR interval* is measured from the start of the P wave
to the start of the QRS complex. It is the time taken for

excitation to pass from the sinus node, through the atrium, atrioventricular node and His–Purkinje system to the ventricle. A prolonged PR interval (>0.22 s) indicates heart block (page 329).

The *ST segment* is the period between the end of the QRS complex and the start of the T wave. ST elevation (>1 mm above the isoelectric line) occurs in the early stages of myocardial infarction (page 354) and with acute pericarditis. ST segment depression (>0.5 mm below the isoelectric line) indicates myocardial ischaemia.

CARDIAC ARRHYTHMIAS

An abnormality of the cardiac rhythm is called a cardiac arrhythmia. Such a disturbance may cause sudden death, syncope, dizziness, palpitations or no symptoms at all. Paroxysmal arrhythmias may not be detected on a single ECG recording. Twenty-four-hour ambulatory ECG monitoring (continuous recording for 24 hours) and event recorders (a portable device activated by the patient to record the ECG when symptoms occur) are outpatient investigations often used to detect arrhythmias causing intermittent symptoms.

There are two main types of arrhythmia:

* *Bradycardia*, where the heart rate is slow (<60 beats/min). The slower the heart rate the more probable that the arrhythmia will be symptomatic
* *Tachycardia*, where the heart rate is fast (>100 beats/min). Tachycardias are more likely to be symptomatic when the arrhythmia is fast and sustained. They are subdivided into *supraventricular tachycardias*, which arise from the atrium or the atrioventricular junction, and *ventricular tachycardias*, which arise from the ventricles.

Arrhythmias and conduction disturbances complicating acute myocardial infarction are discussed on page 359.

Sinus rhythms
Sinus arrhythmia
Fluctuations of autonomic tone result in phasic changes in the sinus discharge rate. Thus, during inspiration

parasympathetic tone falls and the heart rate quickens, and on expiration the heart rate falls. This variation is normal, particularly in children and young adults.

Sinus bradycardia

Sinus bradycardia is normal during sleep and in well trained athletes. During the acute phase of a myocardial infarction it often reflects ischaemia of the sinus node. Other causes include hypothermia, hypothyroidism, cholestatic jaundice, raised intracranial pressure, and drug therapy with β-blockers, digitalis and other antiarrhythmic drugs. Patients with symptomatic bradycardia are treated with a permanent cardiac pacemaker. Intravenous atropine (600 mg i.v.) is used in the acute situation.

Sinus tachycardia

Sinus tachycardia is a physiological response during exercise and excitement. It may also occur with fever, anaemia, cardiac failure, thyrotoxicosis and drugs (e.g. catecholamines and atropine). Treatment is aimed at correction of the underlying cause. If necessary, β-blockers may be used to slow the sinus rate, but not in uncontrolled heart failure.

Pathological bradycardias

There are two main forms of severe bradycardia: sinus node disease and atrioventricular block.

Sinus node disease (sick sinus syndrome)

Most cases of chronic sinus node disease are the result of idiopathic fibrosis occurring in elderly people. Bradycardia is caused by intermittent failure of sinus node depolarization or failure of the sinus impulse to propagate through the perinodal tissue to the atria. This is seen on the ECG as a long pause between consecutive P waves (>2 s). The slow heart rate predisposes to ectopic pacemaker activity and tachyarrhythmias are common (tachy–brady syndrome).

Insertion of a permanent pacemaker is only indicated in symptomatic patients to prevent dizzy spells and blackouts. Antiarrhythmic drugs are used to treat tachycardias. Thromboembolism is common in sick sinus syndrome and patients should be anticoagulated unless there is a contraindication.

Atrioventricular block

There are three forms: first-degree heart block, second-degree (partial) block and third-degree (complete) block. The common causes are ischaemic heart disease, cardiomyopathy and, particularly in elderly people, fibrosis of the conducting tissue.

- *First-degree atrioventricular (AV) block* is the result of delayed atrioventricular conduction and reflected by a prolonged PR interval on the ECG. No change in heart rate occurs and treatment is unnecessary.
- *Second-degree (partial AV) block* occurs when some atrial impulses fail to reach the ventricles. Asymptomatic patients require no treatment other than careful follow-up, because there may be progression to complete heart block. Symptomatic patients are treated with insertion of a permanent pacemaker. There are three forms (Figure 8.5):
  - Mobitz type 1 block (Wenckebach's phenomenon), in which the PR interval gradually increases, culminating in a dropped beat
  - Mobitz type II block occurs when a dropped QRS complex is not preceded by progressive PR prolongation
  - A 2:1 or 3:1 block occurs when every second or third P wave conducts to the ventricles. A 4:1 or 5:1 block can also occur.
- *Third-degree (complete) AV block.* There is no association between atrial and ventricular activity and ventricular contractions are maintained by a spontaneous escape rhythm (usually about 40/min) from an automatic centre below the site of the block. The ECG shows regular P waves and QRS complexes which occur independently of one another. The usual symptoms are dizziness and blackouts (Stokes–Adams attacks). If the ventricular rate is very slow, cardiac failure may occur. Insertion of a permanent pacemaker is always required for sustained complete heart block. In the acute situation, e.g. myocardial infarction, recovery may be expected and intravenous atropine or a temporary pacemaker may be all that is necessary

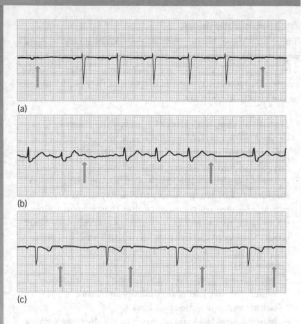

Figure 8.5
Three varieties of second-degree atrioventricular (AV) block. **(a)** Wenckebach (Mobitz-type I) AV block. The PR interval gradually prolongs until the P wave does not conduct to the ventricles (arrows). **(b)** Mobitz-type II AV block. The P waves that do not conduct to the ventricles (arrows) are not preceded by gradual PR interval prolongation. **(c)** Two P waves to each QRS complex. The PR interval prior to the dropped P wave is always the same. It is not possible to define this type of AV block as type I or type II Mobitz block and it is, therefore, a third variety of second-degree AV block (arrows show P waves).

Intraventricular conduction disturbances

The intraventricular conduction system consists of the His bundle, the right and left bundle branches and the anterosuperior and posteroinferior divisions of the left bundle-branch block. Complete block of a bundle branch is associated with a wider QRS complex (0.12 s or more). The shape of the QRS depends on whether the right or the left bundle is blocked.

Pathological tachycardias
Mechanisms of arrhythmia production

The mechanisms responsible for most tachyarrhythmias are abnormal automaticity and re-entry mechanisms.

Abnormal automaticity

Arrhythmias arise if there is enhanced automaticity of the normal conducting tissue or automaticity is acquired by damaged cells of the atria or ventricles; this causes ectopic beats and, if sustained, tachyarrhythmias.

Re-entry Re-entry may occur if there are two separate pathways for impulse conduction (Figure 8.6).

Atrial tachyarrhythmias

Ectopic beats, tachycardia, flutter and fibrillation may all arise from the atrial myocardium. They share common aetiologies, which are listed in Table 8.2.

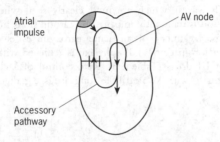

Figure 8.6
A re-entry circuit. The impulse is conducted normally through the AV node and initiates ventricular depolarization. In certain circumstances the accessory pathway is able to transmit the impulse retrogradely back in to the atria, thus completing a circuit and initiating a self-sustaining re-entry tachycardia.

Table 8.2 Causes of atrial arrhythmias

Ischaemic heart disease
Rheumatic heart disease
Thyrotoxicosis
Cardiomyopathy
Lone atrial fibrillation (i.e. no cause discovered)
Wolff–Parkinson–White syndrome
Pneumonia
Atrial septal defect
Carcinoma of the bronchus
Pericarditis
Pulmonary embolus
Acute and chronic alcohol abuse
Cardiac surgery

Atrial ectopic beats

These are caused by premature discharge of an ectopic atrial focus. On the ECG this produces an early and abnormal P wave, usually followed by a normal QRS complex. Treatment is not usually required unless they cause troublesome palpitations or are responsible for provoking more significant arrhythmias.

Atrial flutter

Atrial flutter is almost always associated with organic disease of the heart. The atrial rate is usually about 300 beats/min. The AV node usually conducts every second flutter beat, giving a ventricular rate of 150 beats/min. The ECG (Figure 8.7(a)) characteristically shows 'sawtooth' flutter waves (F waves), which are most clearly seen when AV conduction is transiently impaired by carotid sinus massage or drugs. Treatment of an acute paroxysm is electrical cardioversion (page 641). Prophylaxis is achieved with class Ia, Ic or III drugs (Table 8.3). Rate control of a chronic arrhythmia is with AV nodal blocking drugs, e.g. digoxin.

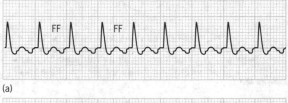

(a)

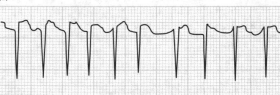

(b)

Figure 8.7
(a) Atrial flutter. The flutter waves are marked with an F, only half of which are transmitted to the ventricles. (b) Atrial fibrillation. There are no P waves, the ventricular response is fast and irregular.

Table 8.3 Vaughan Williams classification of antiarrhythmic drug therapy

Class	Mechanism of action	Individual drugs
Ia	Membrane-stabilizing action	Quinidine, procainamide, disopyramide
Ib		Lignocaine, mexiletine
Ic		Flecainide, propafenone
II	β-Adrenergic blockers	Metoprolol, atenolol, propranolol
III	Increases refractory period of conducting system	Amiodarone, sotalol, bretylium
IV	Calcium channel blocking agents	Verapamil, diltiazem

Adenosine and digoxin are other antiarrhythmic drugs which do not fit into this classification.
These drugs all have proarrhythmic side effects (among others) and should be used with caution.
All except amiodarone are negatively inotropic and may exacerbate heart failure.

Atrial fibrillation (AF)

This is a common arrhythmia, occurring in between 5% and 10% of patients over 65 years of age. It also occurs, particularly in a paroxysmal form, in younger patients. Atrial activity is chaotic and mechanically ineffective. The AV node conducts a proportion of the atrial impulses to produce an irregular ventricular response. There are no clear P waves on the ECG (Figure 8.7(b)), only a fine oscillation of the baseline (so-called fibrillation or f waves).

When AF arises in an apparently normal heart it is sometimes possible to convert to sinus rhythm, either electrically (by cardioversion, page 641) or chemically (with class Ia, Ic or III drugs). When AF is caused by an acute precipitating event, such as alcohol toxicity, chest infection or thyrotoxicosis, the underlying cause should be treated initially. Chronic AF occurring in a diseased heart will usually not respond to cardioversion, and treatment is by control of the ventricular rate, usually with digoxin. Atrial fibrillation is associated with an increased risk of thromboembolism and anticoagulation should be given for at least 3 weeks before (with the exception of those who require emergency cardioversion) and 4 weeks after cardioversion. Most patients with chronic AF should also be anticoagulated (INR 2.0–3.0). The exception is young patients with lone AF who are not diabetic or hypertensive. This group has a low incidence of thromboembolism and is treated with aspirin alone.

Junctional tachycardia

Junctional tachycardias are paroxysmal in nature and usually occur in the absence of structural heart disease. They are re-entrant arrhythmias caused by an abnormal pathway in the AV node or by an accessory pathway (bundle of Kent), as in the Wolff–Parkinson–White syndrome (Figure 8.8). The usual history is of a sudden onset of fast (140–280/min) regular palpitations. On the ECG the P waves may be seen very close to the QRS complex, or are not seen at all. The QRS complex is usually of normal shape because, as with other supraventricular arrhythmias, the ventricles are activated in the normal way, down the bundle of His. Occasionally the QRS complex is wide, because of a rate-related bundle-branch block, and it may be difficult to distinguish from ventricular tachycardia.

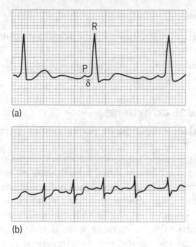

Figure 8.8
(a) An ECG showing Wolff–Parkinson–White syndrome. During sinus rhythm electrical impulses are conducted quickly through the abnormal pathway resulting in a short PR interval and a slurred proximal limb of the QRS complex (δ wave). **(b)** A trace demonstrating the paroxysmal tachycardia which may result from this syndrome.

Termination of an attack

- Manoeuvres that increase vagal stimulation of the sinus node: carotid sinus massage, ocular pressure or the Valsalva manoeuvre
- Drug treatment: Adenosine is a very short-acting AV nodal blocking drug given as a 3 mg bolus dose intravenously. It will terminate most junctional tachycardias. If there is no response after 1–2 minutes a further bolus of 6 mg is given. A third bolus of 12 mg may be given if there is still no response. Transient side effects include complete heart block, hypotension, nausea and bronchospasm. Asthma and second- or third-degree AV block are contraindications to adenosine. An alternative treatment is intravenous verapamil 10 mg i.v. over 5–10 minutes (contraindicated if the QRS complex is wide and therefore differentiation from ventricular tachycardia difficult)
- Rapid atrial pacing or DC cardioversion is used if adenosine fails.

Prophylaxis

- Radiofrequency ablation of the accessory pathway via a cardiac catheter
- Flecainide, disopyramide, amiodarone and β-blockers are the drugs most commonly used.

Ventricular arrhythmias

Ventricular ectopic beats (extrasystoles, premature beats)

Ventricular ectopic beats may be asymptomatic or patients may complain of extra beats, missed beats or heavy beats. The ectopic electrical activity is not conducted to the ventricles through the normal conducting tissue and thus the QRS complex on the ECG is widened, with a bizarre configuration (Figure 8.9). In normal individuals ectopic beats are of no significance, but treatment is sometimes given for symptoms. In patients with heart disease they are associated with an increased risk of sudden death. A recent meta-analysis of published trials suggests that prophylaxis with amiodarone may reduce mortality by preventing arrhythmias and sudden death.

Ventricular tachycardia

Ventricular tachycardia and ventricular fibrillation are usually associated with underlying heart disease, e.g. ischaemia, cardiomyopathy and hypertensive heart disease. Ventricular tachycardia is defined as three or more

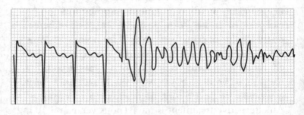

Figure 8.9
A rhythm strip demonstrating four beats of sinus rhythm followed by a ventricular ectopic beat that initiates ventricular fibrillation. The ST segment is elevated owing to acute myocardial infarction.

consecutive ventricular beats occurring at a rate of 120/min or more. The ECG shows a rapid ventricular rhythm with broad abnormal QRS complexes which can sometimes be confused with a broad complex junctional tachycardia. Ventricular tachycardia may produce severe hypotension, when urgent DC cardioversion is necessary. If there is no haemodynamic compromise, treatment is usually with intravenous lignocaine (50–100 mg i.v. over 5 min followed by an intravenous infusion of 2–4 mg/min). Prophylaxis is usually with mexiletine, disopyramide, flecainide or amiodarone. Patients who are refractory to all medical treatment may need an implantable defibrillator (a small device implanted behind the rectus abdominis and connected to the heart; it recognizes ventricular tachycardia or ventricular fibrillation and automatically delivers a defibrillation shock to the heart).

Ventricular fibrillation

This is a very rapid and irregular ventricular activation (see Figure 8.9) with no mechanical effect and hence no cardiac output. Ventricular fibrillation rarely reverts spontaneously and management is immediate cardioversion (Emergency Box 8.1).

Cardiac arrest

In cardiac arrest there is no effective cardiac output. The patient is unconscious and apnoeic with absent arterial pulses (best felt in the carotid artery in the neck). Irreversible brain damage occurs within 3 minutes if an adequate circulation is not established. Management of a cardiac arrest is described below (Emergency Box 8.1).

Prognosis of cardiac arrest In many patients resuscitation is unsuccessful, particularly in those who collapse out of hospital and are brought into hospital in an arrested state. In patients who are successfully resuscitated the prognosis is often poor because they have severe underlying heart disease. The exception is those who are successfully resuscitated from a ventricular fibrillation arrest in the early stages of myocardial infarction, when the prognosis is much the same as for other patients with an infarct.

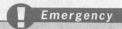

Emergency

Call for help
Thump the chest firmly over the sternum: occasionally reverts VT/VF to sinus rhytem

AIRWAY
- Place patient on his or her back on a firm surface
- Remove obstructing material, e.g. blood and vomit
- Open the airway by flexing the neck and extending the head

BREATHING
- Give four breaths in quick succession of mouth-to-mouth resuscitation. Watch for the rise and fall of the patient's chest, indicating adequate ventilation

CIRCULATION
- Circulation is achieved by external chest compression
- The heel of one hand is placed over the lower half of the victim's sternum and the heel of the second hand is placed over the first with the fingers interlocked. With straight arms the sternum is depressed by 1–2 inches

Compressions: respiration
= 5:1 if two rescuers, 100 compressions per munute
= 15:2 if one rescuer, 80 compressions per minute

Advanced life support
- Institute as soon as help arrives; continue cardiac massage throughtout except during defibrillation
- Defibrillate immediately (ventricular fibrillation is the most common arrhythmia in cardiac arrest)
- Give 100% O_2 via Ambu-Bag, intubate as soon possible and initiate positive pressure ventilation
- Establish intravenous access and connect ECG leads
- If intravenous access not possible give drugs via endotracheal tube (3 × intravenous dose) diluted to 10 ml with 0.9% saline

Management of arrhythmias causing cardiac arrest

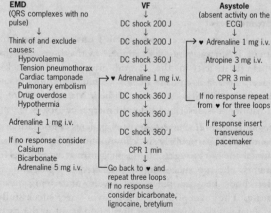

EMD
(QRS complexes with no pulse)
↓
Think of and exclude causes:
    Hypovolaemia
    Tension pneumothorax
    Cardiac tamponade
    Pulmonary embolism
    Drug overdose
    Hypothermia
↓
Adrenaline 1 mg i.v.
↓
If no response consider
    Calsium
    Bicarbonate
    Adrenaline 5 mg i.v.

VF
↓
DC shock 200 J
↓
DC shock 200 J
↓
DC shock 360 J
↓
♥ Adrenaline 1 mg i.v.
↓
DC shock 360 J
↓
DC shock 360 J
↓
DC shock 360 J
↓
CPR 1 min
↓
Go back to ♥ and repeat three loops
If no response consider bicarbonate, lignocaine, bretylium

Asystole
(absent activity on the ECG)
↓
♥ Adrenaline 1 mg i.v.
↓
Atropine 3 mg i.v.
↓
CPR 3 min
↓
If no response repeat from ♥ for three loops
↓
If response insert transvenous pacemaker

EMD, electromechanical dissociation, VF, ventricular fibrillation; VT, ventricular tachycardia.

Emergency box 8.1
Basic life support (ABC)

CARDIAC FAILURE

Cardiac failure occurs when, in spite of normal venous pressures, the heart is unable to maintain sufficient cardiac output to meet the demands of the body. It is a common condition, with an estimated annual incidence of 10% in patients over 65. Although the prognosis has improved in recent years the mortality is still high, with approximately 50% of patients dead within 5 years.

Aetiology

The causes of heart failure are given in Table 8.4.

- *Low-output failure* develops when the heart is unable to generate adequate output.
- *High-output failure* is uncommon and occurs when the heart is unable to meet the perfusion requirements of

Table 8.4 Causes of heart failure: the predominant clinical picture is indicated

	Left heart failure	Right heart failure	Biventricular failure
Myocardial dysfunction			
Ischaemic heart disease	X		
Systemic hypertension	X		
Dilated cardiomyopathy			X
Volume overload			
Ventricular septal defect	X		
Mitral regurgitation	X		
Aortic regurgitation	X		
Pulmonary regurgitation		X	
Tricuspid regurgitation		X	
Outflow obstruction			
Aortic stenosis	X		
Pulmonary hypertension		X	
Pulmonary embolism		X	
Pulmonary stenosis		X	
Compromised ventricular filling			
Constrictive pericarditis		X	
Pericardial tamponade		X	
Restrictive cardiomyopathy			X
Arrhythmia			
Severe bradycardia		X	
Severe tachycardia		X	

tissue metabolism, in spite of an increased cardiac output. Causes include anaemia, systemic to pulmonary shunts, thyrotoxicosis, Paget's disease and beri–beri (page 619).

Pathophysiology

When the heart fails, compensatory mechanisms attempt to maintain cardiac output and peripheral perfusion. However, as heart failure progresses the mechanisms are overwhelmed and become pathophysiological.

Neurohumoral activation

Sympathetic nervous system Activation of the sympathetic nervous system improves ventricular function by increasing heart rate and myocardial contractility. Constriction of venous capacitance vessels redistributes flow centrally and the increased venous return to the heart (preload) further augments ventricular function via the Starling mechanism (Figure 8.10). Sympathetic stimulation, however, also leads to arteriolar constriction, this increasing the afterload which would eventually reduce cardiac output.

Renin–angiotensin system The fall in cardiac output and increased sympathetic tone lead to diminished renal perfusion, activation of the renin–angiotensin system, and hence increased fluid retention. Salt and water retention further increases venous pressure and maintains stroke volume by the Starling mechanism (Figure 8.10). As salt and water retention increases, however, peripheral and pulmonary congestion cause oedema and contribute to dyspnoea. Angiotensin II also causes arteriolar constriction, thus increasing the afterload and the work of the heart.

Atrial natriuretic peptides (ANPs) Distension of the atria leads to release of these peptides, which have vasodilator and natriuretic properties. The effect of their action may represent a beneficial, albeit inadequate, compensatory response leading to reduced cardiac load (preload and afterload).

Ventricular dilatation Myocardial failure leads to a reduction of the volume of blood ejected with each heartbeat, and thus an increase in the volume of blood remaining after systole. The increased diastolic volume

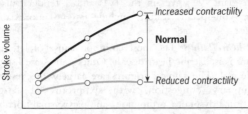

Figure 8.10
The Starling curve. Starling's law states that the stroke volume is directly proportional to the diastolic filling (i.e. the preload or ventricular end-diastolic pressure). Changes in contractility (e.g. increased with sympathetic stimulation) and afterload have an independent effect on ventricular function. In heart failure (bottom line) the ventricular function curve is relatively flat so that increasing the preload has only a small effect on cardiac output.

stretches the myocardial fibres and, as Starling's law would suggest, myocardial contraction is restored. Once cardiac failure is established, however, the compensatory effects of cardiac dilatation become limited by the flattened contour of Starling's curve. Eventually the increased venous pressure contributes to the development of pulmonary and peripheral oedema. In addition, as ventricular diameter increases greater tension is required in the myocardium to expel a given volume of blood, and oxygen requirements increase.

Clinical features

It is clinically useful to divide heart failure into the syndromes of right, left and biventricular (congestive) cardiac failure (see Table 8.4), but it is rare for any one part of the heart to fail in isolation.

Right heart failure The most frequent cause of chronic right heart failure is secondary to left heart failure. Other causes are indicated in Table 8.4. There is jugular venous distension, hepatomegaly and dependent pitting oedema (over the ankles and calves in ambulant patients, over the sacrum in bed-bound patients). Less frequently ascites or pleural transudates occur. Dilatation of the right ventricle may give rise to functional tricuspid incompetence, with giant 'V' waves in the JVP and a tender pulsatile liver. Non-specific features include fatigue, anorexia and nausea.

Left heart failure The most common cause of left heart failure is ischaemic heart disease. Other causes are listed in Table 8.4. The clinical features are largely the result of pulmonary congestion, with symptoms of fatigue, exertional dyspnoea, orthopnoea and paroxysmal nocturnal dyspnoea (page 391). Physical signs include tachypnoea, tachycardia, a displaced apex beat and basal lung crackles. A third heart sound occurs and is the result of rapid filling of the ventricles. In severe failure, dilatation of the mitral annulus results in functional mitral regurgitation.

Biventricular failure (congestive) This term is used variously but is best restricted to cases where right heart failure is a result of pre-existing left heart failure. The physical signs are thus a combination of the above syndromes.

Acute heart failure This is a medical emergency, with left or right heart failure developing over minutes or hours. It most commonly occurs in the setting of myocardial infarction.

Investigations

A clinical diagnosis of heart failure should always be confirmed by objective measures of structure and function. Similarly, the underlying cause should be established in all patients.

- Radiology. The chest radiograph is usually unhelpful in determining the cause of heart failure, but shows cardiac enlargement (cardiothoracic ratio >50% on a posteroanterior chest film) and characteristic appearances in left heart failure (Figure 8.11).
- ECG may show evidence of underlying causes, e.g. arrhythmias, ischaemia, left ventricular hypertrophy in hypertension.
- Echocardiography is the most useful diagnostic investigation. It allows an assessment of left ventricular function, and identifies valvular abnormalities and pericardial effusion. An ejection fraction of <0.45 is usually accepted as evidence for systolic dysfunction.
- Blood tests. These include full blood count, urea and electrolytes, and sometimes thyroid function tests.

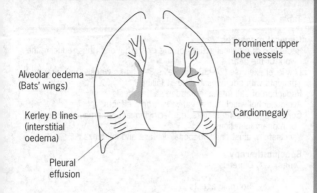

Figure 8.11
The chest radiograph in left ventricular failure.

- Other investigations. Radionuclide ventriculography (technetium-99m (^{99m}Tc) scan) is sometimes performed to quantity ejection fraction (page 699), and identify sections of the left ventricular wall that contract abnormally. Cardiac catheterization is usually reserved for the small proportion of patients with a surgically correctable lesion, e.g. aortic or mitral valve abnormalities. In such cases the surgeon requires precise definition of the lesion and demonstration of the coronary anatomy.

Treatment of chronic heart failure

Treatment is aimed at relieving symptoms, retarding disease progression and improving survival (Table 8.5).

Drug treatment

Diuretics Diuretics are the first line of treatment in patients with heart failure. They act by promoting renal sodium excretion, with enhanced water excretion as a secondary effect. The resulting loss of fluid reduces ventricular filling pressures (preload) and thus decreases pulmonary and systemic congestion.

- *Thiazide diuretics*, e.g. bendrofluazide, are mild diuretics that inhibit sodium reabsorption in the distal renal tubule. The exception is metolazone, which causes a

Table 8.5 The management of chronic heart failure

General measures
Reduction of physical activity during exacerbations, thus reducing the
  work of the heart
Low-level exercise (20–30 min walks 3–5 times weekly) encouraged in
  patients with compensated heart failure
Reduction of salt intake: no added salt at meals
Avoid alcohol which has negative inotropic effects
Correct aggravating factors, e.g. arrhythmias, anaemia, hypertension,
  pulmonary infections
Vaccinate against pneumococcal disease and influenza

Specific therapy

Drugs	Diuretics
	Vasodilators
	Inotropic agents
	Antiarrhythmic drugs
	β-adrenoceptor blockers
Surgery	Replacement of diseased valves
	Cardiac transplantation
	Repair of ventricular septal defect
	Coronary artery bypass graft

profound diuresis and is used in severe heart failure
unresponsive to large doses of loop diuretics. The major
side effects of the thiazides are hypokalaemia,
hyperglycaemia and hyperuricaemia.

- *Loop diuretics*, e.g. frusemide and bumetanide, inhibit
  sodium reabsorption in the ascending limb of the loop
  of Henle. They are potent diuretics used in
  moderate/severe heart failure. These drugs produce
  marked renal potassium loss and promote
  hyperuricaemia.
- *Potassium-sparing diuretics* are relatively ineffective when
  given alone and are usually prescribed in combination
  with a loop diuretic. Spironolactone, an aldosterone
  antagonist, is the most effective but causes
  gynaecomastia. Amiloride and triamterene have a
  direct action on ion transport in the distal renal tubule.
  They increase renal sodium loss and reduce potassium
  loss.

Vasodilator therapy Vasodilators have a beneficial effect in
heart failure by reducing venous constriction (reduction of
preload) and/or arteriolar constriction (reduction of
afterload).

- *Angiotensin-converting enzyme (ACE) inhibitors*, e.g. captopril enalapril and lisinopril, enhance renal salt and water excretion and increase cardiac output by reducing afterload. They not only improve symptoms, but also limit the development of progressive heart failure and prolong survival, and should be given to all patients with heart failure, in addition to diuretic therapy. The major side effect is first-dose hypotension, which is a particular risk in those with severe heart failure receiving large doses of diuretics. These patients should omit the preceding dose of diuretic and begin therapy in hospital, with a test dose given at bedtime. Other side effects are prerenal renal failure (page 299), hyperkalaemia, rash, and persistent cough due to inhibition of bradykinin metabolism.
- *Angiotensin II inhibitors* (e.g. Losartan) have similar haemodynamic effects to ACE inhibitors but do not affect bradykinin metabolism and therefore do not cause coughing. Both these drugs are contraindicated in patients with bilateral renal artery stenosis.
- *Other vasodilators* The combination of isosorbide mononitrate (a vasodilator) and hydralazine (arteriolar vasodilator) improves symptoms and survival, and is used when ACE inhibitors are not tolerated or their use is contraindicated. Calcium channel blockers, e.g. nifedipine, diltiazem, also reduce afterload but may have a detrimental effect on left ventricular function. The second-generation calcium antagonist amlodipine is safe in heart failure and possibly of prognostic benefit.

Other vasodilators, used less commonly, include prazosin, nitroprusside and the calcium channel antagonists.

Inotropic agents

- *Digoxin* is of undoubted benefit in patients with congestive heart failure and atrial fibrillation. A recent study has shown that when combined with ACE inhibitors and diuretics, digoxin reduces death and hospitalization rates from progressive heart failure.
- *Sympathomimetic agents* dopamine and dobutamine are intravenous adrenergic agonists. They are used in the treatment of cardiogenic shock (page 444) or occasionally as a temporary measure in a patient with

severe intractable heart failure. Xamoterol is an orally acting β-adrenoreceptor agonist. It is effective in improving cardiac performance but its use is very limited because it may precipitate an acute deterioration in patients with severe heart failure.

Antiarrhythmic drugs Arrhythmias are frequent in heart failure and are implicated in sudden death. A recent meta-analysis of published trials suggests that the mortality is reduced by prophylactic treatment with amiodarone.

β-blockers Although previous opinion held that β-blockers were contraindicated in heart failure, several studies have shown that these agents can improve symptoms and exercise tolerance in patients with heart failure. This effect is thought to arise through blockade of the chronically activated sympathetic system. A new β-blocker (carvedilol) with additional α_1 blocking effects has recently been shown to significantly improve mortality. At present these drugs should be used only in those who remain symptomatic with diuretics, vasodilators and digoxin.

Prognosis

There is usually a gradual deterioration necessitating increased doses of diuretics, and sometimes admission to hospital. The prognosis is poor in those with severe heart failure (i.e. breathless at rest or on minimal exertion), with a 1-year survival rate of 50%. Younger patients with severe intractable heart failure are usually referred to a specialist cardiothoracic centre for consideration of cardiac transplantation. Eighty per cent of patients survive 1 year; early deaths are the result of operative mortality, organ rejection and overwhelming infection secondary to immunosuppressive treatment. After this time the greatest threat to health is accelerated coronary atherosclerosis, the cause of which is unknown.

Pulmonary oedema

This is a very frightening life-threatening emergency characterized by the rapid onset of extreme breathlessness. Causes include acute, severe left ventricular failure (e.g. myocardial infarction, acute mitral and aortic regurgitation), mitral stenosis and arrhythmias. An acute elevation of left atrial pressure produces corresponding elevation of the pulmonary capillary pressure and increased transudation of fluid into the pulmonary interstitium and alveoli (cardiogenic pulmonary oedema). *Non-cardiogenic pulmonary oedema* is seen in very ill patients and is discussed on page 453.

Clinical features

The patient is acutely breathless, wheezing and anxious. There is usually a cough productive of frothy blood-tinged (pink) sputum. Increased sympathoadrenal activity leads to profuse sweating, tachycardia and peripheral circulatory shutdown. On auscultation there is a gallop rhythm, and wheezes and crackles are heard throughout the chest.

Investigations

- Radiology. The chest radiograph shows distension of the upper lobe veins (indicating a raised pulmonary venous pressure) and bilateral perihilar shadowing in a 'butterfly' or 'bat's wing' distribution caused by alveolar fluid. Interstitial pulmonary oedema produces Kerley B lines (see Figure 8.11).
- ECG and cardiac enzymes may show evidence of a myocardial infarction as the precipitating event.
- Arterial blood gases show hypoxaemia. Initially the P_aCO_2 falls because of overbreathing, but later increases because of impaired gas exchange.

Management

In many cases the patient is so unwell that treatment (Emergency Box 8.2) must begin before investigations are completed. Intravenous opiates, e.g. morphine, and diuretics are the first-line agents. Morphine relieves dyspnoea by a combination of vasodilatation and relief of anxiety. Respiratory depression occurs with large doses (>10 mg). Diuretics produce immediate vasodilatation in addition to the more delayed diuretic response. If the patient does not improve, intravenous nitrates may be used to reduce the preload. Occasionally, in severe cases which do not respond to treatment, ventilation is necessary.

> **! Emergency**

Sit the patient up
60% oxygen by face mask
Frusemide 40–80 mg i.v.
Morphine 2.5–10 mg i.v. + an antiemetic, e.g. metoclopramide
   10 mg i.v.

Consider
   Intravenous GTN infusion (2–10 mg/h)
   Intravenous aminophylline (250 mg over 10 min) to relieve
   bronchospasm

Treat exacerbating and precipitating factors
   Hypertension
   Pulmonary infection
   Arrhythmias

Mechanical ventilation if no response to treatment

Emergency Box 8.2
Management of pulmonary oedema

Cardiogenic shock

Cardiogenic shock (pump failure) is an extreme type of cardiac failure characterized by hypotension, a low cardiac output and signs of poor tissue perfusion, such as oliguria, cold extremities and poor cerebral function. Its most common cause is massive myocardial infarction, and management is discussed on page 444.

ISCHAEMIC HEART DISEASE

Myocardial ischaemia results from an imbalance between the supply of oxygen to cardiac muscle and myocardial demand. The most common cause is coronary artery atheroma, which results in a fixed obstruction to coronary blood flow. Other causes of ischaemia include coronary artery thrombosis, spasm or, rarely, arteritis (e.g. polyarteritis). Increased demand for oxygen due to an increase in cardiac output may occur in thyrotoxicosis or myocardial hypertrophy (e.g. from aortic stenosis or hypertension).

Coronary artery disease is the single largest cause of death in the UK, resulting in approximately 60 deaths per 100 000 population.

Atheroma consists of atherosclerotic plaques (seen post mortem as raised yellow-white areas covering the intimal surface of the artery) rich in cholesterol and other lipids, surrounded by smooth muscle cells and fibrous tissue. A number of risk factors have been identified for coronary atherosclerosis, some of which are irreversible and some which can be modified.

Irreversible risk factors

Age Atherosclerosis is progressively more common as age increases. It rarely presents in the young, except in familial hyperlipidaemia (page 541).

Gender Men are more often affected than women, although the incidence in women after the menopause is similar to that in men. The cause for this difference is poorly understood, but probably relates to the loss of the protective effect of oestrogen.

Family history Coronary artery disease is often present in several members of the same family. It is unclear, however, whether family history is an independent risk factor as so many other factors are familial. A number of genetic risk factors have been associated with coronary artery disease. For example, a specific genotype of the *ACE* gene associated with higher circulating ACE levels may be significantly associated with a predisposition to coronary artery disease and myocardial infarction.

Potentially reversible risk factors

Hyperlipidaemia Elevated cholesterol levels increase the risk of premature atherosclerosis, particularly when associated with low levels of high-density lipoproteins (HDLs). There is increasing evidence that high triglyceride levels are independently linked with coronary atheroma. Lowering serum cholesterol not only slows the progression of coronary atherosclerosis, but may also cause regression of the disease.

Smoking In men the risk of developing coronary artery disease is directly related to the number of cigarettes smoked. In women this relationship, although still important, is less clear. Stopping smoking reduces the risk but does not eliminate it.

Hypertension Both elevated systolic and elevated diastolic hypertension are linked to an increased incidence of coronary artery disease.

Other factors Diabetes mellitus, lack of exercise and obesity have all been linked to an increased incidence of atheroma. Recently a number of factors, including infection with *Chlamydia pneumoniae* and high levels of homocystine in the blood, have been linked to atherosclerosis, although it is unclear whether they are directly linked to the pathogenesis of the disease.

Angina

Angina pectoris is a descriptive term for chest pain arising from the heart as a result of myocardial ischaemia.

Clinical features

Angina is usually described as central crushing chest pain, coming on with exertion and relieved by rest within a few minutes. It is often exacerbated by cold weather, anger and excitement, and it frequently radiates to the arms and neck. Variants of classic angina include:

- Decubitus angina (occurs on lying down)
- Prinzmetal's angina is caused by coronary artery spasm and results in angina that occurs without provocation, usually at rest.
- Unstable angina: Angina which increases rapidly in severity, occurs at rest, or is of recent onset
- Syndrome X refers to those patients with symptoms of angina, a positive exercise test and normal coronary arteries thought to result from functional abnormalities of the coronary microcirculation.

Physical examination in patients with angina is often normal but must include a search for risk factors (e.g. hypertension and xanthelasma occurring in hyperlipidaemia).

Diagnosis

The primary diagnosis is clinical because investigations may be normal. Occasionally chest wall pain or oesophageal reflux causes diagnostic confusion (page 321).

Investigations

- Resting ECG typically shows ST segment depression and T-wave flattening or inversion during an attack. The ECG is normal in up to 80% of people between attacks.
- Exercise ECG testing is positive in about 75% of people with severe coronary artery disease; a normal test does not exclude the diagnosis. ST segment depression (>1 mm) at a low workload or a paradoxical fall in blood pressure with exercise usually indicates severe coronary artery disease, and these patients should be considered for coronary angiography.
- Radioisotope studies (thallium–201 perfusion scan, page 697) are particularly useful in those with equivocal exercise tests. Ischaemic areas show as 'cold spots' during exercise.
- Coronary angiography is occasionally used when the cause of pain is unclear. More commonly the test is performed to delineate the exact coronary anatomy before coronary artery surgery is considered.

Management

General Underlying problems such as obesity, thyrotoxicosis, hypercholesterolaemia, anaemia or aortic valve disease should be treated. Smoking should be discouraged, other risk factors evaluated and steps taken to correct them.

Prognostic therapies

- Aspirin (75 mg daily) reduces the risk of coronary events in patients with coronary artery disease.
- Lipid lowering agents (page 542).

Symptomatic treatment Acute attacks are treated with sublingual glyceryl trinitrate. Patients should be encouraged to use this before exertion, rather than waiting for the pain to develop. The main side effect is a severe bursting headache, which is relieved by inactivating the tablet either by swallowing or spitting it out.

When angina occurs frequently or with only modest exertion, regular prophylactic therapy should be employed. Nitrates or β-blockers are usually used as first-line agents, and calcium antagonists added if necessary.

- *Nitrates* reduce venous and intracardiac diastolic pressure, reduce impedance to the emptying of the left ventricle, and dilate coronary arteries. They are available in a variety of slow-release preparations, including infiltrated skin plasters, buccal pellets and long-acting oral nitrate preparations, e.g. isosorbide mononitrate, isosorbide dinitrate. The major side effect is headache, which tends to diminish with continued use.
- *β-Adrenergic blocking drugs*, e.g. metoprolol 25–50 mg twice daily and atenolol 50–100 mg daily, reduce heart rate and the force of ventricular contraction, both of which reduce the myocardial oxygen demand. They are contraindicated in asthma, and relatively contraindicated in peripheral vascular disease.
- *Calcium antagonists*, e.g. diltiazem, block calcium influx into the cell and the utilization of calcium within the cell. They relax the coronary arteries and reduce the force of left ventricular contraction, thereby reducing oxygen demand. The side effects (postural dizziness, headache, ankle oedema) are the result of systemic vasodilatation. Nifedipine increases mortality and should not be used in this situation.
- *Nicorandil* is a new agent which combines nitrate-like activity with potassium channel blockade. It can be useful when there are contraindications to the above agents.

When angina persists or worsens in spite of general measures and optimal medical treatment, patients should be considered for coronary artery bypass grafting (CABG) or angioplasty.

Coronary angioplasty Localized atheromatous lesions are dilated by cardiac catheterization using small inflatable balloons. This technique is widely applied for angina resulting from isolated, proximal, non-calcified atheromatous plaques. Complications include acute occlusion in 2–4% of cases (necessitating full surgical back-up) and restenosis (30% in the first 6 months).

Intracoronary stents reduce the risk of restenosis but increase the cost of the procedure. Aspirin is routinely given but the use of monoclonal antibodies to the glycoprotein IIb/IIIa platelet receptor (the final common pathway of aggregation) in selected high-risk cases may reduce periprocedural complications.

Surgery The left or right internal mammary artery is used to bypass stenoses in the left anterior descending or right coronary artery respectively. Less commonly, the saphenous vein from the leg is anastamosed to the proximal aorta, and coronary artery distal to the obstruction. Surgery successfully relieves angina in about 90% of cases and, when performed for left main stem obstruction or three-vessel disease, an improved lifespan and quality of life can be expected. Operative mortality rate is less than 1%. In most patients the angina eventually recurs because of accelerated atherosclerosis in the graft (particularly vein grafts), which can be treated by stenting.

Management of unstable angina

This is a medical emergency with a risk of myocardial infarction if treatment is inadequate. Management involves admission to hospital, bed rest, intravenous heparin, aspirin and a combination of all antianginal drugs. Early coronary angiography with a view to surgery or angioplasty is recommended, particularly when symptoms continue in spite of optimum medical treatment.

Prognosis

The average annual mortality rate for patients with stable angina is 4% a year, with the worst prognosis in those with extensive coronary artery disease.

Myocardial infarction

Myocardial infarction (MI) is now the most common cause of death in developed countries. It is almost always the result of rupture of an atherosclerotic plaque, with the development of thrombosis and total occlusion of the artery.

Clinical features

Central chest pain similar to that occurring in angina is the most common presenting symptom. Unlike angina it usually occurs at rest, is more severe and lasts for some hours. The pain is often associated with sweating, breathlessness, nausea, vomiting and restlessness. There may be no physical signs unless complications develop (see later), although the patient often appears pale, sweaty and grey. About 20% of patients have no pain, and such 'silent' infarctions either go unnoticed or present with hypotension, arrhythmias or pulmonary oedema. This occurs most commonly in elderly patients or those with diabetes or hypertension.

Investigations

In most cases the diagnosis is made on the basis of the clinical history and early ECG appearances. Serial changes (over 3 days) in the ECG and cardiac enzymes confirm the diagnosis and allow an assessment of infarct size (on the magnitude of the enzyme rise and extent of ECG changes). A normal ECG in the early stages does not exclude the diagnosis.

The ECG usually shows a characteristic pattern. Within hours there is ST segment elevation (>1 mm in two or more contiguous leads) followed by T-wave flattening or inversion (Figure 8.12). Pathological Q waves are broad (>1 mm) and deep (>2 mm, or >25% of the amplitude of the following R wave) negative deflections that start the QRS complex. They are seen once full-thickness infarction (as opposed to non-Q wave or subendocardial infarction) has occurred. They develop because the infarcted muscle is electrically silent so that the recording leads 'look through' the infarcted area. This means that the electrical activity being recorded (on the opposite ventricular wall) is moving away from the electrode and is therefore negative.

Typically ECG changes are confined to the leads that 'face' the infarct. Leads II, III and AVF are involved in inferior infarcts; I, II and AVL in lateral infarcts; and V2–V6 in anterior infarcts. As there are no posterior leads a posterior wall infarct is diagnosed by the appearance of reciprocal changes in V1 and V2 (i.e. the development of tall initial R waves, ST segment depression and tall upright T waves).

Cardiac enzymes Necrotic cardiac muscle releases enzymes into the systemic circulation. The most commonly measured is creatine kinase (CK), which is also produced by damaged skeletal muscle and brain. The myocardial-bound

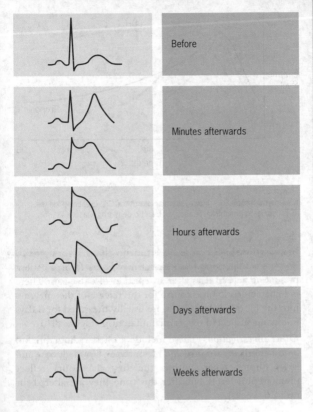

Before

Minutes afterwards

Hours afterwards

Days afterwards

Weeks afterwards

Figure 8.12
Electrocardiographic evolution of myocardial infarction. After the first few minutes the T waves become tall, pointed and upright and there is ST segment elevation. After the first few hours the T waves invert, the R wave voltage is decreased and Q waves develop. After a few days the ST segment returns to normal. After weeks or months the T wave may return to upright but the Q wave remains.

(MB) isoenzyme fraction of CK is, however, specific for heart muscle damage. Elevated levels of troponin T and troponin I are highly specific for cardiac muscle damage and measurement of these regulatory proteins is becoming more widely available. Aspartate aminotransferase (AST) and lactic dehydrogenase (LDH) are now rarely used for the diagnosis

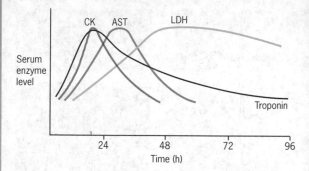

Figure 8.13
The enzyme profile in acute myocardial infarction. CK, creatinine kinase; AST, aspartate aminotransferase; LDH, lactic dehydrogenase.

of infarction, but because levels remain elevated for up to 10 days after infarction measurement may be useful in a patient presenting several days after an episode of chest pain. There is a characteristic time course for the release of the enzymes into the blood, and thus they are usually measured for 3 days following suspected myocardial infarction (Figure 8.13).

Other investigations These include a chest radiograph, full blood count, serum urea and electrolytes, blood glucose and lipids (lipids taken within the first 12 hours reflect preinfarction levels, but after this time they are altered for up to 6 weeks).

Management

The aims of treatment are relief of pain, limitation of infarct size and treatment of complications (Emergency Box 8.3).

Thrombolytic therapy is indicated in patients with chest pain consistent with myocardial infarction and ST segment elevation on the ECG. These agents can achieve early reperfusion in 50–70% of patients (compared to a spontaneous reperfusion of less than 30%) and have been shown to reduce both mortality and the extent of myocardial damage associated with myocardial infarction. They should be given as soon as possible, although benefit may occur for up to 12 hours after the onset of symptoms. Commonly used thrombolytic agents are streptokinase and recombinant tissue-type plasminogen activator (t-PA).

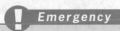

Emergency

Immediate management
- Insert intravenous cannula. Take blood for cardiac enzymes, blood count, urea and electrolytes, glucose and lipids
- Attach patient to a cardiac monitor
- Pain relief: diamorphine (2.5–5 mg i.v). Repeat after 15 minutes if necessary; half the dose in the elderly Antiemetic, e.g. metoclopramide 10 mg i.v prevents nausea and vomiting
- 60% oxygen by face mask or nasal cannula. Discontinue if arterial oxygen saturation is normal
- Aspirin: 300 mg to be chewed
- Streptokinase: 1.5 million units in 100 ml 0.9% sodium chloride over 1 h by intravenous infusion pump
- Metoprolol 5 mg slow i.v.injection if systolic BP >160 mmHg. Repeat every 15 minutes, titrated against heart rate and BP. Do not give if hypotension, heart failure, bradycardia, asthma
- Insulin infusion if admission blood glucose >11 mmol/l, aim for blood glucose of 7–10.9 mmol/l
- Treat complications (pp. 359–361)
- Treat persistent pain with glyceryl trinitrate infusion 2–10 mg/h titrated against the response; consider angiography and possible angioplasty.

Subsequent management of uncomplicated infarction
- Repeat ECG, CK and electrolytes at 24 and 48 hours after admission
- Initiate secondary prevention therapy
  ACE inhibitors, e.g. captopril 6.25 mg with dose titrated up to 25 mg three times daily
  Aspirin 150 mg daily β-Blockers, e.g. metoprolol 25–50 mg three times daily
  Warfarin in selected patients (page 187)
  Stop smoking
- Start lipid-lowering diet if blood cholesterol >4.8 mmol/l. Consider statins if cholesterol very high
- Transfer from CCU to medical ward after 48 h
- Mobilize gradually after 24–48 h if pain-free
- Discharge from hospital after 5 days
- Exercise test 6 weeks later. Consider angiography if ischaemic ECG changes or chest pain in early stages
- Advice to patient: refer to rehabilitation nurse; no driving for one month, unless heavy goods or public service licence holder when special assessment required; usually return to work in 2 months.

Emergency Box 8.3
Summary of the management of myocardial infarction

Streptokinase is the cheapest and most commonly used, but may induce the development of antistreptokinase antibodies. This puts the patient at risk of allergic reactions and reduces the effectiveness of subsequent thrombolysis with streptokinase; t-PA is given to patients previously treated with streptokinase or when the systolic blood pressure is less than 100 mmHg, t-Pa must be followed by intravenous heparin. The side effects and contraindications to thrombolysis are discussed on page 184. Aspirin enhances the benefits of thrombolysis and should be given immediately and continued indefinitely as secondary prophylaxis.

Recanalization of the infarct-related artery may also be achieved by primary (direct) angioplasty without prior or concomitant thrombolytic therapy; in experienced hands the results are equal or superior to thrombolysis. It is only a therapeutic option when rapid access to a catheterization laboratory is possible, the cardiologist is experienced in interventional cardiology and a full support team is immediately available. Therefore, it is not usually used in preference to thrombolysis but should be considered in patients when thrombolytic therapy is contraindicated (page 184), or in patients who have received thrombolysis and who seem on clinical grounds not to have reperfused (ongoing chest pain and persistent ST elevation).

Transfer to coronary care unit (CCU) Fatal cardiac arrhythmias occur most commonly in the period immediately following the infarct. Patients should be admitted as soon as possible to the CCU, where close ECG monitoring and immediate resuscitation are possible. In selected patients, ACE inhibitors reduce mortality and prevent the development of heart failure. They should be started on the first day after MI in patients with extensive anterior infarction, impaired left ventricular ejection fraction (<35%) on echocardiography, or who experience heart failure in the acute event. Treatment is continued indefinitely. Mortality is increased in diabetic patients with MI, largely owing to the high incidence of cardiac failure. This is thought to be due, at least in part, to metabolic changes which occur in the early stages of MI, and may be reduced by rigorous control of blood glucose by insulin infusion, and monitoring with 2-hourly BM stix. This regimen is also indicated in patients not known to be diabetic who have an admission blood glucose of >11 mmol/l. β-Blockers reduce infarct size and the incidence of sudden death. They should initally be given intravenously and continued orally for at least 2–3 years.

Complications

The common complications are listed in Table 8.6.

Table 8.6 Complications associated with myocardial infarction

Early (within 2–3 days)	Late
Arrhythmias	Mitral valve regurgitation
Cardiac failure	Rupture of ventricular septum or wall
Heart block	Dressler's syndrome
Pericarditis	Ventricular aneurysm
Myocardial rupture (usually fatal)	Recurrent arrhythmias
Thromboembolism	Thromboembolism

Disturbances of rate, rhythm and conduction (page 327)

- *Atrial arrhythmias* Sinus tachycardia is common; treatment is that of the underlying cause, particularly pain, anxiety and heart failure. Sinus bradycardia is especially associated with acute inferior wall myocardial infarction. Treatment consists of elevating the foot of the bed and giving intravenous atropine (4 mg) if there are associated symptoms. Atrial fibrillation occurs in about 10% of cases and is usually a transient rhythm disturbance. Treatment with intravenous digoxin or amiodarone is indicated if the fast rate is exacerbating ischaemia or causing heart failure.
- *Ventricular arrhythmias* Ventrciular ectopic beats are very common and may precede the development of ventricular tachycardia or fibrillation. Antiarrhythmic drug treatment has not, however, been shown to affect progression to these more serious arrhythmias. Ventricular tachycardia (VT) may degenerate into ventricular fibrillation (page 337) or may itself produce shock or cardiac failure. Treatment of VT is with intravenous lignocaine (page 337) or direct current cardioversion if there is severe hypotension. Ventricular fibrillation (VF) may be primary (occuring in the first 24–48 hours) or secondary (occurring late after infarction and associated with large infarcts and heart

failure). Treatment is with immediate DC cardioversion. Recurrences may be prevented with intravenous lignocaine or amiodarone. Late VF is associated with a poor prognosis and a high incidence of sudden death, and prophylactic antiarrhythmic treatment must be continued long term.

- *Heart block occurring with inferior infarction* is common and usually resolves spontaneously. Some patients respond to intravenous atropine, but a temporary pacemaker may be necessary if the rhythm is very slow or producing symptoms.

- *Complete heart block occurring with anterior wall infarction* indicates the involvement of both bundle branches by extensive myocardial necrosis, and hence a very poor prognosis. The ventricular rhythm in this case is unreliable and a temporary pacing wire is necessary. Heart block is often permanent and a permanent pacing wire may be necessary.

Cardiac failure in a mild form occurs in up to 40% of patients following myocardial infarction. Extensive infarction may cause pulmonary oedema (see Emergency Box 8.1), which may also occur following rupture of the ventricular septum or mitral valve papillary muscle. Both conditions present with worsening heart failure, a systolic thrill and a loud pansystolic murmur. Mortality is high and urgent surgical correction is often needed. Hypotension with a raised JVP is usually a complication of right ventricular infarction, which may occur with inferior wall infarcts. Initial treatment is with volume expansion and pericardial effusion (which produces similar signs) ruled out on an echocardiogram.

Thromboembolism occurs most commonly following prolonged bed rest and with cardiac failure. Patients at risk of embolism from left ventricular or left atrial clot (those with severe left ventricular dysfunction, persistent AF or mural thrombus on echocardiography) should be anticoagulated with warfarin to achieve a target INR of 2–3.

Pericarditis is characterized by sharp chest pain and a pericardial rub. Treatment is with non-steroidal anti-inflammatory drugs until spontaneous resolution occurs within 1–2 days. Late pericarditis (2–12 weeks after) with fever and a pericardial effusion (Dressler's syndrome) is rare; usually it occurs weeks to months after infarction, and corticosteroids may be necessary in some patients.

Prognosis

Fifty per cent of patients die during the acute event, many before reaching hospital. A further 10% die in hospital, and of the survivors a further 20% die in the next 2 years.

Rheumatic fever

Rheumatic fever is an inflammatory disease that occurs in children and young adults (the first attack usually occurs between 5 and 15 years of age) as a result of infection with group A streptococci. It is a complication of less than 1% of streptococcal pharyngitis, developing 2–3 weeks after the onset of sore throat. It is thought to develop because of an autoimmune reaction triggered by the streptococci, and is not the result of direct infection of the heart.

Epidemiology

The incidence in developed countries has decreased dramatically since the 1920s. This is thought to be the result of improved sanitation, a change in the virulence of the organism and the use of antibiotics.

Clinical features

The disease presents suddenly with fever, joint pains and loss of appetite. The major clinical features are as follows:

- Changing heart murmurs, mitral and aortic regurgitation, cardiac failure and chest pain, caused by carditis affecting all three layers of the heart
- Polyarthritis is classically a fleeting polyarthritis affecting the large joints, e.g. knees, ankles and elbows
- Sydenham's chorea ('St Vitus' dance') refers to involvement of the central nervous system that develops late after a streptococcal infection. Sufferers are noticeably 'fidgety' and display spasmodic, unintentional movements
- Skin manifestations include erythema marginatum (transient pink coalescent rings develop on the trunk) and small non-tender subcutaneous nodules which occur over tendons, joints and bony prominences.

Investigations

Blood count shows a leucocytosis and a raised ESR.
The diagnosis is based on the revised Duckett Jones criteria, which depend on the combination of certain clinical features and evidence of recent streptococcal infection.

Treatment

Treatment is with complete bed rest and high-dose aspirin. Penicillin is given to eradicate residual streptococcal infection, and then long-term to all patients with persistent cardiac damage.

Chronic rheumatic heart disease

More than 50% of those who suffer acute rheumatic fever with carditis will later (after 10–20 years) develop chronic rheumatic valvular disease, predominantly affecting the mitral and aortic valves (see below).

VALVULAR HEART DISEASE

Cardiac valves may be incompetent (regurgitant), stenotic or both. The most common problems are acquired left-sided valvular lesions: aortic stenosis, mitral stenosis, mitral regurgitation and aortic regurgitation. Abnormal valves produce turbulent blood flow, which is heard as a murmur on auscultation; a few murmurs are also felt as a thrill on palpation. Murmurs may sometimes be heard with normal hearts ('innocent murmurs'), often reflecting a hyperdynamic circulation, e.g. in pregnancy, anaemia and thyrotoxicosis. Benign murmurs are soft, short, systolic, may vary with posture, and are not associated with signs of organic heart disease.

Diagnosis of valve dysfunction is made clinically and by echocardiography. The severity can usually be assessed by Doppler echocardiography, which measures the direction and velocity of blood flow and allows a calculation to be made of the pressure across a stenotic valve. Transoesophageal echocardiography and invasive cardiac catheterization are usually only necessary to assess complex situations such as coexisting valvular and ischaemic heart disease, or suspected dysfunction of a prosthetic valve. Treatment of valve dysfunction is both medical and surgical; this may be valve replacement, valve repair (some incompetent valves) or valvotomy (the fused cusps of a stenotic valve are separated along the commissures). The timing of surgery is critical and must not be delayed until there is irreversible ventricular dysfunction or pulmonary hypertension.

Prosthetic heart valves

Prosthetic heart valves may be either tissue or mechanical. Tissue valves are usually fashioned from pig aortic valves (a porcine xenograft), but occasionally human aortic valve is used (homograft). Tissue valves tend to degenerate within about 10 years but patients do not need long-term anticoagulation. These valves are often used in elderly patients. Mechanical valves last much longer but patients need lifelong anticoagulation. There are several types: a ball-and-cage design (Star–Edwards valve), a tilting disc (Björk–Shiley valve) or a double tilting disc (St Jude valve). Valves are susceptible to infection and thrombosis and may cause haemolysis or systemic emboli.

The individual valve lesions are considered separately below, but disease may affect more than one valve (particularly in rheumatic heart disease and endocarditis), when a combination of clinical features is produced. Damaged and prosthetic valves are at risk of infection during an episode of bacteraemia (e.g. after tooth extraction, endoscopy or surgery) and patients should always receive prophylactic antibiotics to cover these procedures (see page 374).

Mitral stenosis
Aetiology
Most cases of mitral stenosis are a sequela of rheumatic heart disease that primarily affects women. However, a reliable history of rheumatic fever is not always obtained.

Pathophysiology
Valve thickening and cusp fusion leads to progressive immobility of the valve cusps and a narrowed (stenotic) valve orifice. Symptoms are the result of increased left atrial

pressure and reduced cardiac output, caused by the mechanical obstruction of filling of the left ventricle. An increase in left atrial pressure leads to left atrial hypertrophy and dilatation. Thrombus may form in the dilated atrium, which is also prone to fibrillate and give rise to systemic emboli (e.g. to the brain, resulting in a stroke). Chronically elevated left atrial pressure leads to an increase in pulmonary capillary pressure and pulmonary oedema. Pulmonary arterial vasoconstriction leads to pulmonary hypertension and eventually right ventricular hypertrophy, dilatation and failure.

Symptoms

Exertional dyspnoea which becomes progressively more severe is usually the first symptom. A cough productive of blood-tinged sputum is common, and frank haemoptysis may occasionally occur. The onset of atrial fibrillation may produce an abrupt deterioration and precipitate pulmonary oedema.

Signs

- Cyanotic or dusky-pink discoloration on the upper cheeks produces the so-called mitral facies or malar flush that occurs with severe stenosis.
- The pulse is often irregular as a result of atrial fibrillation.
- The apex beat is 'tapping' in quality as a result of a combination of a palpable first heart sound and left ventricular backward displacement produced by an enlarging right ventricle.
- Auscultation at the apex reveals a loud first heart sound, an opening snap (when the mitral valve opens) in early diastole, followed by a rumbling mid-diastolic murmur. If the patient is in sinus rhythm the murmur becomes louder when atrial systole occurs (presystolic accentuation), as a result of increased flow across the narrowed valve.

The presence of a loud second heart sound, parasternal heave, elevated JVP, ascites and peripheral oedema indicates that pulmonary hypertension producing right ventricular overload has developed.

Investigations

Investigations are performed to confirm the diagnosis, to estimate the severity of valve stenosis and to look for pulmonary hypertension.

Chest X-ray appearances of mitral stenosis are indicated diagrammatically in Figure 8.14

ECG usually shows atrial fibrillation. In patients in sinus rhythm left atrial hypertrophy results in a bifid P wave ('P mitrale').

Echocardiography is the most useful non-invasive investigation to confirm the diagnosis and to assess the severity.

Management

General Treatment is often not required for mild mitral stenosis. Complications are treated medically, e.g. digoxin for atrial fibrillation, diuretics for heart failure and anticoagulation in patients with atrial fibrillation to prevent clot formation and embolization.

Specific If symptoms are more than mild, or if there is evidence that pulmonary hypertension is beginning to develop, mechanical relief of the mitral stenosis is indicated. In many cases closed balloon valvotomy (access to the mitral valve is obtained via a catheter passed through the femoral vein, right atrium and interatrial septum, and a

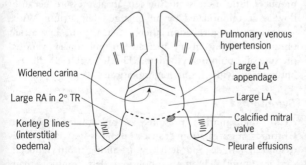

Figure 8.14
The chest radiograph in mitral stenosis. LA, left atrium; RA, right atrium; TR, tricuspid regurgitation.

balloon inflated across the valve to split the commissures) provides relief of symptoms. In other cases open commissurotomy, valve reconstruction or mitral valve replacement is necessary.

Mitral regurgitation

Aetiology

Rheumatic heart disease and a prolapsing mitral valve are the most common causes of mitral regurgitation (Table 8.7).

Table 8.7 Causes of mitral regurgitation

Rheumatic heart disease
Mitral valve prolapse
Infective endocarditis*
Ruptured chordae tendinae*
Rupture of the papillary muscle* complicating myocardial infarction
Papillary muscle dysfunction
Dilating left ventricle disease causing 'functional' mitral regurgitation
Hypertrophic cardiomyopathy
Rarely: systemic lupus erythematosus, Marfan's syndrome
Ehlers–Danlos syndrome

* These disorders may produce acute regurgitation.

Pathophysiology

The circulatory changes depend on the speed of onset and severity of regurgitation. Long-standing regurgitation produces little increase in the left atrial pressure because flow is accommodated by an enlarged left atrium. With acute mitral regurgitation there is a rise in left atrial pressure, resulting in an increase in pulmonary venous pressure and pulmonary oedema. The left ventricle dilates, but more so with chronic regurgitation.

Symptoms

Acute regurgitation presents as pulmonary oedema. Chronic regurgitation causes progressive exertional dyspnoea, fatigue and lethargy (resulting from reduced cardiac output). Thromboembolism is less common than with mitral stenosis, although infective endocarditis is much more common.

Signs

- The apex is displaced laterally, with a diffuse thrusting character.
- The first heart sound is soft.
- There is a pansystolic murmur (palpated as a thrill), loudest at the apex and radiating widely over the precordium and into the axillae.
- A third heart sound is often present, caused by rapid filling of the dilated left ventricle in early diastole.

Investigations

- Chest radiography shows signs of left atrial enlargement and an increased heart size resulting from left ventricular dilatation.
- ECG shows P mitrale before the onset of atrial fibrillation. There may be evidence of left ventricular hypertrophy (page 325).
- Echocardiocardiography confirms the diagnosis and may indicate the cause. The severity of the lesion can usually be assessed from Doppler studies without the need to resort to cardiac catheterization.

Management

Mild mitral regurgitation in the absence of symptoms can be managed conservatively by following the patient with serial echocardiograms. Patients should be referred for surgery (mitral valve replacement or repair) if more than mild symptoms develop or there is evidence of left ventricular dysfunction (ventricular dilatation or reduced ejection fraction).

Prolapsing mitral valve

This is a common condition occurring mainly in young women. One or more of the mitral valve leaflets prolapses back into the left atrium during ventricular systole, producing mitral regurgitation in a few cases.

Aetiology

The cause is unknown but it may be associated with Marfan's syndrome, thyrotoxocosis, rheumatic or ischaemic heart disease.

Clinical features

Most patients are asymptomatic. Atypical chest pain is the most common symptom. Some patients complain of palpitations caused by atrial and ventricular arrhythmias. The typical finding on examination is a midsystolic click, which may be followed by a murmur. Occasionally there are features of mitral regurgitation.

Investigation

Echocardiography is diagnostic and shows the prolapsing valve cusps.

Management

Chest pain and palpitations are treated with β-blockers. Anticoagulation to prevent thromboembolism is indicated if there is significant mitral regurgitation and atrial fibrillation. Prophylaxis against endocarditis is advised if there is significant mitral valve regurgitation.

Aortic stenosis

Aetiology

There are three causes of aortic valve stenosis:

- Degeneration and calcification of a normal tricuspid valve – presenting in the elderly
- Calcification of a congenital bicuspid valve – presenting in middle age
- Rheumatic heart disease.

Pathophysiology

Obstruction to left ventricular emptying results in left ventricular hypertrophy. In turn this results in increased myocardial oxygen demand, relative ischaemia of the myocardium and consequent angina, arrhythmias and eventually left ventricular failure.

Symptoms

There are usually no symptoms until the stenosis is moderately severe (aortic orifice reduced to a third of its normal size). The classic symptoms are angina, exertional syncope and the symptoms of congestive heart failure. Ventricular arrhythmias may cause sudden death.

Signs

The most common sign of aortic stenosis is a harsh systolic ejection murmur (palpated as a thrill), best heard in the aortic area and radiating to the neck. The murmur may be preceded by an ejection click, which is the result of sudden opening of a deformed but mobile valve. The pulse is slow rising and the apex beat thrusting.

Investigations

* Chest radiograph shows a normal heart size, prominence of the ascending aorta (poststenotic dilatation) and there may be valvular calcification.
* ECG may show evidence of left ventricular hypertrophy.
* Echocardiography is diagnostic in most cases. Doppler examination of the valve allows an assessment of the pressure gradient across the valve during systole.
* Cardiac catheterization and coronary angiography is used particularly in patients with angina to exclude coronary artery disease, which may coexist in this predominantly elderly population.

Management

The onset of symptoms in a patient with aortic stenosis is an ominous sign: 75% of patients will be dead within 3 years unless the valve is replaced. Thus aortic valve replacement is usually indicated in symptomatic patients or for severe stenosis (valve gradient of more than 50 mmHg), irrespective of symptoms. Balloon aortic valvotomy is sometimes used as a 'bridge' to valve replacement in very sick patients.

Aortic regurgitation

Aetiology

Aortic regurgitation results from either disease of the valve cusps or dilatation of the aortic root and valve ring. The most common causes are rheumatic fever, and infective endocarditis complicating an already damaged valve (Table 8.8).

Pathophysiology

Chronic regurgitation volume loads the left ventricle and results in hypertrophy and dilatation. The stroke volume is

Table 8.8 Causes and associations of aortic regurgitation

Damage to the aortic valve cusps
  Infective endocarditis*
  Acute rheumatic fever*
  Chronic rheumatic heart disease
  Bicuspid aortic valve

Dilatation of aorta and valve ring
  Dissection of the aorta*
  Syphilis
  Arthritides
    Reiter's syndrome
    Ankylosing spondylitis
    Rheumatoid arthritis
  Severe hypertension
  Aortic endocarditis
  Marfan's syndrome
  Osteogenesis imperfecta

* These conditions may produce acute aortic regurgitation.

increased, which results in an increased pulse pressure and the myriad clinical signs described below. Eventually contraction of the ventricle deteriorates, resulting in left ventricular failure. The adaptations to the volume load entering the left ventricle do not occur with acute regurgitation and patients may present with pulmonary oedema and a reduced stroke volume (hence many of the signs of chronic regurgitation are absent).

Symptoms

In chronic regurgitation patients remain asymptomatic for many years before developing dyspnoea, orthopnoea and fatigue as a result of left ventricular failure.

Signs

- A 'collapsing' (water-hammer) pulse with wide pulse pressure is pathognomonic. Rare manifestations of this sign, which also indicate severe disease are:
  - Quincke's sign (visible capillary pulsation in the nailbed)
  - De Musset's sign (head bobbing)
  - Durozier's sign (systolic bruit heard on compression of the femoral artery).
- The apex beat is displaced laterally and is thrusting in quality.

- A blowing early diastolic murmur is heard at the left sternal edge in the fourth intercostal space. It is accentuated when the patient sits forward with the breath held in expiration. Increased stroke volume produces turbulent flow across the aortic valve, heard as a midsystolic murmur.
- A mid-diastolic murmur (Austin Flint murmur) may be heard over the cardiac apex and is thought to be produced as a result of the aortic jet impinging on the mitral valve, producing premature closure of the valve and physiological stenosis.

Investigations

- Chest radiograph shows a large heart and dilatation of the ascending aorta.
- ECG shows evidence of left ventricular hypertrophy.
- Echocardiography with Doppler examination of the aortic valve helps estimate the severity of regurgitation.
- Aortography during cardiac catheterization helps confirm the severity of the disease.

Management

Mild symptoms may respond to the reduction of afterload with vasodilators and diuretics. The timing of surgery and valve replacement is critical and must not be delayed until there is irreversible left ventricular dysfunction.

Tricuspid and pulmonary valve disease

Tricuspid and pulmonary valve disease are both uncommon. Tricuspid stenosis is almost always the result of rheumatic fever and is frequently associated with mitral and aortic valve disease, which tends to dominate the clinical picture.

Tricuspid regurgitation is usually functional and secondary to dilatation of the right ventricle (and hence tricuspid valve ring) in severe right ventricular failure. Much less commonly it is caused by rheumatic heart disease, infective endocarditis or carcinoid syndrome (page 68). On examination there is a pansystolic murmur heard at the lower left sternal edge, the jugular venous pressure is elevated, with giant 'v' waves (produced by the regurgitant jet through the tricuspid valve in systole), and the liver is enlarged and pulsates in systole. There may be severe peripheral oedema and ascites. In functional tricuspid regurgitation these signs improve with diuretic therapy.

Pulmonary regurgitation results from pulmonary hypertension and dilatation of the valve ring. Occasionally it is the result of endocarditis (usually in intravenous drug abusers). Auscultation reveals an early diastolic murmur heard at the upper left sternal edge (Graham Steell murmur), similar to that of aortic regurgitation. Usually there are no symptoms and treatment is rarely required. Pulmonary stenosis is usually a congenital lesion but may present in adult life with fatigue, syncope and right ventricular failure.

Infective endocarditis

Infective endocarditis is an infection of the endocardium or vascular endothelium of the heart. It may occur as a fulminating or acute infection, but more commonly runs an insidious course and is known as subacute (bacterial) endocarditis (SBE).

Infection occurs in the following:

- On valves which have a congenital or acquired defect (usually on the left side of the heart). Right-sided endocarditis is more common in intravenous drug addicts
- On normal valves (acute infection only)
- On prosthetic valves, when infection may be 'early' (acquired at surgery) or 'late' (following bacteraemia). Infected prosthetic valves often need to be replaced
- In association with a ventricular septal defect or persistent ductus arteriosus.

Aetiology

The most common organisms causing endocarditis are:

- *Streptococcus viridans* (in 50% of cases): this organism is a normal commensal of the upper respiratory tract; bacteraemia occurs following dental extractions, tonsillectomy and bronchoscopy. However, most patients have no history of recent surgery.

- *Enterococcus faecalis*: implicated in endocarditis affecting older men with prostatic disease or following pelvic surgery.
- *Staphylococcus aureus*: this often produces an acute fulminating illness, seen particularly in intravenous drug addicts (using dirty needles) and in patients with central venous lines.

Uncommon organisms: other bacteria, fungi, *Coxiella burnetii* (causative organism of Q fever, page 413) and *Chlamydia psittaci*.

Pathology

A mass of fibrin, platelets and infectious organisms forms vegetations along the edges of the valve. Virulent organisms destroy the valve, producing regurgitation and worsening heart failure.

Clinical features

Symptoms and signs result from:

- Infection, producing an insidious onset of malaise, fever, night sweats, weight loss and anaemia. Slight splenomegaly is common. Clubbing is rare and occurs late.
- Valve destruction, leading to heart failure and new or changing heart murmurs (in 90% of cases).
- Embolization of vegetations and metastatic abscess formation in the brain, spleen and kidney. Embolization from right-sided endocarditis causes pulmonary infarction and pneumonia.
- Immune complex deposition in blood vessels producing a vasculitis and petechial haemorrhages in the skin, under the nails (splinter haemorrhages) and on the retinae (Roth's spots). Osler's nodes (tender subcutaneous nodules in the fingers) and Janeway lesions (painless erythematous macules on the palms) are uncommon. Immune complex deposition in the joints causes arthralgia and, in the kidney, acute glomerulonephritis. Microscopic haematuria occurs in 70% of cases but renal failure is uncommon.

Endocarditis should always be considered in any patient with a heart murmur and fever.

Investigation

- Blood count shows a normochromic/normocytic anaemia with a raised ESR and often a leucocytosis.
- Blood cultures must be taken before antibiotics are started. Six sets taken over 24 hours will identify the organism in 75% of cases. Special culture techniques and serological tests are occasionally necessary if blood cultures are negative and unusual organisms suspected.
- Serum immunoglobulins are increased and complement levels decreased as a result of immune complex formation.
- Urine stix testing shows haematuria in most cases.
- Echocardiography identifies vegetations and underlying valvular dysfunction. Small vegetations may be missed and a normal echocardiogram does not exclude endocarditis. Transoesophageal echocardiography is more sensitive (but not 100%) and is being increasingly used, particularly in cases of suspected prosthetic valve endocarditis.
- Chest X-ray may show heart failure or emboli in right-sided endocarditis.
- ECG may show myocardial infarction (emboli) or conduction defects.

Management

Drug therapy Treatment is with bactericidal antibiotics. Treatment given intravenously for the first 2 weeks and oral treatment continued for a further 2–4 weeks. While awaiting the results of blood cultures a combination of intravenous benzylpenicillin and gentamicin will cover most organisms. In acute fulminating cases the initial treatment should include flucloxacillin and fusidic acid to cover *Staph. aureus*. Subsequent treatment depends on the results of blood cultures and the antibiotic sensitivity of the organism. Antibiotic doses are adjusted to ensure adequate bactericidal activity (microbiological assays of minimum bactericidal concentrations). Surgery to replace the valve should be considered when there is severe heart failure, early infection of prosthetic material, worsening renal failure and extensive damage to the valve.

Prophylaxis

Patients at risk of endocarditis should receive antibiotic therapy before undergoing a procedure likely to result in bacteraemia. The choice of antibiotic depends on the procedure and the likelihood of endocarditis.

···

PULMONARY HEART DISEASE

Pulmonary hypertension

Elevation of the pulmonary artery pressure (pulmonary hypertension) occurs with chronic lung disease, increased pulmonary blood flow (which occurs with atrial septal defect, ventricular septal defect and patent ductus arteriosus), left ventricular failure, mitral stenosis, recurrent pulmonary emboli and primary pulmonary hyptertension. The latter is a rare condition of unkown aetiology predominantly affecting young women. Medial hypertrophy, intimal proliferation and fibrosis, and thrombotic lesions are distributed throughout the pulmonary vasculature.

Clinical features

Chest pain, fatigue, dyspnoea and syncope are common symptoms. The physical signs include a right parasternal heave (caused by right ventricular hypertrophy) and a loud pulmonary second sound. In advanced disease there is right heart failure. There are also features of the underlying disease.

Investigations

- Chest radiograph shows enarged proximal pulmonary arteries which taper distally. It may also reveal the underlying cause (e.g. emphysema, calcified mitral valve).
- ECG shows right ventricular hypertrophy and P pulmonale. Echocardiography shows right ventricular hypertrophy and dilatation, and may reveal the underlying cause of pulmonary hypertension. Pulmonary artery pressure can be measured indirectly with Doppler echocardiography.

Management

The treatment is that of the cause. In primary pulmonary hypertension there is a progressive downhill course which in some patients can be slowed by a combination of warfarin and oral calcium channel blockers as pulmonary vasodilators. Continuous (a year or more) intravenous infusion of epoprostenol (prostacyclin) reduces pulmonary resistance and improve symptoms. However, many patients ultimately require heart and lung transplantation.

Pulmonary embolism

Pulmonary embolism is a common condition and usually a consequence of thrombosis in the ileofemoral veins (deep venous thrombosis, page 390). More rarely it results from clot formation in the right atrium in patients with right-sided cardiac failure, particularly if there is atrial fibrillation.

Pathology

After pulmonary embolism lung tissue is ventilated but not perfused, resulting in impaired gas exchange. A massive embolism suddenly increases pulmonary vascular resistance, causing acute right heart failure. A small embolus may be clinically silent unless it causes pulmonary infarction.

Clinical features

- Massive pulmonary embolism presents as a medical emergency: the patient has severe central chest pain and suddenly becomes shocked, pale and sweaty, with marked tachypnoea and tachycardia. Syncope and death may follow rapidly. On examination the patient is shocked, with central cyanosis. There is elevation of the jugular venous pressure, a right ventricular heave, accentuation of the second heart sound and a gallop rhythm.
- Small/medium pulmonary emboli presents with dyspnoea and, if there is pulmonary infarction, haemoptysis, pleuritic chest pain and a pleural rub.
- Multiple recurrent pulmonary emboli present with symptoms and signs of pulmonary hypertension (see below), developing over weeks to months.

Investigations

- Chest radiograph is often normal but may show decreased vascular markings and a raised hemidiaphragm

(caused by loss of lung volume). With pulmonary infarction a late feature is the development of a wedge-shaped opacity adjacent to the pleural edge, sometimes with a pleural effusion.
- ECG is usually normal except for sinus tachycardia. The features of acute right heart strain may be seen: tall peaked P waves in lead II, right axis deviation and right bundle-branch block.
- Blood gases may show hypoxaemia and hypocapnia.
- Radionuclide lung scan (V/Q scan) demonstrates areas of ventilated lung with perfusion defects (ventilation–perfusion defects). However, up to 50% of V/Q scans are non-diagnostic and may be normal, or show matched defects which can also be seen with some chronic lung diseases, e.g. emphysema.
- Ultrasound can be performed for the detection of clots in pelvic or ileofemoral veins.
- Spiral CT images the pulmonary vessels directly and has approximately 90% sensitivity and specificity for medium/large pulmonary emboli. This technique is currently unable to detect small emboli.
- MRI gives similar results and is used if CT is contraindicated.
- Plasma D–dimers are a subset of fibrinogen degradation products released into the circulation when a clot begins to dissolve. Undetectable levels exclude a diagnosis of pulmonary embolism.
- Pulmonary angiography is the definitive method of diagnosis and is sometimes undertaken if surgery is considered in acute massive embolism. It shows obstructed vessels or obvious filling defects in the artery.

Management

Treatment (Emergency Box 8.4) can be started on the basis of clinical suspicion pending investigation. Immediate surgical embolectomy is considered in preference to thrombolysis for severe cases of acute massive embolism.

Chronic cor pulmonale

Cor pulmonale is right heart failure resulting from chronic pulmonary hypertension.

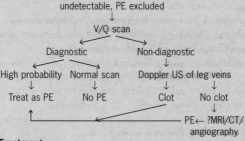

Emergency

Investigation and diagnosis

Clinically suspected PE
↓
Plasma D-dimers (fibrin
degradation product): if
undetectable, PE excluded
↓
V/Q scan

Diagnostic   Non-diagnostic

High probability   Normal scan   Doppler US of leg veins
↓   ↓   ↓   ↓
Treat as PE   No PE   Clot   No clot
↓
PE← ?MRI/CT/
angiography

Treatment
60% oxygen if hypoxaemic
Dissolution of the thrombus
    Consider for massive embolism with hypotension and signs of
    acute right heart strain
    Streptokinase: 250 000 U by i.v. infusion over 30 minutes,
    followed by 100 000 U/h for 24 h
Analgesia
    Morphine (5–10 mg i.v.) to relieve pain and anxiety
Prevention of further thrombi
    Intravenous heparin and oral warfarin (page 186).
Intravenous fluids (to raise the filling pressure) +/– inotropes for
patients present with moderate/severe embolism

Emergency Box 8.4
Management of pulmonary embolism (PE)

Aetiology

Chronic obstructive pulmonary disease caused by
bronchitis and emphysema is responsible for most cases
(Table 8.9). Pulmonary vascular resistance is increased
because of destruction of the pulmonary vascular bed and
pulmonary vasoconstriction caused by acidosis and hypoxia.
Eventually, increased resistance leads to right heart strain
and right ventricular failure.

Treatment

Treatment is directed towards the underlying pulmonary
disease as well as right ventricular failure. Acute chest

Table 8.9 Causes of cor pulmonale

Intrinsic lung disease, e.g. COPD, pulmonary fibrosis
Recurrent pulmonary emboli
Skeletal abnormalities, e.g. kyphoscoliosis
Hypoventilation, e.g. morbid obesity
Neuromuscular disease, e.g. poliomyelitis, myasthenia gravis
Obstruction, e.g. sleep apnoea syndrome

infections must be treated promptly. Oxygen therapy over a long period may reduce established pulmonary hypertension, with an improvement in overall prognosis (page 406).

MYOCARDIAL DISEASE

Myocarditis

Myocarditis is an inflammation of the myocardium. The most common cause in the UK is viral, particularly Coxsackie virus infection, but it may also occur with diphtheria, rheumatic fever, radiation injury and some drugs.

Clinical features

Patients present with an acute illness characterized by fever and varying degrees of biventricular failure. Cardiac arrhythmias and pericarditis may also occur.

Investigations

* Chest radiograph may show cardiac enlargement.
* ECG shows non-specific T-wave and ST changes.
* The diagnosis is supported by demonstration of an increase in serum viral titres and inflammation on cardiac biopsy. The findings rarely influence management and biopsy is not usually performed.

Management

Treatment is with bed rest and treatment of cardiac failure. The prognosis is generally good.

CARDIOMYOPATHY

Cardiomyopathies are myocardial disorders that are not secondary to coronary disease or hypertension, or to congenital, valvular or pericardial abnormalities.

There are four main types:

- Dilated
- Hypertrophic
- Restrictive
- Arrhythmogenic right ventricular.

Dilated cardiomyopathy

Dilated cardiomyopathy (DCM) is characterized by a dilated left ventricle which contracts poorly. In about 25% of patients it is a familial disease.

Clinical features

Shortness of breath is usually the first complaint; less often patients present with embolism (from mural thrombus) or arrhythmia. Subsequently there is progressive heart failure with the symptoms and signs of biventricular failure.

Investigations

- Chest X-ray may show cardiac enlargement.
- ECG is often abnormal. The changes are non-specific and include arrhythmias and T-wave flattening.
- Echocardiography shows dilated ventricles with global hypokinesis (compare with ischaemia with regional contractile impairment).

Other tests such as coronary arteriography, viral and autoimmune screen, and endomyocardial biopsy may be needed to exclude other diseases (Table 8.10) which present with the clinical features of DCM.

Management

Heart failure and atrial fibrillation are treated in the conventional way (pages 334, 344). Ventricular tachycardia is

Table 8.10 Heart muscle disease presenting with features of DCM

Ischaemia
Hypertension
Congenital heart disease
Peripartum cardiomyopathy
Alcohol
Muscular dystrophy
Amyloidosis
Haemochromatosis

not prevented with antiarrythmic drugs and is best treated with an internal cardioverter defibrillator. A history of embolization or AF is an indication for anticoagulation. Severe cardiomyopathy is treated with cardiac transplantation.

Hypertrophic cardiomyopathy

Hyertrophic cardiomyopathy is characterized by marked ventricular hypertrophy of unknown cause, usually with disproportionate involvement of the interventricular septum. The hypertrophic non-compliant ventricles impair diastolic filling, so that stroke volume is reduced. Most cases are familial, autosomal dominant, and caused by mutations in genes coding for proteins that regulate contraction e.g. troponin T and β-myosin.

Clinical features

Patients may be symptomless or have dyspnoea, angina or syncope. Atrial and ventricular arrhythmias are common; ventricular tachyarrhythmias are the major cause of sudden death, which is most common in adolescence and young adulthood. The carotid pulse is jerky because of rapid ejection and sudden obstruction to the ventricular outflow during systole. An ejection systolic murmur occurs because of left ventricular outflow obstruction, and the pansystolic murmur of functional mitral regurgitation may also be heard.

Investigations

- ECG is almost always abnormal. A pattern of left ventricular hypertrophy with no discernable cause is diagnostic.
- Echocardiography shows ventricular hypertrophy with disproportionate involvement of the septum.

Management

The risk of arrhythmias and sudden death is reduced by amiodarone, but survivors of cardiac arrest need to be fitted with an internal defibrillator. Chest pain and dyspnoea are treated with β-blockers and verapamil. In selected cases outflow tract gradients are reduced by surgical resection or alcohol ablation of the septum, or by dual-chamber pacing.

Family members should be screened for evidence of disease by ECG and echocardiography.

Restrictive cardiomyopathy

The rigid myocardium restricts diastolic ventricular filling and the clinical features resemble those of constrictive pericarditis (see later). In the UK the most common cause is amyloidosis. The ECG, chest radiograph and echocardiogram are often abnormal, but the findings are non-specific. Diagnosis is by cardiac catheterization, which shows characteristic pressure changes. An endomyocardial biopsy may be taken during the catheter procedure, thus providing histological diagnosis. There is no specific treatment and the prognosis is poor, with most patients dying less than a year after diagnosis. Cardiac transplantation is performed in selected cases.

Arrhythmogenic right ventricular cardiomyopathy

There is progressive fibroadipose replacement of the wall of the right ventricle. The typical presentation is ventricular tachycardia or sudden death in a young man.

PERICARDIAL DISEASE

Acute pericarditis

Aetiology

Acute inflammation of the pericardium is usually caused by Coxsackie viral infection or follows acute myocardial infarction. Other causes include uraemia, connective tissue diseases, trauma, tuberculosis and malignancy (breast, lung, leukaemia and lymphoma).

Clinical features

There is sharp retrosternal chest pain which is characteristically relieved by leaning forward. Pain may be worse on inspiration and radiate to the neck and shoulders. The cardinal clinical sign is a pericardial friction rub, which may be transient.

Diagnosis

ECG shows ST segment elevation in all the leads except AVR and V1. The elevated ST segments are characteristically concave upwards (convex upwards in infarction) and return towards baseline as inflammation subsides.

Management

Treatment is of the underlying disorder plus NSAIDs. Systemic corticosteroids are used in resistant cases.

Pericardial effusion and tamponade

Pericardial effusion is an accumulation of fluid in the pericardial sac which may result from any of the causes of pericarditis. Pericardial tamponade is a medical emergency and occurs when a large amount of pericardial fluid (which has often accumulated rapidly) restricts diastolic ventricular filling and causes a marked reduction in cardiac output.

Clinical features

The effusion obscures the apex beat and the heart sounds are soft. The signs of pericardial tamponade are hypotension, tachycardia and an elevated jugular venous pressure, which paradoxically rises with inspiration (Kussmaul's sign). There is invariably pulsus paradoxus (a fall in blood pressure of more than 10 mmHg on inspiration). This is the result of increased venous return to the right side of the heart during inspiration. The increased right ventricular volume thus occupies more space within the rigid pericardium and impairs left ventricular filling.

Investigations

- Chest radiograph shows a large globular heart.
- ECG shows low voltage complexes.
- Echocardiography is diagnostic, showing an echo-free space around the heart.

Management

The treatment of tamponade is emergency pericardiocentesis. Pericardial fluid is drained percutaneously by introducing a needle into the pericardial sac. If the effusion recurs, in spite of treatment of the underlying cause, excision of a pericardial segment may be necessary. Fluid is then absorbed through the pleural and mediastinal lymphatics.

Constrictive pericarditis

In the UK most cases of constrictive pericarditis are idiopathic in origin or result from intrapericardial haemorrhage during heart surgery. Tuberculous infection is no longer the most common cause.

Clinical features

The heart becomes encased within a rigid fibrotic pericardial sac which prevents adequate diastolic filling of the ventricles. The clinical features resemble those of right-sided cardiac failure, with jugular venous distension, dependent oedema, hepatomegaly and ascites. Kussmaul's sign (JVP rises paradoxically with inspiration) is usually present and there may be pulsus paradoxus, atrial fibrillation and, on auscultation, a pericardial knock caused by rapid ventricular filling.

Investigations

A chest radiograph shows a normal heart size and pericardial calcification (best seen on the lateral film). Diagnosis is made by CT, which shows pericardial thickening and calcification.

Management

Treatment is by surgical excision of the pericardium.

....

SYSTEMIC HYPERTENSION

The level of blood pressure can be said to be abnormal when it is associated with a clear increase in morbidity and mortality from heart disease, stroke and renal failure. This level varies with age, sex, race and country. The definition varies, but recent guidelines from the USA recommend a definition of hypertension as 140/90 mmHg, based on at least two readings on separate occasions. The validity of a single blood pressure measurement is unclear (blood pressure rises acutely in certain situations, e.g. visiting the doctor) and usually several readings are required to confirm a diagnosis of hypertension. Occasionally, ambulatory blood pressure monitoring (blood pressure measured throughout the day using a non-invasive technique) is used if there is doubt as to the level of blood pressure.

Aetiology

Essential hypertension More than 90% of cases of hypertension have no known underlying cause, and the terms 'primary' or 'essential' hypertension are used. Several factors may play an aetiological role:

- Familial tendency
- Low birthweight
- Obesity   ✓exercise
- High alcohol intake
- High salt intake – controversial
- Insulin resistance (syndrome X).

Secondary hypertension This should always be considered, particularly in those presenting under the age of 35. Causes of secondary hypertension are the following:

- Renal disease, which accounts for over 80% of cases of secondary hypertension. Chronic glomerulonephritis, chronic pyelonephritis, congenital polycystic kidneys and renal artery stenosis are the diseases usually involved
- Endocrine disease (page 511): Conn's syndrome, Cushing's syndrome, phaeochromocytoma and acromegaly
- Coarctation of the aorta
- Pre-eclampsia occurring in the third trimester of pregnancy
- Drugs, including oestrogen-containing oral contraceptives, other steroids and vasopressin.

Clinical features

Hypertension is generally asymptomatic, although malignant or accelerated hypertension (usually BP >200/140 mmHg) may present with characteristic symptoms. These include visual impairment, nausea, vomiting, fits, headaches or symptoms of acute cardiac failure. Secondary causes of hypertension may be suggested by specific features, such as attacks of sweating and tachycardia in phaeochromocytoma.

Examination In most patients the only finding is high blood pressure, but in others signs relating to the cause (e.g. abdominal bruit in renal artery stenosis, delayed femoral pulses in coarctation of the aorta) or the end-organ effects of hypertension may be present, e.g. loud second heart sound, left ventricular heave, fourth heart sound in hypertensive heart disease, and retinal abnormalities. The latter are graded according to severity:

- Grade 1 – increased tortuosity and reflectiveness of the retinal arteries (silver wiring)
- Grade 2 – grade 1 plus arteriovenous nipping
- Grade 3 – grade 2 plus flame-shaped haemorrhages and soft 'cotton-wool' exudates
- Grade 4 – grade 3 plus papilloedema.

Investigations

Investigations are carried out to identify end-organ damage and those patients with secondary causes of hypertension.

- Chest radiograph may show heart failure. Rib notching indicates coarctation of the aorta.
- Serum urea and electrolytes may show evidence of renal impairment, in which case more specific renal investigations are indicated. Hypokalaemia occurs in Conn's syndrome.
- ECG may show evidence of left ventricular hypertrophy or myocardial ischaemia.
- Urine stix testing is performed to look for haematuria and proteinuria, which may indicate renal disease (either the cause or the effect of hypertension).

Young patients with hypertension (<35 years) or those where a secondary cause is suspected (e.g. from clinical examination or abnormal baseline investigations) should undergo further investigation, e.g. urinary catecholamines for phaeochromocytoma, full renal investigation for renovascular hypertension.

Management

Treatment of moderate-to-severe hypertension reduces the incidence of stroke, heart failure and renal damage but has less effect on coronary artery disease. Indications for drug treatment are:

- Diastolic BP ≥100 mmHg on repeated measurement
- Diastolic blood pressure 90–100 mmHg if there is evidence of end-organ damage *or* other risk factors, e.g. diabetes, *or* age >60 years

- Systolic blood pressure ≥160 mmHg except if diastolic ≤95 mmHg + no end-organ damage + systolic BP ≤200 mmHg.

General measures include:

- Weight reduction
- Reduction of heavy alcohol consumption
- No added salt diet
- Regular exercise.

Drug therapy A large number of drugs may be used in treatment and these are usually selected on the basis of efficacy, tolerance and compliance. Calcium channel blockers and ACE inhibitors are replacing thiazide diuretics and β-blockers as first-line agents. Single agents are used initially, but combination treatment may be needed in patients not controlled with one drug. Particularly effective combinations include an ACE inhibitor or β-blocker with a diuretic, and the combination of a calcium antagonist with a β-blocker.

Diuretics increase renal sodium and water excretion and directly dilate arterioles. Loop diuretics, e.g. frusemide, and thiazide diuretics, e.g. bendrofluazide, are equally effective in lowering blood pressure, although thiazides are usually preferred as the duration of action is longer, the diuresis is not so severe and they are cheaper. The major concern with thiazide diuretics is their adverse metabolic effects: increased serum cholesterol, hypokalaemia, hyperuricaemia (may precipitate gout) and impairment of glucose tolerance.

β-Adrenergic blocking agents The mechanism of action of these agents is unclear. Although they reduce the force of cardiac contraction and renin production, they probably act predominantly via the central nervous system. There are a wide range of β-blocking agents with different properties, such as cardioselectivity, intrinsic sympathomimetic activity and lipid solubility. Complications include aggravation of left ventricular failure, bradycardia, cold extremities, fatigue and weakness.

ACE inhibitors, e.g. captopril, enalapril and lisinopril, block the conversion of angiotensin I to angiotensin II, which is a potent vasoconstrictor, and block degradation of bradykinin, which is a vasodilator. Side effects include first-dose hypotension and cough, proteinuria, rashes and leucopenia in high doses. ACE inhibitors are contraindicated in renal artery stenosis because inhibition of the renin–angiotensin system in this instance may lead to loss of renal blood flow and infarction of the kidney.

Angiotensin II receptor antagonists, e.g. losartan and valsartan, selectively block receptors for angiotensin II. They share some of the actions of ACE inhibitors and may be useful in patients who cannot tolerate ACE inhibitors because of cough.

Calcium antagonists, e.g. amlodipine and nifedipine, are increasingly used and act predominantly by dilatation of peripheral arterioles. Side effects are few and include bradycardia and cardiac conduction defects (verapamil and diltiazem), headaches, flushing and fluid retention.

Other agents α-Blocking agents (e.g. doxazosin), hydralazine, and centrally acting agents (e.g. moxonidine) may be indicated in specific circumstances.

Management of severe hypertension

Patients with severe hypertension (diastolic BP >140 mmHg) are treated with oral antihypertensives, e.g. atenolol 25 mg or nifedipine retard 10 mg. If unsuccessful, a second dose can be given after 6 hours. The aim should be to reduce the diastolic blood pressure slowly (over 24–48 hours) to about 100–110 mmHg. Sublingual and intravenous antihypertensives are not recommended because they may produce a precipitous fall in blood pressure leading to cerebral infarction.

Patient with severe hypertension complicated by hypertensive encephalopathy (altered consciousness, seizures or transient focal neurological signs), acute pulmonary oedema or aortic dissection (page 389) require a more urgent reduction in blood pressure. Treatment is with intravenous sodium nitroprusside (starting dose 0.3 μg/kg/min, i.e. 100 mg nitroprusside in 250 ml saline at 2–5 ml/h) and/or a β-blocker.

ARTERIAL AND VENOUS DISEASE
Aortic aneurysms

Aortic aneurysms are usually abdominal and result from atheroma.

Abdominal Abdominal aortic aneurysms may be asymptomatic and found as a pulsating mass on abdominal examination or as calcification on a plain radiograph. An expanding aneurysm may cause epigastric or back pain. A ruptured aortic aneurysm is a surgical emergency presenting with epigastric pain radiating to the back, and hypovolaemic shock. Diagnosis is by ultrasonography or CT scan. Surgery is indicated for a symptomatic aneurysm or large asymptomatic aneurysms (>5 cm).

Thoracic Cystic medial necrosis and atherosclerosis are the usual causes of thoracic aneurysms. Cardiovascular syphilis is no longer a common cause.

Clinical features

Thoracic aneurysms may be asymptomatic, cause pressure on local structures (causing back pain, dysphagia and cough) or result in aortic regurgitation if the aortic root is involved. Aortic dissection results from a tear in the intima: blood under high pressure creates a false lumen in the diseased media. Typically there is an abrupt onset of severe, tearing central chest pain, radiating through to the back. Involvement of branch arteries may produce neurological signs, absent pulses and unequal blood pressure in the arms.

Management

The chest radiograph shows a widened mediastinum in dissection. The diagnosis is made by CT scanning and transoesophageal echocardiography or MRI. Management involves urgent control of blood pressure (page 388) and surgical repair for proximal aortic dissection.

Raynaud's disease and phenomenon

Intermittent spasm occurs in the arteries supplying the fingers and toes. There is initial pallor (resulting from vasoconstriction) followed by cyanosis and, finally, redness from hyperaemia. Raynaud's disease (no underlying disorder) occurs most commonly in young women and must be differentiated from secondary causes of Raynaud's phenomenon, e.g. connective tissue diseases and β-blockers. Treatment is by keeping the hands and feet warm, stopping smoking, and in some cases nifedipine.

Venous disease

Superficial thrombophlebitis This usually occurs in the leg. The vein is painful, tender and hard, with overlying redness. Treatment is with simple analgesia, e.g. NSAIDs. Anticoagulation is not necessary as embolism does not occur.

Deep venous thrombosis Thrombosis can occur in any vein, but those of the pelvis and leg are the most common sites. Deep vein thrombosis (DVT) is often a result of prolonged immobility in bed, particularly following abdominal or pelvic surgery. Other risk factors are cardiac failure, pregnancy and childbirth, oral contraceptive drugs, malignant disease, chronic pulmonary disease and hypercoagulable states.

Clinical features

DVT is often asymptomatic but the leg may be warm and swollen, with calf tenderness and superficial venous distension.

Investigations

Diagnosis of iliofemoral thrombosis is made by Doppler ultrasonography. This method is not reliable for calf vein thrombosis, which is diagnosed by venography.

Management

This is discussed on page 186.

The main aim of therapy is to prevent pulmonary embolism, and all patients with thrombi above the knee must be anticoagulated. Anticoagulation for below-knee thrombi is controversial but is usually recommended for 6 weeks to reduce proximal extension.

Anticoagulation is initially with heparin and subsequently with warfarin, continued for 3 months in the absence of a definite risk factor, e.g. bed rest, when treatment is usually for 4 weeks. Thrombolytic therapy is occasionally used for patients with a large iliofemoral thrombosis.

Permanent pain, swelling, oedema and sometimes venous eczema may result from destruction of the deep-vein valves. Elastic support stockings are then required for life.

Respiratory disease

SYMPTOMS OF RESPIRATORY DISEASE

The common symptoms of respiratory disease are cough, sputum production, chest pain (page 321), breathlessness, haemoptysis and wheeze.

Cough is a non-specific symptom and the most common manifestation of lower respiratory tract disease. It may be the only symptom of asthma, when it is typically worse at night, on waking and after exercise. A chronic cough, sometimes accompanied by sputum production, is common in smokers; however, a worsening cough may be the presenting symptom of bronchial carcinoma and needs investigation.

Dyspnoea This is the subjective sensation of shortness of breath. *Orthopnoea* is breathlessness that occurs when lying flat and is the result both of abdominal contents pushing the diaphragm into the thorax and of redistribution of blood from the lower extremities to the lungs. *Paroxysmal nocturnal dyspnoea* is a manifestation of left heart failure: the patient wakes up gasping for breath and finds some relief by sitting upright. The mechanism is similar to orthopnoea, but because sensory awareness is depressed during sleep, severe interstitial pulmonary oedema can accumulate.

The speed of onset of breathlessness is useful when formulating a differential diagnosis (Table 9.1). The clinical history and examination will often suggest a probable cause, particularly with sudden and acute breathlessness. Simple lung function tests and a chest X-ray are the initial investigations for most patients with breathlessness.

Wheeze Wheezing is the result of airflow limitation of any cause. It may be due to localized obstruction of the airways, e.g. cancer, foreign body, or to generalized obstruction, of which the commonest causes are asthma and chronic obstructive pulmonary disease. Rarer causes are cystic

Table 9.1 Differential diagnosis of dyspnoea

Sudden	Acute: over hours	Over days	Over months/years	Intermittent
Inhaled foreign body	Asthma	Pleural effusion	COPD	Asthma
Pneumothorax	Pneumonia	Cancer of the	Pulmonary fibrosis	Pulmonary oedema
Pulmonary embolism	Pulmonary oedema	bronchus/trachea	Anaemia	
	Extrinsic allergic alveolitis			

COPD, chronic obstructive pulmonary disease.

fibrosis and bronchiectasis. Wheeze should be distinguished from stridor which is a harsh inspiratory wheezing sound caused by obstruction of the trachea or major bronchi, e.g. by tumour.

Haemoptysis (coughing blood) requires thorough investigation. The common causes are bronchiectasis, bronchial carcinoma, pulmonary infarction, bronchitis and pneumonia. Pulmonary oedema is associated with the production of pink frothy sputum. Rust-coloured sputum may occur with pneumococcal pneumonia but haemoptysis should not be attributed to infection without investigation. Less common causes include benign tumour, bleeding disorder and, rarely, Wegener's granulomatosis (page 425) and Goodpasture's syndrome (page 277). A chest radiograph should be performed in all patients and subsequent investigations (e.g. bronchoscopy, CT, isotope lung scan) decided from the history and examination.

Massive haemoptysis, which is usually due to bronchiectasis or cancer (more than 200 ml in 24 h), may be life-threatening and is an indication for hospital admission.

Respiratory function tests

Respiratory function tests can be simple outpatient investigations carried out to assess airflow limitation and lung volumes. The normal values vary for age, sex and height, and between individuals.

Peak expiratory flow rate (PEFR) is measured with a peak flow meter. This records the maximum expiratory flow rate during a forced expiration after full inspiration. It is useful in detecting airflow limitation and in monitoring the response to treatment of acute asthma.

Forced expiratory volume (FEV) and forced vital capacity (FVC) are measured with a spirometer. The patient exhales as fast and as long as possible from a full inspiration; the volume expired in the first second is the FEV_1 and the total volume expired is the FVC. The ratio FEV_1:FVC is a measure of airflow limitation and is normally about 75%.

- Airflow limitation: FEV_1:FVC <75%
- Restrictive lung disease: FEV_1:FVC >75%.

More sophisticated techniques allow the measurement of total lung capacity (TLC) and residual volume (RV). These are increased in obstructive lung disease, e.g. asthma or COPD, because of air trapping, and reduced in lung fibrosis.

Transfer factor (T_{CO}) measures the transfer of a low concentration of added carbon monoxide in the inspired air to haemoglobin. The transfer coefficient (K_{CO}) is the value corrected for differences in lung volume. Gas transfer is reduced early on in emphysema and lung fibrosis.

Assessment of lung function is also made by measuring arterial blood gases (page 638) and with exercise tests to assess walking distance in a 6-minute period.

DISEASES OF THE UPPER RESPIRATORY TRACT

The common cold (acute coryza)

The common cold is caused by infection with one of the many strains of rhinovirus. Spread is by droplets and close personal contact. After an incubation period of 12 hours to 5 days the major symptoms are malaise, slight pyrexia, a sore throat and a watery nasal discharge, which becomes mucopurulent after a few days. Treatment is symptomatic. The differential diagnosis is mainly from rhinitis.

Sinusitis

Sinusitis is an infection of one of the paranasal sinuses (maxillary, frontal or ethmoid) and may complicate allergic rhinitis or an upper respiratory tract infection (caused by mucosal oedema and blockage of the ostium). Acute infections are usually caused by *Streptococcus pneumoniae* or *Haemophilus influenzae*. Symptoms are frontal headache, facial pain and tenderness, and nasal discharge. The diagnosis is usually clinical and treatment is with antibiotics and nasal decongestants. Rare complications include local and cerebral abscesses.

Rhinitis

The symptoms of rhinitis are sneezing, a watery nasal discharge and nasal blockage. *Perennial rhinitis* occurs throughout the year and may be allergic (the allergens are similar to those for asthma) or non-allergic. *Seasonal allergic rhinitis* (hay fever) occurs during the summer months and is caused by allergy to grass and tree pollen and a variety of mould spores (e.g. *Aspergillus fumigatus*) which grow on cultivated plants. The diagnosis of rhinitis is clinical. Skin-prick testing and measurement of specific serum IgE antibody in conjunction with a detailed clinical history will identify causal antigens. The management involves avoidance of allergens if practical, and topical antihistamines, decongestants and topical steroids. A low dose of oral prednisolone may be necessary when other treatments fail.

Acute pharyngitis

Viruses, particularly from the adenovirus group, are the most common cause of acute pharyngitis. Symptoms are a sore throat and fever which are self-limiting and only require symptomatic treatment. More persistent and severe pharyngitis may imply bacterial infection, often secondary invaders, of which the most common organisms are haemolytic *Streptococcus*, *Haemophilus influenzae* and *Staphylococcus aureus*. This requires appropriate antibiotic therapy.

Acute laryngotracheobronchitis

This is usually the result of infection with one of the parainfluenza viruses or measles virus. Symptoms are most severe in children under 3 years of age. Inflammatory oedema involving the larynx causes a hoarse voice, barking cough (croup) and stridor. Tracheitis produces a burning retrosternal pain. Treatment is with oxygen and inhaled steam; tracheostomy is needed in severe cases.

Influenza

The influenza virus belongs to the orthomyxovirus group and exists in two main forms, A and B. The surface of the virion is coated with haemagglutinin (H) and an enzyme, neuraminidase (N), which are important for attachment to the host respiratory epithelium. Human immunity develops against the H and N antigens. Influenza A has the capacity to undergo antigenic 'shift', and major changes in the H and N antigens are associated with pandemic infections which may cause millions of deaths worldwide. Minor antigenic 'drifts' are associated with less severe epidemics.

Clinical features

After an incubation period of 1–3 days there is an abrupt onset of fever, myalgia, headache, sore throat and dry cough, which may last several weeks.

Diagnosis

Laboratory diagnosis is not always necessary, but serology shows a fourfold rise in antibody titre over a 2-week period.

Management

Treatment is usually symptomatic (aspirin, bed rest, maintenance of fluid intake), together with amantadine and antibiotics for individuals with chronic bronchitis, or heart or renal disease.

Complications

Pneumonia is the most common complication. This is either viral or the result of secondary infection with bacteria, of which *Staphylococcus aureus* is the most serious, with a mortality rate of up to 20%.

Prophylaxis

Influenza vaccine is prepared from current strains. It is effective in 70% of people and lasts for about a year. It is offered annually to the chronically sick, the elderly, immunosuppressed individuals, residents of long-stay facilities (where rapid spread is likely to follow the introduction of infection), and medical staff during a pandemic.

Inhalation of foreign bodies

Children inhale foreign bodies – frequently peanuts – more often than adults. In adults inhalation is usually associated with a depressed conscious level, such as after an alcoholic binge. A large object may totally occlude the airways and rapidly result in death. Smaller objects impact more peripherally (usually the right main bronchus, because it is more vertical than the left) and cause choking, or patients may present at a later stage with persistent suppurative pneumonia or lung abscess. In an emergency the foreign body is dislodged from the airway using the Heimlich manoeuvre: the subject is gripped from behind with the arms around the upper abdomen, a sharp forceful squeeze pushes the diaphragm into the thorax and the rapid airflow generated may be sufficient to force the foreign body out of the trachea or bronchus. In the non-emergency situation bronchoscopy is used to remove the foreign body.

. . . .

DISEASES OF THE LOWER RESPIRATORY TRACT

Asthma

Asthma is a common chronic inflammatory condition of the lung airways, the cause of which is incompletely understood. It has three characteristics: reversible airflow limitation, airway hyperresponsiveness to a range of stimuli, and inflammation of the bronchi.

Epidemiology

The prevalence of asthma is increasing, particularly in the second decade of life, when 10–15% of the population are affected. There is a geographical variation: asthma is more common in New Zealand and much rarer in Far Eastern countries.

Aetiology

There are two major factors involved in the development of asthma:

- *Atopy* This is the term used in individuals who readily develop antibodies of immunoglobulin E (IgE) class against common environmental antigens such as the house dust mite, grass pollen and fungal spores from *Aspergillus fumigatus*.
- *Increased responsiveness of the airways of the lung* (as measured by a fall in FEV_1) to stimuli such as inhaled histamine and methacholine (bronchial provocation tests).

Asthma has traditionally been divided into extrinsic (atopic) and intrinsic (non-atopic) on the basis that in extrinsic asthma allergens can be identified by positive skin-prick reactions to common inhaled allergens. It is now recognized that almost all asthmatic patients show some degree of atopy, and this classification is used less often. The development of atopy is determined by both environmental and genetic factors. Environmental factors include pre- and postnatal exposure to allergens, childhood exposure to respiratory irritants such as tobacco smoke, and some viral infections. Asthma and atopy run in families, the inheritance being estimated to be between 40% and 60%. A number of possible gene linkages to asthma have been identified and some of these have been shown to mediate the switch to IgE production, differentiation into T-helper cells with production of IL-4 and IL-5, and also to influence eosinophil production and recruitment to the lung.

Pathogenesis and precipitating factors

The pathogenesis of asthma is complex and not fully understood. It involves a number of cells, mediators, nerves and vascular leakage which can be activated by several mechanisms, of which exposure to allergens is the most relevant.

The cellular component of the inflammatory response includes eosinophils, T lymphocytes, macrophages and mast cells, which release a number of inflammatory mediators. Mast cell degranulation is produced by the union of antigen with IgE antibody which is bound to the mast cell surface.

Precipitating factors The major allergen (Der p1) is contained in the faecal particles of the house dust mite, *Dermatophagoides pteronnysinus*, which is found in dust throughout the house. Non-specific factors which may cause wheezing are viral infections, cold air, exercise, irritant dusts, vapours and fumes (cigarette smoke, perfume, exhaust fumes), emotion and drugs (NSAID, aspirin and β-blockers).

Over 200 materials encountered at the workplace may give rise to wheezing, which typically improves on days away from work and during holidays (occupational asthma). Common occupations associated with asthma are veterinary medicine and animal handling (allergens are mouse, rat and rabbit urine and fur), bakery (wheat, rye) and laundry work (biological enzymes).

A rare cause of asthma is the airborne spores of *Aspergillus fumigatus*, a soil mould. There are fleeting shadows on the chest radiograph and peripheral blood eosinophilia (allergic bronchopulmonary aspergillosis, not to be confused with the severe aspergillus pneumonia occurring in the immunocompromised).

Clinical features

Symptoms are episodic wheezing, cough and shortness of breath which are typically worse at night and in the early morning. A cough may be the only presenting symptom. Some patients have just one or two attacks a year, whereas others have chronic symptoms. On examination, during an attack, there is reduced chest expansion, prolonged expiratory time and expiratory polyphonic wheezes.

Investigations

The diagnosis of asthma is often made on the history and response to bronchodilators. There is no single satisfactory diagnostic test for all asthmatic patients.

- Lung function tests: Demonstration of a greater than 15% improvement in FEV_1 or PEFR following inhalation of a bronchodilator.
- Peak flow charts: Measurement of PEFR by the patient on waking, during the day and before bed shows the characteristic variability in airflow limitation. Most asthmatic individuals will show obvious diurnal variation, with lowest values occurring in the early morning (the 'morning dip', Figure 9.1).
- Chest radiograph is performed at diagnosis and usually only repeated in an acute severe asthma attack.
- Skin-prick tests are used to identify allergens to which the patient is sensitive. A weal develops 15 minutes after allergen injection in the epidermis of the forearm.
- Histamine or methacholine bronchial provocation tests are usually reserved for difficult diagnostic cases. Bronchial hyperreactivity is demonstrated by asking the patient to inhale gradually increasing doses of histamine or methacholine and demonstrating a fall in FEV_1. Patients with clinical symptoms of asthma respond to very low doses.
- Serum: *Aspergillus* antibody titres should be measured in those with a marked blood eosinophilia or transient shadowing on the chest X-ray.

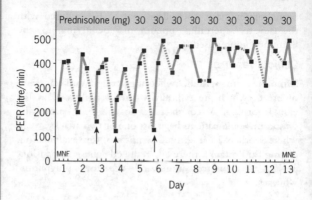

Figure 9.1
Classic diurnal variation of asthma, showing the effect of steroids. The arrows indicate the morning 'dips'. M, morning; N, noon; E, evening.

Management

The effective treatment of asthma centres on patient education, the avoidance of precipitating factors and specific drug treatment.

Avoidance of precipitating factors Patients should be discouraged from smoking and avoid allergens, e.g. household pets, which have been shown to provoke attacks. Avoidance of the house dust mite may be possible with frequent house cleaning and the use of effective covers for bedding. It is necessary to identify occupational asthma because early diagnosis and removal of the patient from exposure may cure the asthma. Continued exposure may lead to severe asthma, which continues even when exposure ceases.

Specific drug treatment Most drugs are delivered directly into the lungs as aerosols or powders, which means that lower doses can be used and systemic side effects are reduced compared to oral treatment. Asthma is now managed on a stepwise approach which depends partly on repeated measurements of PEFR by the patient (Table 9.2). The aim is that the patient starts treatment at the step most appropriate to the initial severity, and when control of symptoms is achieved treatment is gradually reduced to the

Table 9.2 The stepwise management of chronic asthma in adults

Step	PEFR (% predicted)	Treatment
1.	100	Inhaled short-acting β-agonist as required If needed > once daily move to step 2
2.	≤80	Low-dose inhaled corticosteroid: Beclomethasone or budesonide up to 400 µg twice daily Fluticasone up to 200 µg twice daily
3.	50–80	High-dose inhaled corticosteroid via a large volume spacer: Beclomethasone or budesonide up to 1000 µg twice daily Fluticasone up to 500 µg twice daily or low-dose inhaled corticosteroid plus salmeterol 50 µg twice daily
4.	50–80	High-dose inhaled corticosteroid plus either inhaled salmeterol, slow-release theophylline, inhaled ipratropium, cromoglycate or nedocromil
5.	≤50	Add in oral steroids once daily

• Patient measures PEFR at home to guide treatment
• Short-acting inhaled β-agonist taken at any step as required
• A rescue of oral steroids may be needed at any time and at any step

next step over a period of 3–6 months. The aim is to have minimal symptoms with few exacerbations and minimal need for relieving bronchodilators. Ideally a PEFR >80% of predicted or the patient's best should be achieved with less than 20% circadian variation.

• β_2-Adrenoreceptor agonists, e.g. salbutamol, terbutaline and the longer-acting salmeterol, relax bronchial smooth muscle and cause bronchial dilatation.
• Anticholinergic bronchodilators, e.g. ipratropium bromide or oxitropium bromide, cause bronchodilatation and may be additive to adrenoreceptor stimulants.
• Corticosteroids are powerful anti-inflammatory agents. Inhaled steroids e.g. beclomethasone diptopionate, budesonide and fluticasone propionate, are used as maintenance treatment in all but very mild asthmatic individuals.
• Anti-inflammatory agents, e.g. sodium cromoglycate, prevent activation of inflammatory cells and may be useful in mild asthma.

- Slow-release theophylline may be useful in some patients. The side effects (tachycardia, arrhythmias and nausea) are seen less than with rapid-release preparations. Intravenous aminophylline (a water-soluble preparation of theophylline and ethylenediamine) is sometimes used in acute severe asthma.
- The immunosuppressive drug methotrexate in low doses has been used in severely asthmatic individuals as a steroid-sparing agent.
- Leukotriene receptor antagonists e.g. montelukast, are a new class of asthma medication. (Leukotrienes are inflammatory mediators whose effects include bronchoconstriction and increased mucous production.) Regular use of these agents with an inhaled steroid in mild to moderate asthma improves pulmonary function and clinical symptoms, and appears to be safe and well tolerated.

Acute severe asthma Acute severe asthma is diagnosed when a patient has severe progressive asthmatic symptoms over a number of hours or days. It is a medical emergency that must be recognized and treated immediately at home, with subsequent transfer to hospital (Emergency Box 9.1). In the UK, 1500 patients still die annually from this condition.

Clinical features

Features of acute severe asthma are:

- Inability to complete a sentence in one breath
- Pulse >110 beats/min
- Respiration ≥25 breaths/min
- PEFR 33–50% of predicted value or 33–50% of patient's best.

Life-threatening features are:

- Silent chest, cyanosis or feeble respiratory effort
- Bradycardia or hypotension
- Exhaustion, confusion or coma
- PEFR <33% of predicted or best
- Blood gas markers of a very severe attack are $P_a\text{CO}_2$ >6 kPa, $P_a\text{O}_2$ <8 kPa, and pH <7.35.

The management of acute severe asthma is summarized in Emergency Box 9.1 Patients with moderate asthma

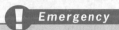

Emergency

Emergency Box 9.1 - Management of acute severe asthma in hospital

- 60% oxygen
- Salbutamol 5 mg or terbutaline 10 mg via oxygen-driven nebuliser
- Hydrocortisone 200 mg intravenously
- No sedatives of any kind
- Antibiotics only if definite evidence of infection
- Chest X-ray to exclude a pneumothorax

Monitor in all patients:
- Arterial oxygen saturation
- Arterial blood gases if PaO_2 < 92% or life-threatening features
- PERF 30 minutes after starting treatment, and then before and after β agonist treatment
- Consider repeat blood gases 2 hours after starting treatment

If improved – continue
60% oxygen
Hydrocortisone 200 mg 6 hourly
iv change to oral prednisolone
40 mg after 24 hours
Nebulised β agonist 4 hourly

After 24 hours – consider
Adding in high dose inhaled corticosteroid
Change nebulised to inhaled β-agonist

Discharge from hospital
When PEF > 75% predicted or patient's best and diurnal variability < 25%
When stable on discharge treatment for 24 hours
Check inhaler technique
Determine reason for exacerbation

Life threatening features present or poor response to treatment
60% oxygen
Hydrocortisone 200 mg 6 hourly
Repeat nebulised β agonist every 15 – 30 mins
Add in nebulised ipatropium 0.5mg
Consider intravenous:

salbutamol (250 µg bolus/10 mins followed by infusion) or aminophylline (250 mg bolus over 20 mins followed by infusion 750 – 1500 mg/24 hours). Do not give initial bolus to patient taking oral aminophylline, monitor blood concentrations if continued for 24 hours

If poor response within 1 hour transfer to ITU for possible intubation and mechanical ventilation

Emergency box 9.1
Management of acute severe asthma in hospital

(defined as a PEFR 50–75% of predicted and with none of the above features) who present to hospital are treated with a nebulized β-agonist. Provided they improve and are then stable for at least 1 hour, they may be discharged with a tapering dose of predisolone (e.g. starting at 40 mg daily).

Acute bronchitis

Acute bronchitis is usually viral but may be complicated by bacterial infection, particularly in smokers and in patients with chronic airflow limitation. Symptoms are cough, retrosternal discomfort, chest tightness and wheezing, which usually resolve spontaneously over 4–8 days.

Chronic obstructive pulmonary disease – COPD

COPD is the term used to describe patients with chronic bronchitis and emphysema. Chronic bronchitis is defined *symptomatically* as cough productive of sputum on most days for at least 3 months of the year for more than 1 year. Emphysema is a *pathological diagnosis* and is defined as dilatation and destruction of the lung tissue distal to the terminal bronchioles. Although it has been suggested that these definitions separate patients into two different clinical groups (the 'pink puffers' with predominant emphysema and the 'blue bloaters' with predominant chronic bronchitis), most have both emphysema and chronic bronchitis, irrespective of the clinical signs. Chronic obstructive pulmonary disease (COPD) is the collective term used for this group of patients.

Epidemiology

COPD develops over many years and patients are rarely symptomatic before middle age. It is common (18% of male and 14% of female smokers) in the UK, where it is one of the leading causes of lost working days.

Pathology

In chronic bronchitis there is airway narrowing, and hence airflow limitation, as a result of hypertrophy and hyperplasia of mucous glands, bronchial wall inflammation and mucosal oedema. The epithelial cell layer may ulcerate and, when the ulcers heal, squamous epithelium may replace columnar epithelium (squamous metaplasia).

Emphysematous changes lead to loss of elastic recoil, which normally keeps airways open during expiration; this is associated with expiratory airflow limitation and air trapping.

Aetiology and pathogenesis

- *Smoking* is the dominant causal agent. Persistent irritation by cigarette smoke causes hypertrophy of the mucus glands. In addition, the lungs of smokers are infiltrated by granulocytes, which may damage lung tissue by releasing proteases. In addition α_1-antitrypsin (see below) is inactivated by cigarette smoke.
- *Atmospheric pollution* plays a minor role compared to smoking.
- α_1-Antitrypsin deficiency (page 124) is a rare cause of early-onset emphysema. α_1-Antitrypsin is normally present in lung secretions and inhibits proteases. In theory, deficiency allows lung damage from proteases to proceed unchecked.

Clinical features

The main symptoms are cough, sputum production, wheeze and breathlessness. Frequent infective exacerbations (from *Streptococcus pneumoniae* or *Haemophilus influenzae*) occur, giving purulent sputum. On examination the patient with severe disease is breathless at rest, with prolonged expiration and using the accessory muscles of respiration; chest expansion is poor and the lungs are hyperinflated. There may be a wheeze or quiet breath sounds. In 'pink puffers' breathlessness is the predominant problem; they are not cyanosed. 'Blue bloaters' hypoventilate; they are cyanosed, may be oedematous and have features of CO_2 retention (warm peripheries with a bounding pulse, flapping tremor of the outstretched hands and confusion in severe cases).

Investigations

The diagnosis is made clinically in a lifetime smoker.

- Lung function tests. The ratio of FEV_1 to FVC is reduced (<70%) and the PEFR is low. Lung volumes are normal or increased, and the loss of alveoli with emphysema results in a decreased gas transfer coefficient of carbon monoxide.
- Chest radiograph. Typical features are hyperinflation, a flat diaphragm, reduced peripheral lung markings and bullae, although the chest radiograph may be normal.

- Haemoglobin and PCV may be high as a result of secondary polycythaemia (page 168).
- Arterial blood gases may be normal or show hypoxia and hypercapnia.

Complications

- Respiratory failure (page 449)
- Cor pulmonale, i.e. right heart failure secondary to lung disease (page 377).

Management

The most important aspect of management is to persuade the patient to stop smoking, which will slow down the rate of deterioration. Drug therapy is similar to that for asthma.

Assessment of reversibility is made with a 2-week course of oral prednisolone (30 mg daily), with measurement of lung function before and after the treatment period. If there is objective evidence of benefit (>15% improvement in FEV_1) oral steroids are gradually reduced and replaced with inhaled steroids.

Bronchodilators Inhaled β_2-agonists and the anticholinergic agent ipratropium bromide may produce symptomatic improvement even with little change in lung function tests.

Long-term domiciliary oxygen therapy will reduce mortality if given for 19 hours per day (every day) at a flow rate of 1–3 l/min to increase arterial oxygen saturation to >90%. It is prescribed to patients who no longer smoke and who have an FEV_1<1.5 l/min and a P_aO_2<7.3 kPa.

Additional treatments include venesection for polycythaemia (page 168), diuretics for oedema, and vaccination against influenza and pneumococcus. Exacerbations of COPD are usually the result of a superimposed respiratory infection (often *Haemophilus influenzae*) and are treated in a similar manner to asthma. However, these patients often depend on a degree of hypoxaemia to maintain respiratory drive and therefore, if oxygen is necessary, low concentrations (24%) are given, via a Venturi mask (fixed-performance mask), so as not to reduce respiratory drive. The oxygen concentration may be increased in increments (28% and then 35%) if clinical examination and repeated arterial blood gases do not show hypoventilation and carbon dioxide retention. Antibiotics, e.g. amoxycillin, should be given promptly for all exacerbations and patients should be encouraged to cough up sputum, initially with the help of a physiotherapist. Exacerbations are occasionally the result of pneumothorax, heart failure or pulmonary embolism, and these must be considered and excluded. Some patients with an acute exacerbation and respiratory failure will require respiratory support (page 451).

Prognosis

Fifty per cent of patients with severe breathlessness due to COPD die within 5 years.

Obstructive sleep apnoea

Obstructive sleep apnoea (OSA) is characterized by repetitive apnoea (cessation of breathing for 10 seconds or more) as a result of obstruction of the upper airway during sleep.

Epidemiology

OSA affects about 2% of the population and is most common in overweight middle-aged men. It can also occur in children, particularly those with large tonsils.

Aetiology

Apnoea occurs if the upper airway at the back of the throat is sucked closed when the patient breathes in. This occurs during sleep because the muscles that hold the airway open are hypotonic. Airway closure continues until the patient is woken up by the struggle to breathe against a blocked throat. Contributing factors include alcohol ingestion before sleep, obesity and COPD. It is more common in hypothyroidism and acromegaly.

Clinical features

The major symptoms are snoring, apnoeas witnessed by bed partners, and excessive daytime sleepiness, which may lead to impairment of work performance and driving. Other symptoms are irritability, personality change, morning headaches, impotence and nocturnal choking. Patients with sleep apnoea have an increased risk of hypertension, heart failure, myocardial infarction and stroke.

Diagnosis

Overnight oximetry (transcutaneous measurement of oxygen saturation) shows frequent falls in arteriolar oxygen saturation in some, but not all, patients.

Polysomnography is a detailed sleep study performed in a sleep laboratory and provides a definitive diagnosis. It includes measurement of sleep quality, nasal and oral airflow, thoracoabdominal movements and arterial oxygen saturation.

Management

- Predisposing factors, e.g. obesity, tonsillar hypertrophy and facial deformities, should be treated. Alcohol and sedatives should be avoided.
- CPAP (continuous positive airway pressure) to the airway via a tight-fitting nasal mask – nasal CPAP – during sleep keeps the pharyngeal walls open and is a very effective treatment.

Bronchiectasis

Bronchiectasis is defined as dilatation of the bronchi. It may be localized to a lobe or generalized throughout the bronchial tree. There is impaired clearance of bronchial secretions with secondary bacterial infection.

Aetiology

- *Idiopathic*: in which there is progressive bronchiectasis with no underlying cause
- *Inflammatory*: infective processes, e.g. measles, whooping cough, Klebsiella pneumonia, may damage and weaken the bronchial wall, leading to dilatation and ciliary damage
- *Obstruction*: proximal obstruction of an airway, e.g. inhaled foreign body, enlarged tuberculous lymph nodes, leads to distal accumulation of secretions which then become infected, resulting in localized bronchiectasis.
- *Congenital factors*: these include cystic fibrosis (page 410), Kartagener's syndrome (bronchiectasis associated with immotile cilia, transposition of viscera and sinusitis) and immunoglobulin deficiencies which lead to recurrent infections.

Epidemiology

Most cases arise in childhood, but the incidence has decreased in all age groups with effective antibiotic treatment of pneumonia.

Clinical features

Cough and sputum production are the most common symptoms. In severe bronchiectasis there is production of copious amounts of thick, foul-smelling green sputum. Other symptoms are haemoptysis (which may be massive and life-threatening), breathlessness and wheeze. On examination there is clubbing and coarse crackles over the affected area, usually the lung bases.

Investigations

- Radiology. The chest radiograph may be normal or show dilated bronchi with thickened bronchial walls, and sometimes multiple cysts containing fluid. High-resolution CT (slices are between 1 and 2 mm thick, compared to conventional CT slice of 10 mm) is the investigation of choice and may show bronchial wall thickening that is not shown on a standard chest radiograph. Inspiratory and expiratory scans show air trapping in small airways. Bronchography is only used to assess the extent of disease before surgery (see Management).
- Sputum culture is essential during an infective exacerbation. The common organisms are *Staphylococcus aureus*, *Pseudomonas aeruginosa* and *Haemophilus influenzae*.
- Further investigations, e.g. serum immunoglobulins, sweat test, in patients where an underlying cause is suspected.

Management

- Physiotherapy and daily postural drainage are of vital importance. The patient is taught to carry them out at home.
- Antibiotics, e.g. amoxycillin, for infective exacerbations. If there is no improvement it is probable that there is infection with *Pseudomonas aeruginosa*, which requires specific antibiotics, e.g. ceftazidime, administered by

aerosol or parenterally. Oral ciprofloxacin is an alternative.

- Bronchodilators are used for those with demonstrable airflow limitation.
- Surgery is reserved for the very small minority with localized disease. Severe disease sometimes requires lung or heart–lung transplantation.

Complications

The main complications are pneumonia, haemoptysis which may be life-threatening, and cerebral abscess.

Cystic fibrosis

Cystic fibrosis (CF) is an autosomal recessive condition occurring in 1:2000 live births. It is caused by mutations in a single gene on the long arm of chromosome 7 that encodes the cystic fibrosis transmembrane conductance regulator (CFTR). Mutations in the *CFTR* gene result in the production of a defective transmembrane protein which is involved in chloride transport across epithelial cell membranes in the pancreas and respiratory, gastrointestinal and reproductive tracts. The decreased chloride transport is accompanied by decreased transport of sodium and water, resulting in dehydrated viscous secretions that are associated with luminal obstruction and destruction and scarring of exocrine glands. The most common mutation is ΔF_{508} (deletion, phenylalanine at position 508).

Clinical features

Neonates may present with meconium ileus. Although the lungs of babies born with CF are normal at birth, respiratory symptoms are usually the presenting features. Bronchiectasis and obstructive pulmonary disease are the primary causes of morbidity and mortality in patients with CF. Infants with CF have persistent endobronchial infections due initially to *Staphylococcus aureus*, *Haemophillus influenzae* and Gram-negative bacilli. By the end of the first decade of life *Pseudomonas aeruginosa* is the predominant pathogen (page 416). The resultant inflammatory response damages the airway, leading to progressive bronchiectasis and eventually respiratory failure. Other abnormalities in the respiratory system include pansinusitis and nasal polyps. There may be steatorrhoea and diabetes mellitus as a result of pancreatic insufficiency. Males are infertile because of failure of development of the vas deferens. Chronic ill health in children leads to impaired growth and delayed puberty.

Investigations

- Sweat testing alone (a high sweat sodium >60 mmol/l) may be sufficient to diagnose or rule out cystic fibrosis in patients with typical gastrointestinal or pulmonary disease (classic cystic fibrosis). In patients with suspicious clinical findings and a normal sweat test genotyping is indicated; the commercially available probes will identify more than 90% of all CF genes.
- Genetic screening for the carrier state should be offered to persons or couples with a family history of CF, together with counselling.

Management

Management of bronchiectasis and exocrine pancreatic insufficiency has been described previously. More recently, an understanding of the basic defect and pathogenesis of cystic fibrosis has led to newer treatments, which are described in Table 9.3. Some patients with severe respiratory disease have received lung or heart/lung transplantations (CM page 785).

The emergence of *Burkholderia cepacia* is a problem for patients and doctors alike. It is associated with accelerated lung disease and resistance to antibiotics in some strains. Close contact promotes cross-infection, so siblings and fellow sufferers with cystic fibrosis may pass the organism from one to another.

Prognosis

Ninety per cent of children now survive into their teens and the median survival is 30 years. Most mortality is the result of pulmonary disease.

....

DISEASES OF THE LUNG PARENCHYMA

Pneumonias

Pneumonia may be defined as an inflammation of the substance of the lung and is usually caused by bacteria.

Table 9.3 Pathogenesis and approaches to treatment of respiratory disease in cystic fibrosis. Amiloride, ATP, UTP, DNAase and α_1-antitrypsin are given by aerosol

Pathogenesis	Treatment
Defective gene	Introduction of the normal *CFTR* gene into respiratory epithelium. BUT, trials hampered by suboptimal delivery of gene into cells and local immune response to the gene-carrying viral vector
↓	
Defective protein – CFTR	
↓	
Abnormal epithelial cell transport	Amiloride inhibits excessive sodium absorption. ATP and UTP stimulate chloride secretion through channels other than CFTR
↓	
Viscous intraluminal secretions	
↓	
Chronic bacterial colonization and infections	Prompt treatment with antibiotics for exacerbations
↓	
Accumulation of chronic inflammatory cells and release of proteolytic enzymes	Oral steroids for anti-inflammatory effects. Antiproteases
↓	
Release of DNA from degraded cells	DNAase to digest extracellular DNA

Pneumonia can be classified both anatomically, e.g. lobar (affecting the whole of one lobe) and bronchopneumonia (affecting the lobules and bronchi), or on the basis of aetiology. However, the most useful classification to guide management is based on the clinical circumstances under which the pneumonia is acquired (Table 9.4). *Mycobacterium tuberculosis* is an important cause of pneumonia; it is considered separately, as both mode of presentation and treatment are different from the infective agents shown in Table 9.4.

Clinical features

Precipitating factors for pneumonia are underlying lung disease, smoking, alcohol abuse, immunosuppression and

Table 9.4 Aetiology of pneumonia in the UK

Microbial agent or cause	Prevalence (%)
Community acquired	
Bacteria	
Streptococcus pneumoniae	60–75
Haemophilus influenzae	4–5
Legionella	2–5
Staphylococcus aureus	1–5
Gram-negative bacilli	0–8
Miscellaneous	1–2
Other agents	
Mycoplasma pneumoniae	5–18
Chlamydia sp.	5
Coxiella burnetti	rare
Viruses	uncommon†
Aspiration	
Hospital acquired (nosocomial)	
Gram-negative bacteria	50
Staphyloccocus aureus	<25
Anaerobes	
In the immunosuppressed	
Pneumocystis carinii	
Aspergillus fumigatus	
Cytomegalovirus	
Bacteria (as in other groups)	

† Pneumonia due to viral infection per se is uncommon, most is due to secondary bacterial infection.

other chronic illnesses. The clinical history should enquire about contact with birds (possible psittacosis), contact with farm animals (*Coxiella burnetti*), recent stays in large hotels or institutions (*Legionella pneumophila*) and contact with other patients with pneumonia. Symptoms and signs vary according to the infecting agent and to the immune state of the patient. Most commonly there is pyrexia, combined with respiratory symptoms such as cough, sputum production, pleurisy and dyspnoea. Signs of consolidation and a pleural rub may be present. Signs associated with severe pneumonia and a poor prognosis include a respiratory rate >30/min, diastolic blood pressure <60 mmHg, and confusion. Elderly patients often have fewer symptoms than younger patients.

Investigations

Many otherwise fit patients with community-acquired pneumonia are treated as outpatients and the only investigation needed is a chest X-ray, which should be repeated 6–8 weeks after clinical recovery to confirm resolution. Patients admitted to hospital require investigations to identify the cause and severity of the pneumonia.

- Sputum should be sent for Gram stain and culture, although negative results are reported for 30–60% of cultures of expectorated sputum.
- Blood count. A white cell count above $15 \times 10^9/l$ suggests bacterial infection; very high ($>30 \times 10^9/l$) and low values ($<4 \times 10^9/l$) are found in the very ill and are a poor prognostic sign. The white cell count is $>15 \times 10^9/l$ in only 10% of patients with *Legionella* pneumonia, and sometimes there is lymphopenia. Marked red cell agglutination on the blood film suggests the presence of cold agglutinins (immunoglobulins that agglutinate reds cells at $4°C$), which are raised in 50% of patients with *Mycoplasma* pneumonia.
- Liver biochemistry and serum electrolytes. Liver biochemistry may be abnormal. Raised serum urea and creatinine, hyponatraemia or hypoalbuminaemia indicate severe pneumonia.
- Blood culture is positive in 15–25% of case even if the sputum is negative, and indicates a poorer prognosis.
- Serology. Other organisms causing pneumonia can be diagnosed by detection of a raised IgM antibody by immunofluorescent tests or by a fourfold rise in antibody titre from blood taken early in the clinical course and 10–14 days later.
- Chest radiography confirms consolidation, but these changes may lag behind the clinical course. A chest radiograph which remains persistently abnormal (>6 weeks) suggests an underlying abnormality, usually a carcinoma.
- Arterial blood gases. P_aO_2 <8 kPa or rising P_aCO_2 indicates severe pneumonia.

Management

In mild cases of community-acquired pneumonia treatment can be started immediately with oral amoxycillin and erythromycin for 7 days. More severe cases should be admitted to hospital and treated with intravenous cefuroxime (750 mg to 1.5 g 6 hourly) and clarithromycin (500 mg 12 hourly). Pleuritic pain requires analgesia, and oxygen therapy should be given if there is severe hypoxaemia. Fluids should be encouraged to avoid dehydration. Treatment should be modified in the light of subsequent investigations. Patients with severe pneumonia are best managed on an intensive care unit.

Prognosis

Complications of pneumonia include lung abscess and empyema. In elderly patients the mortality rate may be as high as 25%.

Specific forms of pneumonia

Mycoplasma pneumoniae *Mycoplasma* pneumonia commonly presents in young adults with generalized features such as headaches and malaise, which may precede chest symptoms by 1–5 days. Physical signs in the chest may be scanty, and chest radiographic appearances frequently do not correlate with the clinical state of the patient. Treatment is with erythromycin to clarithromycin. Extrapulmonary complications (myocarditis, erythema multiforme, haemolytic anaemia and meningoencephalitis) will occasionally dominate the clinical picture.

Haemophilus influenzae This is commonly the cause of pneumonia in patients with COPD. There are no other features to differentiate it from other causes of bacterial pneumonia. Treatment is with oral cefaclor.

Chlamydia *Chlamydia pneumoniae* is a more common cause of pneumonia than previously thought. Patients with *C. psittaci* pneumonia may give a history of contact with infected birds, particularly parrots. Symptoms include malaise, fever, cough and muscular pains, which may be low grade and protracted over many months. Occasionally the presentation mimics meningitis, with a high fever, prostration, photophobia and neck stiffness. Diagnosis is confirmed by demonstrating a rising serum titre of complement-fixing antibody, and treatment is with erythromycin or tetracycline.

Staphylococci *Staphylococcus aureus* usually causes pneumonia only after a preceding influenza viral illness or in intravenous drug users. It results in patchy areas of consolidation which can break down to form abscesses that appear as cysts on the radiograph. Pneumothorax, effusions and empyemas are frequent, and septicaemia may develop with metastatic abscesses in other organs. All patients with this form of pneumonia are extremely ill and the mortality rate is in excess of 25%. Treatment is with intravenous flucloxacillin.

Legionellosis Legionnaire's disease can be acquired by the inhalation of aerosols or microaspiration of infected water containing legionella. Infection is linked to contamination of water distribution systems in hotels, hospitals and workplaces. Most cases of legionellosis are due to infection with *L. pneumophilia* which causes more severe disease than most other pathogens associated with community-acquired pneumonia. The clinical and radiological presentation of legionnaire's disease cannot be reliably distinguished from other forms of pneumonia, although a temperature of up to 40°C and the presence of diarrhoea, confusion, lymphopenia and hyponatraemia can be clues. Diagnosis is by direct fluorescent antibody staining of the organism in the pleural fluid, sputum or bronchial washings, or by detection of *L. pneumophilia* antigen in the urine. Treatment is with clarithromycin or rifampicin for 14–21 days.

Pseudomonas aeruginosa *Pseudomonas aeruginosa* is seen in the immunocompromised and in patients with cystic fibrosis, in whom its presence is associated with a worsening of the clinical condition and increasing mortality. Treatment includes intravenous ceftazidime, ciprofloxacin, tobramycin or ticarcillin. Tobramycin and ticarcillin can be inhaled directly into the lung in patients with CF.

Pneumocystis carinii *Pneumocystis carinii* is the most common opportunistic infection in patients with AIDS. The clinical features and treatment are described on page 35.

Aspiration pneumonia Aspiration of gastric contents into the lungs can produce a severe destructive pneumonia as a result of the corrosive effect of gastric acid – the Mendelson's syndrome. Aspiration usually occurs into the posterior segment of the right lower lobe because of the bronchial anatomy. It is associated with periods of impaired consciousness, structural abnormalities, such as tracheo-oesophageal fistulae or oesophageal strictures, and bulbar palsy. Infection is often due to anaerobes and treatment must include metronidazole.

Lung abscess and empyema

A lung abscess results from localized suppuration of the lung associated with cavity formation, often with a fluid level on the chest radiograph. Empyema means the presence of pus in the pleural cavity, usually from rupture of a lung abscess into the pleural cavity, or from bacterial spread from a severe pneumonia.

A lung abscess develops in the following circumstances:

- Complicating aspiration pneumonia or bacterial pneumonia caused by *Staphylococcus* or *Klebsiella pneumoniae*
- Secondary to bronchial obstruction by tumour or foreign body
- From septic emboli from a focus elsewhere (usually staphylococcus)
- Secondary to infarction.

Clinical features

Lung abscess presents with persisting or worsening pneumonia, often with the production of copious amounts of foul-smelling sputum. With empyema the patient is usually very ill, with a high fever and neutrophil leucocytosis. There may be malaise, weight loss and clubbing of the digits.

Investigations

Bacteriological investigation is best conducted on specimens obtained by transtracheal aspiration, bronchoscopy or percutaneous transthoracic aspiration.

Management

Antibiotics are given to cover both aerobic and anaerobic organisms. Intravenous cefuroxime, erythromycin and metronidazole are given for 5 days, followed by oral cefaclor and metronidazole for several weeks. Empyemas should be treated by prompt tube drainage or rib resection and drainage of the empyema cavity. Abscesses occasionally require surgery.

Tuberculosis ND

Epidemiology

Tuberculosis (TB) is now the most common cause of death worldwide from a single infectious disease, and is on the increase in most parts of the world. This results primarily from inadequate programmes for disease control, multiple drug resistance, coinfection with HIV and a rapid rise in the world population of young adults, the group with the highest mortality from tuberculosis. In the UK the incidence of tuberculosis is 40 times greater in Asian immigrants than in the native white population.

Pathology

The initial infection with *Mycobacterium tuberculosis* is known as primary tuberculosis. It usually occurs in the lung but may occur in the gastrointestinal tract, particularly the ileocaecal region. The primary focus in the lung is subpleural in the mid to upper zones (Figure 9.2), and is characterized by exudation and infiltration with neutrophil granulocytes. These are replaced by macrophages which engulf the bacilli and result in the typical granulomatous lesions, which consist of central areas of caseation surrounded by epithelioid cells and Langhans' giant cells (both derived from the macrophage). The primary focus is almost always accompanied by caseous lesions in the regional lymph nodes (mediastinal and cervical). In most people the primary infection and the lymph nodes heal completely and become calcified. Some of these calcified primary lesions harbour tubercle bacilli, which may become reactivated if there is depression of the host defence system. Occasionally there is dissemination of the primary infection, producing miliary tuberculosis.

Reactivation results in typical postprimary tuberculosis. Postprimary tuberculosis refers to all forms of tuberculosis that develop after the first few weeks of the primary infection when immunity to the mycobacteria has developed.

Clinical features

Primary TB is usually symptomless; occasionally there may be erythema nodosum (page 632), a small pleural effusion or pulmonary collapse caused by compression of a lobar

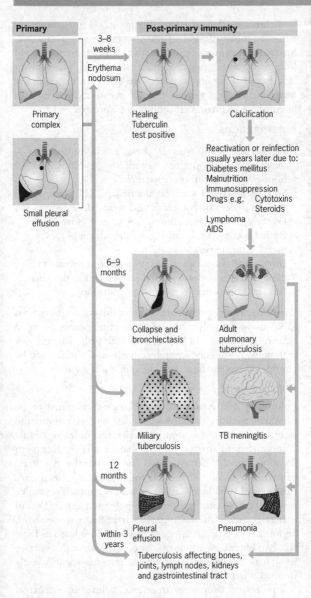

Primary

Primary complex

Small pleural effusion

3–8 weeks
Erythema nodosum

Post-primary immunity

Healing
Tuberculin test positive

Calcification

Reactivation or reinfection usually years later due to:
Diabetes mellitus
Malnutrition
Immunosuppression
Drugs e.g.   Cytotoxins
              Steroids
Lymphoma
AIDS

6–9 months

Collapse and bronchiectasis

Adult pulmonary tuberculosis

Miliary tuberculosis

TB meningitis

12 months

Pleural effusion

Pneumonia

within 3 years

Tuberculosis affecting bones, joints, lymph nodes, kidneys and gastrointestinal tract

Figure 9.2
The manifestations of primary and postprimary tuberculosis.

bronchus by enlarged nodes (Figure 9.2). Most commonly clinical tuberculosis represents delayed reactivation. Symptoms begin insidiously, with malaise, anorexia, weight loss, fever and cough. Sputum is mucoid purulent or bloodstained, but night sweats are uncommon. There are often no physical signs, although occasionally signs of a pneumonia or pleural effusion may be present.

Investigations

- Chest radiography typically shows patchy or nodular shadows in the upper zones, with loss of volume and fibrosis with or without cavitation.
- Sputum is stained with Ziehl–Nielsen (ZN) stain for acid- and alcohol-fast bacilli and cultured on Dover's or Lowenstein–Jensen medium. This takes 4–8 weeks.
- Bronchoscopy with washings of the affected lobes is useful if no sputum is available.
- Biopsy with histological examination and culture of pleura, lymph nodes and solid lesions within the lung (tuberculomas) may be required for diagnosis.

Direct testing of sputum and other fluids for *M. tuberculosis* DNA using the polymerase chain reaction may allow rapid diagnosis (within 48 hours) of infection, though the technique is still not entirely reliable and should not be considered diagnostic in the 'difficult' case.

Management

Pulmonary and lymph node tuberculosis assumed to be caused by sensitive organisms is treated with rifampicin and isoniazid for 6 months, along with pyrazinamide for the first 2 months until drug sensitivities are available. Treatment duration should be extended to 9 months for bone tuberculosis and to 12 months for tuberculous meningitis. Ethambutol is included in a treatment regimen if resistance is suspected. Streptomycin is now rarely used in the UK, but it may be added if the organism is resistant to isoniazid. Significant side effects are uncommon and are listed in Table 9.5. A transient asymptomatic rise in the serum transferase level may occur with rifampicin, but treatment is only stopped if hepatitis develops.

The major causes of treatment failure are incorrect prescribing by the doctor and inadequate compliance by

Table 9.5 Side effects of drug treatment

Rifampicin	Stains body secretions and urine pink
	Induces liver enzymes and accelerates metabolism of some drugs including phenytoin, warfarin and oestrogens. Oestrogen-containing contraceptive pills are thus unreliable
	Hepatitis
	Rarely thrombocytopenia
Isoniazid	Polyneuropathy; prophylactic pyridoxine is recommended
	Allergic reactions
	Hepatitis
Pyrazinamide	Hepatitis
	Hyperuricaemia and gout
	Rash and arthralgia
Ethambutol	Dose-related retrobulbar neuritis. Patients are asked to report visual problems and to undergo regular specialist ophthalmic examination

the patient. Treatment should be supervised by a specialist physician. All cases of TB must be notified to the local Public Health Authority so that contact tracing and screening can be arranged. Close contacts of a case are screened for evidence of disease with a chest radiograph and a Mantoux test (intradermal injection of purified protein derivative of *M. tuberculosis* produces induration and inflammation in individuals with active infection, or who have previously been immunized with BCG). Antituberculous treatment is given if the chest X-ray shows evidence of disease, or if the tuberculin test is negative initially but becomes positive on repeat testing 6 weeks later. In adults, an initial positive tuberculin test with a normal chest X-ray is not usually taken as indication of infection.

Prevention

Immunization with BCG (Bacille Calmette–Guérin) reduces the risk of developing tuberculosis by about 15–70%. It is a bovine strain of *M. tuberculosis* which has lost its virulence after growth in the laboratory for many years. Routine immunization is becoming less common in the UK as the incidence of tuberculosis is decreasing in the indigenous population. Immunization produces cellular immunity and a positive tuberculin test, and is the main reason why the Mantoux test is now of little value for diagnosis of active disease in the UK. BCG immunization of the new born is still given in developing countries, where TB is more prevalent.

Chemoprophylaxis

Patients with chest radiographic changes compatible with previous tuberculosis and who are about to undergo treatment with an immunosuppressive agent should receive chemoprophylaxis with isoniazid.

GRANULOMATOUS LUNG DISEASE

A granuloma is a mass or nodule of chronic inflammatory tissue and is characterized by the presence of epithelioid multinucleate giant cells. Sarcoidosis is the most common cause of lung granulomas.

Sarcoidosis

Sarcoidosis is a multisystem granulomatous disorder that commonly affects young adults and usually presents with bilateral hilar lymphadenopathy (BHL), pulmonary infiltrations and skin or eye lesions.

Epidemiology

The disease has been identified in all ethnic groups, but is much more common in patients of African origin than in caucasians. The disease may also be clinically more severe in this group. It is most common in young adults and is more prevalent in females than in males.

Aetiology

The exact aetiology is unknown. However, it appears likely that genetically predisposed hosts are exposed to antigens that trigger an exaggerated cellular immune response and the formation of granulomas.

Immunopathology

- The typical non-caseating (compare TB) sarcoid granuloma consists of a focal accumulation of epithelioid cells, macrophages and lymphocytes, mainly T cells.

- There is a depressed cell-mediated immunity to antigens, such as tuberculin and *Candida albicans*, and an overall lymphopenia with low circulating T cells, as a result of sequestration of lymphocytes within the lung and slightly increased B cells.
- There is an increased number of cells in the bronchoalveolar lavage, particularly CD4 helper cells.
- Transbronchial biopsies show infiltration of alveolar walls and interstitial spaces with mononuclear cells before granuloma formation.

Clinical features

The most common presentation is with bilateral hilar lymphadenopathy, which may be found incidentally on a routine chest radiograph or be associated with mild fever, malaise, arthralgia and erythema nodosum (page 632). Pulmonary infiltration may predominate, and, in a minority of patients there is progressive fibrosis resulting in increasing effort dyspnoea, cor pulmonale and death. The chest radiograph is negative at presentation in up to 20% of non-respiratory cases. Skin and ocular sarcoidosis are the most common extrapulmonary problems (Table 9.6). Asymptomatic hypercalcaemia is found on routine blood tests in 10% of established cases, but is less commonly a clinical problem. Hepatitis and hepatosplenomegaly are uncommon, but granulomas may often be found if a liver biopsy is performed. Cardiac involvement is rare.

Table 9.6 Extrapulmonary features of sarcoidosis

Skin	Erythema nodosum, skin papules, lupus pernio (red/blue infiltration of the nose)
Eye	Anterior uveitis, conjunctivitis, keratoconjunctivitis sicca, uveoparotid fever (bilateral uveitis, parotid gland enlargement and facial nerve palsy)
Bone	Arthralgias, bone cysts
Metabolic	Hypercalcaemia as a result of high circulating levels of 1,25-(OH$_2$)D$_3$ from activated sarcoid macrophages
Liver	Granulomatous hepatitis, hepatosplenomegaly
CNS	VIIth cranial nerve palsy, hypothalamic involvement, hypopituitarism
Heart	Ventricular arrhythmias, conduction defects, cardiomyopathy with cardiac failure

Investigations

Diagnosis depends on a compatible clinical picture, exclusion of other causes of granulomatous diseases, such as tuberculosis and beryllium poisoning, and histological evidence of non-caseating granulomas.

- Chest X-ray may show typical features (see above). CT scanning is useful for assessment of diffuse lung involvement.
- Transbronchial biopsy is the most useful investigation and gives positive histological evidence in 90% of cases of pulmonary sarcoidosis.
- Lung function tests in pulmonary infiltration show a restrictive lung defect with a decreased total lung capacity, FEV_1, FVC and gas transfer.
- Serum angiotensin-converting enzyme (ACE) is raised in 75% of patients. It is useful in assessing the activity of disease, but is not of diagnostic value because it is also elevated in patients with lymphoma, tuberculosis, asbestosis, silicosis and Gaucher's disease.
- Tuberculin test is negative in 80% of patients. It is of no diagnostic value.
- Biopsy and histological examination of involved lymph nodes, liver or skin lesions is sometimes necessary for diagnosis.
- The Kveim test involves an intradermal injection of sarcoid spleen and subsequent (4–6 weeks later) histological examination for non-caseating granulomas. It should no longer be used because of the risk of transmission of infection and the reduced sensitivity and specificity compared to other tests.

Differential diagnosis

The differential diagnosis of bilateral hilar lymphadeno-pathy includes lymphoma, pulmonary tuberculosis and bronchial carcinoma with secondary spread. The combination of symmetrical bilateral hilar lymphadenopathy and erythema nodosum only occurs in sarcoidosis.

Management

The requirement for treatment and the role of steroids are presently contested in many aspects of this disease. Hilar lymphadenopathy with no other evidence of lung involvement does not require treatment. Infiltration or abnormal lung function test that persists for 6 months after diagnosis should be treated with 30 mg prednisolone for 6 weeks, reducing to 15 mg on alternate days for 6–12 months. Most patients with hypercalcaemia or other evidence of extrapulmonary sarcoidosis probably require treatment with prednisolone. Topical steroids are used for eye involvement.

Prognosis

In patients of African origin the mortality rate may be up to 10%, but is less than 5% in caucasians. Death is mainly as a result of respiratory failure or renal damage from hypercalciuria. The prognosis is best in those with BHL and no infiltration on the chest radiograph: more than 90% recover spontaneously.

WEGENER'S GRANULOMATOSIS

Wegener's granulomatosis is a vasculitis of unknown aetiology characterized by lesions involving the upper respiratory tract, the lungs and the kidneys. The disease often starts with rhinorrhoea, with subsequent nasal mucosal ulceration, cough, haemoptysis and pleuritic pain. Chest radiography shows nodular masses or pneumonic infiltrates with cavitation which often show a migratory pattern. Antineutrophil cytoplasmic antibodies are found in the serum in over 90% of cases with active disease, and measurement is useful both diagnostically and as a guide to disease activity in the treated patient. Typical histological changes are best shown in the kidney, where there is a necrotizing glomerulonephritis. Treatment is with cyclophosphamide.

PULMONARY FIBROSIS AND HONEYCOMB LUNG

Pulmonary fibrosis is the end result of many diseases of the respiratory tract. It may be one of the following types:

- Localized, e.g. following unresolved pneumonia
- Bilateral, e.g. in TB
- Widespread, e.g. in cryptogenic fibrosing alveolitis.

Honeycomb lung is the radiological appearance seen with widespread fibrosis. Dilated and thickened terminal and respiratory bronchioles produce cystic airspaces, giving a honeycomb appearance on chest radiography.

Cryptogenic fibrosing alveolitis

Cryptogenic fibrosing alveolitis is a rare disorder of unknown aetiology which causes gradual diffuse fibrosis throughout the lung fields, usually in late middle age.

Clinical features

There is progressive breathlessness, cough and cyanosis, leading eventually to respiratory failure. Finger clubbing occurs in two-thirds of cases, and fine bilateral basal crackles are heard on auscultation. Rarely, an acute form known as the Hamman–Rich syndrome occurs.

Investigation

- Chest radiographic appearances are initially of a ground-glass appearance, progressing to fibrosis and honeycomb lung. However, the chest X-ray may be entirely normal in up to 10% of cases.
- High-resolution CT scan is the most sensitive imaging technique, and shows irregular linear opacities and honeycombing.
- Respiratory function tests show a restrictive defect (page 393) with low lung volumes and impaired gas transfer.
- Blood gases show hypoxaemia with a normal $P_a\text{CO}_2$.
- Histological confirmation with transbronchial or open lung biopsies may be required in younger people.
- Autoantibodies, such as antinuclear factor and rheumatoid factor, may be positive.

Differential diagnosis

This is from other causes of lung fibrosis: connective tissue disease, sarcoidosis, radiation, pneumoconiosis, chronic extrinsic allergic alveolitis and drugs (amiodarone, busulphan, methylsergide).

Treatment

Large doses of prednisolone are used (30 mg daily); azathioprine and cyclophosphamide may also be tried.

Single lung transplantation is now an established treatment for some individuals, and current survival rate figures are 60% at 1 year after transplantation.

Prognosis

The median survival is approximately 5 years.

Extrinsic allergic alveolitis

Extrinsic allergic alveolitis is characterized by a widespread diffuse inflammatory reaction in the alveoli and small airways of the lung as a response to inhalation of a range of different antigens (Table 9.7). By far the most common is farmers' lung, which affects up to one in 10 of the farming community in poor wet areas around the world.

Table 9.7 Extrinsic allergic bronchiolar alveolitis

Disease	Situation	Antigens
Farmers' lung	Forking mouldy hay or other vegetable material	*Faenia rectivirgula* (*Micropolyspora faeni*)
Bird fanciers' lung	Handling pigeons, cleaning lofts or budgerigar cages	Proteins present in feathers and excreta
Malt workers' lung	Turning germinating barley	*Aspergillus clavatus*
Humidifier fever	Contaminated humidifying systems in air conditioners or humidifiers	A variety of bacteria or amoebae

Clinical features

There is fever, malaise, cough and shortness of breath several hours after exposure to the causative antigen. Physical examination reveals tachypnoea, and coarse end–inspiratory crackles and wheezes. Continuing exposure leads to a chronic illness with weight loss, effort dyspnoea, cough and the features of fibrosing alveolitis.

Investigations

- Chest radiograph shows fluffy nodular shadowing with the subsequent development of streaky shadows, particularly in the upper zones.

- Full blood count shows a raised white cell count in acute cases.
- Lung function tests show a restrictive defect with a decrease in gas transfer.
- Precipitating antibodies to causative antigens are present in the serum (these are evidence of exposure and not disease).
- Bronchoalveolar lavage shows increased lymphocytes and granulocytes.

Management

Prevention is the aim, with avoidance of exposure to the antigen if possible. Prednisolone in large doses (30–60 mg daily) may be required to cause regression of the disease in the early stages.

PNEUMOCONIOSIS

Most inhaled particles cause no damage to the lung because they are trapped in the nose, removed by the mucociliary clearance system or destroyed by alveolar macrophages. Small inorganic dust particles that reach the acinus and damage macrophages initiate an inflammatory reaction and subsequent fibrosis. Pneumoconiosis (Table 9.8) is the term used for the lung disease that develops. The incidence of pneumoconiosis has decreased since the introduction of improved working conditions.

Table 9.8 The common pneumoconioses

Disease	Cause	Occupation
Coal workers' pneumoconiosis	Coal dust	Coal mining
Asbestosis	Asbestos	Building trade, pipe fitters
Silicosis	Silica	Mining, sand blasting, stone masons
Berylliosis	Beryllium	Atomic reactors, electronics

Coal workers' pneumoconiosis

The disease is subdivided into simple pneumoconiosis and progressive massive fibrosis (PMF). Simple pneumoconiosis produces small (<1.5 mm) pulmonary nodules on the chest radiograph. The importance of simple pneumoconiosis is that it may lead to the development of PMF with continued exposure. PMF is characterized by large (1–10 cm), often confluent, fibrotic masses, predominantly in the upper lobes. Unlike simple pneumoconiosis the disease may progress after exposure to coal dust has ceased. Symptoms are dyspnoea and cough productive of black sputum. Eventually respiratory failure may supervene. There is no specific treatment and further exposure must be prevented. Patients with PMF and some with simple pneumoconiosis (depending on the severity of chest radiographic changes) are eligible for disability benefit.

Asbestosis

Asbestos is a mixture of fibrous silicates which have the common properties of resistance to heat, acid and alkali, hence their widespread use at one time. Chrysotile or white asbestos comprises 90% of the world production and is less fibrogenic than the other forms – crocidolite (blue asbestos) and amosite (brown asbestos). The diseases caused by asbestos (Table 9.9) are all characterized by a long latency period (20–40 years) between exposure and disease.

CARCINOMA OF THE LUNG
Epidemiology

Bronchial carcinoma is the most common malignant tumour in the western world and in the UK is the third most common cause of death after heart disease and pneumonia. There is a 3.5:1 male:female ratio, but although the rising mortality of this disease has levelled off in men, it continues to rise in women.

Aetiology

Smoking is by far the most important aetiological factor, although there is a higher incidence in urban areas than in rural areas even when allowances are made for smoking. Other aetiological factors are passive smoking, exposure to asbestos, and possibly also contact with arsenic, chromium, iron oxides and the products of coal combustion.

Table 9.9 The effects of asbestos on the lung

Disease	Pathology and clinical features
Asbestos bodies in the lung	They produce no symptoms or change in lung function and serve only as a marker of exposure
Pleural plaques	Fibrotic plaques on the parietal pleura which usually produce no symptoms
Pleural effusion	Recurrent effusions produce pleuritic pain and dyspnoea
*Bilateral diffuse pleural thickening	Thickening of the parietal and visceral pleura which produces effort dyspnoea and a restrictive ventilatory defect
*Mesothelioma	Tumour arising from mesothelial cells of the pleura, peritoneum and pericardium. Often presents with a pleural effusion. There is no treatment and median survival is 2 years
*Asbestosis	Characterized by progressive dyspnoea associated with finger clubbing and bilateral basal end-inspiratory crackles. There is a restrictive ventilatory defect on lung function testing
*Lung cancer, often adenocarcinoma	Presentation and treatment is that of lung cancer (see below)

* The diseases indicated are all eligible for compensation under the Social Security Act of 1975.

Pathology

These are broadly divided into small cell and non-small cell cancer. Non-small cell tumours are further subdivided as shown in Table 9.10.

Clinical features

Local effects of tumour within a bronchus Cough, chest pain, haemoptysis and breathlessness are typical symptoms.

Spread within the chest Tumour may directly involve the pleura and ribs, causing pain and bone fractures. Spread to involve the brachial plexus causes pain in the shoulder and inner arm (Pancoast's tumour), spread to the sympathetic ganglion causes Horner's syndrome (page 563), and spread to the left recurrent laryngeal nerve causes hoarseness and a

Table 9.10 Types of bronchial carcinoma

Cell type	Percentage lung tumours	Characteristics
Non-small cell		
Squamous	40	The most common cancer, occasionally cavitates, widespread metastases occur late
Large cell	25	Less well-differentiated tumour that metastasizes early
Adenocarcinoma	10	More common in non-smokers and as a result of asbestos exposure. Usually occurs peripherally
Alveolar cell	1–2	Presents as a peripheral nodule or as diffuse nodular lesions of multicentric origin
Small cell	20–30	Arises from endocrine cells (Kulchitsky cells) which often secrete polypeptide hormones. Rapidly growing and highly malignant, but the only bronchial cancer that responds to chemotherapy

bovine cough. In addition the tumour may directly involve the oesophagus, heart or superior vena cava (causing upper limb oedema, facial congestion and distended neck veins).

Metastatic disease Metastases present as bone pain, epilepsy or with focal neurological signs.

Non-metastatic manifestations These are rare apart from finger clubbing (Table 9.11). There may, in addition, be non-specific features such as malaise, lethargy and weight loss. On examination of the chest there are often no physical signs, although lymphadenopathy, signs of a pleural effusion, lobar collapse or unresolved pneumonia may be present.

Investigations

The aim of investigation is to confirm the diagnosis, determine the histology and assess tumour spread as a guide to treatment.

Table 9.11 Non-metastatic extrapulmonary manifestations of bronchial carcinoma

Endocrine	Ectopic ACTH secretion (Cushing's syndrome)
	Ectopic antidiuretic hormone secretion (dilutional hyponatraemia)
	Secretion of PTH-like substance (hypercalcaemia)
Neurological	Cerebellar degeneration
	Myopathy, polyneuropathies
	Myasthenic syndrome (Eaton–Lambert syndrome)
Vascular/haematological	Thrombophlebitis migrans
	Non-bacterial thrombotic endocarditis
	Anaemia
	Disseminated intravascular coagulation
Skeletal	Clubbing (30%)
	Hypertrophic osteoarthropathy (clubbing with painful wrists and ankles)
Cutaneous	Dermatomyositis
	Acanthosis nigricans (pigmented overgrowth of skin in axillae or groin)
	Herpes zoster

Confirm the diagnosis Chest radiography is the most valuable initial test, although tumours need to be between 1 and 2 cm to be recognized reliably. They usually appear as a round shadow, the edge of which often has a fluffy or spiked appearance. There may be evidence of cavitation, lobar collapse, a pleural effusion or secondary pneumonia. Spread through the lymphatic channels gives rise to lymphangitis carcinomatosis, appearing as streaky shadowing throughout the lung.

Determine the histology Sputum is examined for malignant cells. Bronchoscopy is used to obtain samples for histological investigation and for obtaining washings for cytology. Transthoracic fine needle aspiration biopsy under radiographic or CT screening is useful for obtaining tissue diagnosis from peripheral lesions.

Assess spread of the tumour At bronchoscopy involvement of the first 2 cm of either main bronchus or of the recurrent laryngeal nerve (vocal cord paresis) indicates inoperability. CT is useful for assessing the mediastinum and the extent of tumour spread. Magnetic resonance imaging is also being increasingly used for staging. Mediastinoscopy and lymph node biopsy may be necessary before surgery if the scan shows lymphadenopathy, which can be reactive or involved by tumour. The presence of bony and liver metastases is determined by serum alkaline phosphatase and other liver biochemistry. Liver ultrasonography and isotope bone scanning are only necessary if these screening tests are abnormal.

Determine patient suitability for major operation Physical examination and respiratory function tests.

Treatment

- Surgery is the only treatment of any value for non-small cell cancer. In the 20% of cases that are suitable for resection the 5-year survival rate is 25–30%.
- Radiotherapy in high doses can produce results that are equal to surgery in patients with localized tumours but who are otherwise unfit for surgery, e.g. poor lung function testing. Palliative radiotherapy is useful for bone pain, haemoptysis and superior vena cava obstruction. Continuous hyperfractionated accelerated radiotherapy (CHART) is showing promising results for non-small cell lung cancer.
- Chemotherapy. In small cell cancer this has resulted in a fivefold increase in median survival, from 3 to 15 months. A small number of patients achieve several years of remission.

  In non-small cell lung cancer the response is less satisfactory, though newer agents achieve response rates of greater than 20% and significantly extend median survival.
- Local treatment. Endoscopic laser therapy, endobronchial irradiation and transbronchial stenting are being increasingly employed to deal with distressing symptoms in inoperable cases. Malignant pleural effusions should be aspirated to dryness and a sclerosing agent (e.g. tetracycline, bleomycin) instilled into the pleural space. In the terminal stages the quality of life must be maintained as far as possible. In addition to general nursing and medical care, patients may need oral or

intravenous opiates for pain (given with laxatives to prevent constipation), and prednisolone may improve the appetite.

Differential diagnosis

In most cases the diagnosis is straightforward. A solitary round shadow on the radiograph may also be the result of a benign growth, a secondary deposit, tuberculoma or hydatid cyst.

Metastatic tumours in the lung

Metastases in the lung are common, usually presenting as round shadows 1.5–3 cm in diameter. The most common primary sites are the kidney, prostate, breast, bone, gastrointestinal tract, cervix or ovary.

DISEASES OF THE PLEURA

Dry pleurisy

Dry pleurisy is the term used to describe inflammation of the pleura when there is no effusion. This results in localized sharp pain made worse on deep inspiration, coughing and bending or twisting movements. Common causes are pneumonia, pulmonary infarct and carcinoma.

Epidemic myalgia (Bornholm's disease) is the result of infection with Coxsackie B virus. It is characterized by an upper respiratory tract infection followed by pleuritic pain and abdominal pain with tender muscles. The chest radiograph remains normal and the illness clears in 1 week.

Pleural effusion

A pleural effusion is an excessive accumulation of fluid in the pleural space. It can be detected clinically when there are more than 500 ml present, and by radiography when there are more than 300 ml. The physical signs and chest radiographic appearances are shown in Figure 9.3.

Aetiology

Serous effusions may be transudates (protein content <30 g/l) or exudates (>30 g/l). The causes of a serous effusion

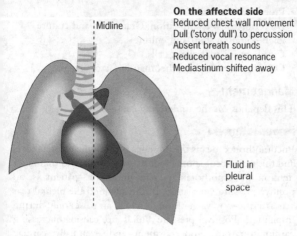

On the affected side
Reduced chest wall movement
Dull ('stony dull') to percussion
Absent breath sounds
Reduced vocal resonance
Mediastinum shifted away

Midline

Fluid in pleural space

Figure 9.3
The physical signs and chest radiographic appearances of a pleural effusion.

are shown in Table 9.12. More rarely, effusions consist of blood (haemothorax), pus (empyema) or lymph (chylothorax). Chylous effusions are caused by leakage of lymph from the thoracic duct as a result of trauma or infiltration by carcinoma.

Table 9.12 Causes of a pleural effusion

Transudates	Exudates
Heart failure	Bacterial pneumonia
Hypoproteinaemia	Carcinoma of the bronchus
Constrictive pericarditis	Pulmonary infarction
Hypothyroidism	Tuberculosis
Meigs' syndrome (ovarian fibroma	Connective tissue disease
with right-sided pleural effusion	Post-myocardial infarction
and ascites)	syndrome
	Acute pancreatitis
	Mesothelioma
	Sarcoidosis (rarely)

Investigations

Diagnosis is by pleural aspiration and biopsy. Fluid is sent for the following:

- Protein estimation
- Bacteriological examination: Gram stain and culture, Ziehl–Nielsen stain and culture
- Cytology for malignant cells
- Occasionally: amylase, rheumatoid factor, glucose.

Management

This depends on the underlying cause.

Pneumothorax

Pneumothorax means the presence of air in the pleural space, and this may occur spontaneously or secondary to trauma. A 'tension pneumothorax' is rare unless the patient is on positive pressure ventilation. In this situation the pleural tear acts as a one-way valve through which air passes only during inspiration. Positive pressure builds up, causing increasing cardiorespiratory embarrassment and eventually cardiac arrest. Treatment is immediate intercostal tube drainage.

Aetiology

Spontaneous pneumothorax usually occurs in young men as a result of rupture of a pleural bleb, usually in the apex of the lung. A bleb is thought to be a congenital defect in the connective tissue of the alveolar wall, which may occur in both lungs with equal frequency. Often these patients are tall and thin. In patients over 40 years of age the usual cause is underlying COPD.

Clinical features

There is a sudden onset of pleuritic pain with increasing breathlessness.

The physical signs, chest radiographic appearances and management are shown in Figures 9.4 and 9.5.

....

DISORDERS OF THE DIAPHRAGM

The most common cause of unilateral diaphragmatic paralysis is the result of involvement of the phrenic nerve (C2–C4) in the thorax by a bronchial carcinoma. Other common causes of phrenic paralysis are trauma, surgery and motor neuron disease. Unilateral paralysis produces no symptoms.

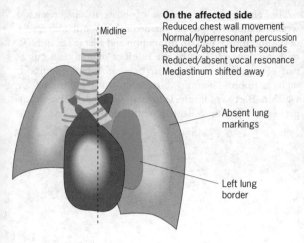

On the affected side
Reduced chest wall movement
Normal/hyperresonant percussion
Reduced/absent breath sounds
Reduced/absent vocal resonance
Mediastinum shifted away

Midline

Absent lung
markings

Left lung
border

Figure 9.4
The physical signs and chest radiographic appearances of pneumothorax.

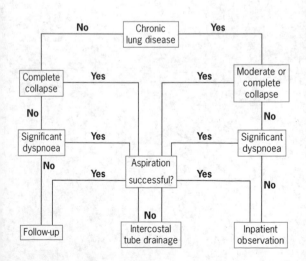

Figure 9.5
Management of a pneumothorax.

The characteristic features of bilateral diaphragmatic weakness are orthopnoea, paradoxical (inward) movement of the abdominal wall on inspiration and a large fall in FVC on lying down. It may be the result of trauma or occur as part of a generalized muscular or neurological condition, such as motor neuron disease, muscular dystrophy or Guillain–Barré syndrome. Treatment is either diaphragmatic pacing or night-time assisted ventilation.

Intensive care medicine (or 'critical care medicine') is concerned mainly with the management of patients with acute life-threatening conditions ('the critically ill') in a specialized unit. It also encompasses the resuscitation and transport of those who become acutely ill, or are injured, either elsewhere in the hospital or in the community. An intensive care unit (ICU) has the facilities and expertise to provide cardiorespiratory support to these sick patients, some of whom also have kidney or liver failure, and management of this is described in the relevant chapters.

All patients admitted to the ICU require skilled nursing care (patient to nurse ratio of 1:1) and physiotherapy. Many require nutritional support. General medical management includes the prevention of venous thrombosis (page 185), pressure sores and constipation. A number of scoring systems, such as the APACHE score, are in use to evaluate the severity of the patient's illness.

ACUTE DISTURBANCES OF HAEMODYNAMIC FUNCTION (SHOCK)

The term 'shock' is used to describe acute circulatory failure with inadequate or inappropriately distributed tissue perfusion resulting in generalized cellular hypoxia. The causes of shock are listed in Table 10.1. Shock is often the result of a combination of these factors.

Pathophysiology

Sympathoadrenal In response to hypotension there is a reflex increase in sympathetic nervous activity and catecholamine release from the adrenal medulla. The resulting vasoconstriction, increased myocardial contractility and heart rate help restore blood pressure and cardiac

Table 10.1 Causes of shock

Hypovolaemic
    Exogenous losses (e.g. haemorrhage, burns)
    Endogenous losses (e.g. sepsis, anaphylaxis)

Cardiogenic
    Myocardial infarction
    Myocarditis
    Rupture of a valve cusp

Obstructive
    Obstruction to outflow (e.g. pulmonary embolus)
    Restricted cardiac filling (e.g. cardiac tamponade)

Distributive
    Vascular dilatation (e.g. drugs, sepsis)
    Arteriovenous shunting
    Maldistribution of flow (e.g. sepsis, anaphylaxis)

output. Activation of the renin–angiotensin system leads to vasoconstriction and salt and water retention, which help to restore circulating volume.

Neuroendocrine response There is release of anterior pituitary hormones and glucagon, which are insulin antagonists. They raise blood sugar and may be responsible for some of the cardiovascular changes.

Release of mediators In septic shock components of microorganisms (e.g. endotoxin of Gram-negative bacteria) release cytokines (tumour necrosis factor, interleukin-1 and interferon-γ) from macrophages and white cells, activate the complement system and cause the release of vasoactive mediators (e.g. prostacyclin, endothelin-1 and nitric oxide) from vascular endothelium. The end result of these processes is vasodilatation, increased vascular permeability, endothelial cell damage and platelet aggregation. Vasodilatation and increased vascular permeability are also seen in shock secondary to anaphylaxis.

A similar widespread inflammatory response may occur with non-infectious processes, e.g. trauma and acute pancreatitis, and is referred to as the *systemic inflammatory response syndrome* (SIRS). The clinical features are pyrexia, tachycardia, tachypnoea and a raised white cell count.

Microcirculatory changes In the early stages of septic shock there is vasodilatation, increased capillary permeability with interstitial oedema, and arteriovenous shunting.

Vasodilatation and increased capillary permeability also occur in anaphylactic shock. In the initial stages of other forms of shock, and in the later stages of sepsis and anaphylaxis, there is capillary sequestration of blood. Fluid is forced into the extravascular space, causing interstitial oedema, haemoconcentration and an increase in plasma viscosity.

In all forms of shock there may be activation of the coagulation pathway, with the development of disseminated intravascular coagulation (DIC, see page 182). The disseminated inflammatory response and microcirculatory changes may lead to progressive organ failure (*multiple organ dysfunction syndrome* (MODS), also known as multiple organ failure (MOF)), the lungs are usually affected first, with the development of the *acute respiratory distress syndrome* (ARDS). The mortality in MODS is high and treatment is supportive.

Clinical features

The history will often indicate the cause of shock, e.g. a patient with major injuries (often internal and thus concealed) will often develop hypovolaemic shock. A patient with a history of peptic ulceration may now be bleeding into the gastrointestinal tract, and rectal examination will show melaena. Anaphylactic shock may develop in susceptible individuals after insect stings and eating certain foods, e.g. peanuts.

Hypovolaemic shock Inadequate tissue perfusion causes blue cold skin with slow capillary refill. The blood pressure (particularly when supine) may be maintained initially, but later hypotension supervenes (systolic BP <100 mmHg) with oliguria (<30 ml of urine/h), confusion and restlessness. Increased sympathetic tone causes tachycardia (pulse >100/min) and sweating.

Cardiogenic shock Additional clinical features are those of myocardial failure, e.g. raised jugular venous pressure (JVP), pulsus alternans (alternating strong and weak pulses) and/or a 'gallop' rhythm (page 342).

Mechanical shock Muffled heart sounds, pulsus paradoxus (pulse fades on inspiration), elevated JVP and Kussmaul's sign (JVP increases on inspiration) occur in cardiac tamponade. In pulmonary embolism there are signs of right heart strain, with a raised JVP with prominent '*a*' waves, right ventricular heave and a loud pulmonary second sound.

Anaphylactic shock Profound vasodilatation leads to warm peripheries and low blood pressure. Erythema, urticaria, angio-oedema, bronchospasm, and oedema of the face and larynx may all be present.

Septic shock In the early stages there is vasodilatation, pyrexia and rigors. At a later stage there are features of hypovolaemic shock. Sepsis in elderly people or in the immunosuppressed is common without the classic clinical features.

Management

This is summarized in Emergency Box 10.1. The underlying cause must be identified and treated appropriately. Whatever the aetiology of shock, tissue blood flow and blood pressure must be restored as quickly as possible to avoid the development of MOF.

Expansion of the circulating volume Volume replacement is obviously important in hypovolaemic shock, but also in anaphylactic and septic shock, where there is vasodilatation, sequestration of blood and loss of circulating volume secondary to capillary leakage. High filling pressures may also be needed in mechanical shock. Care must be taken to prevent volume overload, which leads to a reduction in stroke volume and a rise in left atrial pressure with a risk of pulmonary oedema. The choice of fluid depends on the clinical situation:

- Whole blood is the fluid of choice for haemorrhage. Cross-matched blood must be used if possible, but in extreme emergencies the 'universal donor' group O rhesus-negative blood is used. Complications of massive blood transfusion are hypothermia, thrombocytopenia, hypocalcaemia and depletion of clotting factors.
- Colloidal solutions increase colloid osmotic pressure and produce a greater and more sustained increase in plasma volume than crystalloid solutions. They are used to replace fluid in hypovolaemic patients and are useful for the maintenance of blood volume, but have no oxygen-carrying capacity. Polygelatin solutions (e.g. Gelofusine and Haemaccel) are the most widely used. Human

Emergency

Restore delivery of oxygen to the tissues

Ensure adequate oxygenation and ventilation

- Maintain patent airway: use an oropharyngeal airway or an endotracheal tube if necessary
- Administer 100% oxygen via a tight-fitting face mask
- Maintain respiratory function

Monitor
- Respiratory rate
- Arterial blood gases
- Chest radiograph

Restore cardiac output and BP

- Lay the patient flat or head down
- Expand circulating volume. Give appropriate fluids quickly via 1 or 2 large-bore cannulae (16 G) placed in antecubital vein or via a central vein.
- Support cardiovascular function

Monitor
- Skin colour
- Capillary refill time
- Peripheral temperature
- Urine flow
- Pulse and blood pressure
- ECG
- CVP in most cases
- Swan–Ganz catheter in selected cases

Investigations	**Treat underlying cause**	**Treat complications**
All cases	Control haemorrhage	e.g. coagulopathy,
FBC and coagulation screen	Sepsis	renal failure
Urea and electrolytes	Anaphylaxis	
Blood glucose		
Liver biochemistry		
Blood gases		
Selected cases		
Infection screen		
Blood lactate		
Fibrinogen degradation products		
Cross-match blood		

Emergency Box 10.1
Management of shock

albumin solution and dextrans are less commonly used because of the expense (albumin) and higher complication rate (dextrans). Colloid solutions are often used for acute blood loss before whole blood becomes available, and for volume replacement in anaphylactic and septic shock.

- Crystalloids, e.g. 5% dextrose, 0.9% saline, are readily available and cheap. Once in the circulation they quickly redistribute into the interstitial fluid, therefore large volumes are needed to restore circulating volume and the excess fluid in the interstitial space may contribute to pulmonary oedema. Large volumes of crystalloid (>2 litres) as a treatment for shock are best avoided. However, crystalloids are frequently used for volume replacement with diarrhoea and vomiting, and sometimes with burns.

Myocardial contractility and inotropic agents Myocardial contractility is impaired in cardiogenic shock and at a later stage in other forms of shock as a result of hypoxaemia, acidosis and the release of mediators. It is recommended that the treatment of acidosis should concentrate on correcting the cause; intravenous bicarbonate should only be administered to correct extreme (pH <7.0) persistent metabolic acidosis. When a patient remains hypotensive despite adequate volume replacement inotropic agents are administered. This must be via a large central vein and the effects carefully monitored. The inotropic agents used and their clinical effects are shown in Table 10.2. Many consider dopamine to be the inotrope of choice in critically ill patients, but dobutamine is a better choice when vasconstriction caused by dopamine could be dangerous. Noradrenaline in combination with dobutamine (depending on the cardiac output) is used for shocked patients with a low peripheral resistance, e.g. septic patients.

Additional treatment Vasodilators, e.g. sodium nitroprusside and isosorbide dinitrate, may be useful in selected patients who remain vasoconstricted and oliguric despite adequate volume replacement and a satisfactory blood pressure. Finally, in patients with a potentially reversible depression of left ventricular function (e.g. cardiogenic shock secondary to a ruptured interventricular septum), intra-aortic balloon counterpulsation (IABCP) may be used as a temporary measure to maintain life until definitive surgical treatment can be carried out.

Specific treatment of the cause In all cases the cause of shock must be identified if possible and specific treatment given when indicated.

- Septic shock: antibiotic therapy should be directed towards the probable cause. In the absence of helpful clinical guidelines, 'blind' intravenous antibiotic therapy (e.g. cefuroxime and gentamicin) should be started after performing an infection screen: chest radiograph and culture of blood, urine and sputum. Lumbar puncture, ultrasonography and CT of the chest and abdomen are useful in selected cases. Abscesses require drainage. Steroids have no role in the treatment of septic shock.
- Anaphylactic shock must be identified and treated immediately (Emergency Box 10.2).

! Emergency

Remove the precipitating cause, e.g. stop administration of the drug. Administer:
    0.5 mg adrenaline intramuscularly,* i.e. 0.5 ml of a 1 in 1000 solution
    Colloid, e.g. Haemaccel, 1 litre rapid i.v. infusion and continue depending on response
    Antihistamine, e.g. chlorpheniramine 10 mg i.v.
    Hydrocortisone 200 mg i.v.
    Repeat adrenaline every 10 minutes until improvement occurs

Give intravenous adrenaline (0.5 mg over 5 minutes) with full ECG monitoring if patient is extremely unwell with hypotension and severe dyspnoea.

There is a risk of relapse even after full recovery. Admit patient to hospital for 24 hours for monitoring and treatment with hydrocortisone and chlorpheniramine.

Patients who have had an attack of anaphylaxis and who are at risk of developing another should carry a preloaded syringe of adrenaline for subcutaneous self-administration.

Emergency Box 10.2
Management of anaphylactic shock

Table 10.2 Inotropic agents used in the management of shock: the effect of each inotrope on the adrenergic and dopaminergic receptors is shown

(Dose, µg/kg/min)	β_1	β_2	α_1	α_2	DA_1	DA_2	Comments
Adrenaline							A potent inotrope used in patients not responding to dobutamine or dopamine. At high doses vasoconstriction may increase renal perfusion pressure and urine output, but as dose is further increased marked vasoconstriction leads to decreased cardiac output, oliguria and peripheral gangrene. Agent of choice in septic shock when haemodynamic monitoring not available
Low dose (0.06–0.1)	++	+	+	+	–	–	
Moderate dose (0.1–0.18)	++	+	++	+	–	–	
High dose (>0.18)	++(+)	+	++++	+++	–	–	
Noradrenaline	++	0	+++	+++	–	–	Particularly useful in septic shock as administration leads to increased inotropy and an increase in peripheral vascular resistance. Requires full haemodynamic monitoring
Isoprenaline	+++	+++	0	0	–	–	Rarely used
Dopamine							At low dose general vasodilatory action which may increase urine output and preserve function of vital organs. Increases cardiac output at all doses, but at high doses this beneficial effect may be offset by vasoconstriction, thus increasing afterload and ventricular filling pressures
Low dose (1–3)	±	±	±	?	++	?	
Moderate dose (3–10)	++	+	++	?	++(+)	?	
High dose (>10)	+++	++	+++	?	++(+)	?	

Dopexamine	+	+++	0	0	++	Dopamine analogue. Most useful in patients with a low cardiac output and peripheral vasoconstriction
Dobutamine	++	+	±	?	0	Similar actions to dopexamine, useful in patients with cardiogenic shock
Enoximone	Phosphodiesterase inhibitor with inotropic and vasodilator actions					Occasionally useful in acute heart failure

0, no agonism; +, mild agonism; ++, moderate agonism; +++, profound agonism; α, α-adrenergic receptors; β, β-adrenergic receptors; DA, dopamine receptors.

Monitoring

This is by both clinical and invasive means.

Clinical An assessment of skin perfusion, measurement of pulse, BP, JVP and urinary flow rate will guide treatment in a straightforward case. Additional invasive monitoring will be required in seriously ill patients who do not respond to initial treatment.

Invasive

- Blood pressure: a continuous recording may be made with an intra-arterial cannula, usually in the radial artery.
- Central venous pressure (CVP) is related to right ventricular end-diastolic pressure, which depends on circulating blood volume, venous tone, intrathoracic pressure and right ventricular function. CVP is measured by inserting a catheter percutaneously into the superior vena cava and connecting it to a manometer system (page 639). The normal range is 0–4 cmH_2O above the manubriosternal angle in a supine patient. In shock CVP may be normal, because in spite of hypovolaemia there is increased venous tone. A better guide to circulating volume is the response to a fluid challenge (Figure 10.11).
- Left atrial pressure: in uncomplicated cases the CVP is an adequate guide to the filling pressures of both sides of the heart. However, if there is disparity in function

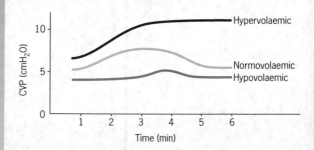

Figure 10.1
The effect of rapid administration (200 ml of 0.9% saline over 1–3 minutes) of a fluid challenge to patients with a CVP within the normal range.

between the two ventricles (e.g. infarction of the left ventricle), left atrial pressure must be measured. A Swan–Ganz catheter is introduced percutaneously into a central vein and then guided through the chambers of the heart into the pulmonary artery. By inflating a balloon at the tip of the catheter, pulmonary artery wedge pressure (PAWP) is measured, which is a reflection of left atrial pressure.

- Cardiac output is measured, using a modified Swan–Ganz catheter, by recording temperature changes in the pulmonary artery after injecting a bolus of cold dextrose into the right atrium.

RESPIRATORY FAILURE

Respiratory failure occurs when pulmonary gas exchange is sufficiently impaired to cause hypoxaemia with or without hypercapnia.

It can be divided into two types (Table 10.3):

- Type 1 respiratory failure is caused by a diffusion defect in the gas exchange area of the lung, ventilation/ perfusion mismatch or right to left shunts (e.g. with cyanotic congenital heart disease). The P_aO_2 is low (<8 kPa) and the P_aCO_2 is normal or low.
- Type 2 respiratory failure is caused by hypoventilation. The P_aO_2 is low and the P_aCO_2 is high (>7 kPa).

Table 10.3 Causes of respiratory failure

Type 1	Type 2
Pulmonary oedema	COPD
Pneumonia	Severe asthma
Asthma	Muscle weakness, e.g.
Pulmonary embolism	Guillain–Barré syndrome
COPD	Respiratory centre depression,
Acute respiratory distress syndrome	e.g. with sedatives
Fibrosing alveolitis	Chest wall deformities
Right to left shunts	

Monitoring

Clinical Assessment should be made on the following criteria: tachypnoea, tachycardia, sweating, pulsus paradoxus, use of accessory muscles of respiration, and inability to speak. Signs of carbon dioxide retention may be present, such as asterixis (coarse tremor), bounding pulse, warm peripheries and papilloedema.

Pulse oximetry Lightweight oximeters placed on an earlobe or finger can give a continuous reading of oxygen saturation by measuring the changing amount of light transmitted through arterial blood. In general, if the saturation is greater than 90% oxygenation can be considered to be adequate. Although simple and reliable, these instruments are not very sensitive to changes in oxygenation. They also give no indication of carbon dioxide retention.

Arterial blood gas analysis Analysis of arterial blood gives definitive measurements of P_aO_2, P_aCO_2; oxygen saturation, pH and bicarbonate (page 638). In type 2 respiratory failure, retention of carbon dioxide causes P_aCO_2 and [H^+] to rise, resulting in respiratory acidosis. The kidney compensates by retaining bicarbonate, reducing the [H^+] towards normal. In type 1 respiratory failure or in hyperventilation there may be a fall in P_aCO_2 and [H^+], resulting in respiratory alkalosis. Other abnormalities of acid–base balance are discussed on page 266.

Management

This includes the administration of supplemental oxygen, control of secretions, treatment of pulmonary infection, control of airway obstruction and limiting pulmonary oedema. In most patients oxygen is given by a face mask or nasal cannulae. With these devices, inspired oxygen concentration varies from 35% to 55%, with flow rates between 6 and 10 litres. However, in patients with chronically elevated carbon dioxide (e.g. COPD), hypoxia rather than hypercapnia maintains the respiratory drive and thus fixed-performance masks (e.g. Venturi masks) should be used, in which the concentration of oxygen can be accurately controlled. Respiratory stimulants such as doxapram have a very limited role in treatment.

Respiratory support Respiratory support should be considered when the above measures are not sufficient. The type depends on the underlying disorder and its clinical severity. Careful consideration should be given to ventilating patients with severe chronic lung disease, as those who are severely incapacitated may be difficult to wean from the ventilator.

- Continuous positive airway pressure (CPAP). Oxygen is delivered to the spontaneously breathing patient under pressure via a tightly fitting face mask (non-invasive positive-pressure ventilation, NIPPV) or endotracheal tube. Oxygenation and vital capacity improves and the lungs become less stiff.
- NIPPV has been shown to be of use in patients with hypercapnic respiratory failure secondary to acute exacerbations of COPD who do not require immediate intubation and ventilation. NIPPV should be instituted at an early stage in the hospital admission when the pH falls below 7.35 and the respiratory rate exceeds 30 breaths per minute. NIPPV is usually given for at least 6 hours a day, and oxygen is administered to maintain arterial oxygen saturation above 90%. NIPPV reduces the need for intubation, complications, mortality and hospital stay.
- Intermittent positive-pressure ventilation (IPPV) IPPV requires tracheal intubation and therefore anaesthesia if the patient is conscious. The beneficial effects of IPPV (Table 10.4) include improved carbon dioxide elimination, improved oxygenation, and relief from exhaustion as the work of ventilation is removed. High concentrations of oxygen (up to 100%) may be administered accurately. If adequate oxygenation cannot be achieved, a positive airway pressure can be maintained at a chosen level throughout expiration by attaching a threshold resistor valve to the expiratory limb of the circuit. This is known as positive end-expiratory pressure (PEEP), and its primary effect is to re-expand underventilated lung areas, thereby reducing shunts and increasing P_aO_2.
- Intermittent mandatory ventilation (IMV). This technique allows the ventilated patient to breathe

Table 10.4 Indications for IPPV

Indication	Comment
Acute respiratory failure	Particularly when exhaustion, confusion, agitation or decreased consciousness are present
Acute ventilatory failure e.g. myasthenia gravis, Guillain–Barré syndrome	Institute when vital capcity fallen to 10–15 ml/kg
Prophylactic postoperative ventilation	In poor-risk patients
Head injury	With acute brain oedema. Intracranial pressure is decreased by elective hyperventilation as this reduces cerebral blood flow
Trauma	e.g. Chest injury and lung contusion
Severe left ventricular failure	
Coma with breathing difficulties	e.g. following drug overdose

spontaneously between mandatory tidal volumes delivered by the ventilator. These coincide with the patient's own respiratory effort. It is used as a method of weaning patients from artificial ventilation, or as an alternative to IPPV.

The major complications of intubation and assisted ventilation are:

– Trauma to the upper respiratory tract from the endotracheal tube;
– Secondary pulmonary infection;
– Barotrauma: overdistension of the lungs and alveolar rupture may present with pneumothorax (page 436) and surgical emphysema;
– Reduction in cardiac output: the increase in intrathoracic pressures during controlled ventilation impedes cardiac filling and lowers cardiac output.

ACUTE RESPIRATORY DISTRESS SYNDROME (ARDS)

ARDS is defined as diffuse bilateral pulmonary infiltrates, refractory hypoxaemia, stiff lungs and respiratory distress in the presence of a recognized precipitating cause and in the absence of cardiogenic pulmonary oedema (i.e. the pulmonary capillary wedge pressure is less than 16 mmHg).

Aetiology

The commonest precipitating factor is sepsis. Other causes include trauma, burns, pancreatitis, fat or amniotic fluid embolism, aspiration pneumonia or cardiopulmonary bypass.

Pathophysiology

The cardinal feature is pulmonary oedema as a result of increased vascular permeability caused by the release of inflammatory mediators. Oedema may induce vascular compression resulting in pulmonary hypertension, which is later exacerbated by vasoconstriction in response to increased autonomic nervous activity. A haemorrhagic intra-alveolar exudate forms which is rich in platelets, fibrin and clotting factors. This inactivates surfactant, stimulates inflammation and promotes hyaline membrane formation. These changes may result in progressive pulmonary fibrosis.

Clinical features

Tachypnoea, increasing hypoxia and laboured breathing are the initial features. The chest radiograph shows diffuse bilateral shadowing, which may progress to a complete 'white-out'.

Management

This is based on the treatment of the underlying condition. Pulmonary oedema should be limited with fluid restriction, diuretics, and haemofiltration if these measures fail.

Steroids currently have no role in the prophylaxis of this condition, but may be beneficial when administered during the late fibroproliferative phase. Aerosolized surfactant, inhaled nitric oxide and aerosolized prostacyclin are experimental treatments whose exact role in the management of ARDS is unclear.

Prognosis

Overall there is a 50% mortality rate, most patients dying from sepsis. The prognosis is very dependent on the underlying cause, and rises steeply with age and with the development of multiorgan failure.

Poisoning, drug and alcohol abuse

11

In most hospitals in the western world the commonest reason for acute admission of young people to a medical ward is acute poisoning. Such poisoning is usually by deliberate self-administration of an excess quantity of prescribed or over-the-counter medicines. Self-poisoning is the most common way by which people commit or attempt suicide (these categories are encompassed by the term 'deliberate self-harm'); other means are usually by violent methods, e.g. hanging, shooting or drowning. Attempted suicide by a violent method is associated with future suicide and these patients must be assessed by a psychiatrist. In adults with self-poisoning admitted to hospital in the UK the most common drugs taken are paracetamol and benzodiazepines, followed by antidepressants and aspirin. In many cases more than one substance is taken; alcohol is frequently a secondary poison. Outside hospital, where most deaths occur, the commonest causes are deliberate carbon monoxide poisoning from inhalation of vehicle exhaust fumes. This is also seen in cases of accidental poisoning with faulty appliances using natural gas.

The majority of cases (80%) of self-poisoning do not require intensive medical management but all require a sympathetic and caring approach to their problems. Both the patient and the family may require psychiatric help (see page 459) and the social services should be contacted to help with social and domestic problems.

Clinical features

Eighty per cent of adults are conscious on arrival at hospital and the diagnosis of self-poisoning can usually be made easily from the history. In the unconscious patient a history from friends or relatives is helpful, and the diagnosis can often be inferred from tablet bottles or a suicide note brought by the ambulance attendants. In any patient with an

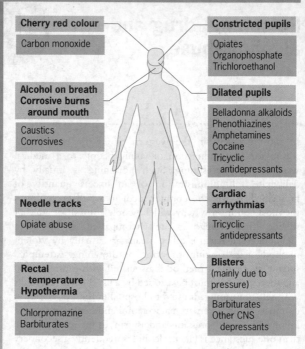

Cherry red colour

Carbon monoxide

Constricted pupils

Opiates
Organophosphate
Trichloroethanol

**Alcohol on breath
Corrosive burns
around mouth**

Caustics
Corrosives

Dilated pupils

Belladonna alkaloids
Phenothiazines
Amphetamines
Cocaine
Tricyclic
    antidepressants

Needle tracks

Opiate abuse

**Cardiac
arrhythmias**

Tricyclic
    antidepressants

**Rectal
    temperature
Hypothermia**

Chlorpromazine
Barbiturates

Blisters
(mainly due to
pressure)

Barbiturates
Other CNS
depressants

Figure 11.1
Physical signs of poisoning.

altered conscious level drug overdose must always be considered in the differential diagnosis. On arrival at hospital the patient must be assessed urgently in the accident and emergency department. A full physical examination must include an assessment of cardiorespiratory status and conscious level (page 572).

The physical signs that may aid identification of the agents responsible for poisoning are shown in Figure 11.1.

Investigations

Blood and urine samples should always be taken on admission for the determination of drug levels, as these are invaluable for the management of certain poisons, e.g. paracetamol and salicylates, and are helpful in legal disputes. Drug screens of blood and urine are also occasionally indicated in the seriously ill unconscious patient in whom the cause of coma is unknown. Further investigations depend on the drugs ingested and clinical assessment of the patient, e.g. arterial blood gases in the comatose patient.

Management

Most patients with self-poisoning require only general care and support of the vital systems. However, for a few drugs additional therapy is required. In the UK the Regional Poisons Centre provides a round-the-clock service for advice about the management of overdose; the telephone number is to be found in the *British National Formulary*. The management of a patient with overdose is summarized in Table 11.1.

Table 11.1 Principles of management of patients with self-poisoning

1. Emergency resuscitation
2. Prevent further drug absorption
3. Increase drug elimination
4. Administration of specific drug antidotes
5. Psychiatric assessment

Emergency resuscitation

- Nurse the patient in the lateral position with the lower leg straight and the upper leg flexed; this reduces the risk of aspiration.
- Clear the airway and intubate if the gag reflex is absent.
- Administer 60% oxygen by face mask in patients not intubated.
- Artificial ventilation is sometimes necessary if ventilation is inadequate (page 451).
- Treat hypotension (page 442), arrythmias (page 327) and convulsions (page 589).
- Respiratory function (arterial blood gas analysis or pulse oximetry) and ECG monitoring in selected patients.
- Treat hypothermia (<35°C) with 'space blankets', warm (37°C) intravenous fluids and inspired gases.

Prevention of further drug absorption
Most patients coming to hospital after an overdose are not at serious risk. These

measures are usually reserved for those who have taken a potentially serious overdose.

- *Gastric lavage* is used to remove the drug from the stomach. It is of little value after 4 hours except in the case of salicylates and tricyclic antidepressants, which remain within the stomach for many hours. The main danger of gastric lavage is aspiration, and the unconscious patient must be intubated with a cuffed endotracheal tube if the gag reflex is absent. Lavage is contraindicated for some poisons, e.g. corrosives, petrol or paraffin.
- *Whole bowel lavage* is used for the treatment of poisoning with iron and lithium and other metallic compounds, slow-release preparations of theophylline and propranolol, and packets of illicit drugs. Isotonic saline is infused (2 l/h) via a nasogastric tube until the rectal effluent is clear.
- *Induction of vomiting* with ipecacuanha syrup may be useful in small children as they are more difficult to lavage. It is rarely used in adults, as only small amounts of drug are recovered.
- *Activated charcoal* (50 g, followed by 50 g every hour for 3 hours) administered by mouth or nasogastric tube adsorbs unabsorbed poison still present in the gut. It is useful given after lavage, or when lavage is contraindicated.

Increasing drug elimination

- *Forced alkaline diuresis* depends on the principle that ionization of acid drugs (e.g. salicylates) is increased in alkaline urine and thus renal tubular reabsorption is reduced (as only lipophilic non-ionized drugs cross the lipid membrane readily). It is a potentially dangerous procedure which is usually only undertaken in cases of severe salicylate poisoning (Figure 11.2). Careful clinical and laboratory monitoring is necessary.
- *Dialysis* (peritoneal or haemodialysis) is used with some drugs in cases of severe poisoning, e.g. lithium, methyl or ethyl alcohols, and patients with severe salicylate poisoning (blood salicylate level >700 mg/l, or 5.1 mmol/l) refractory to urine alkalization.

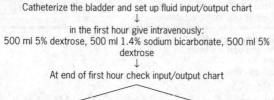

Catheterize the bladder and set up fluid input/output chart
↓
in the first hour give intravenously:
500 ml 5% dextrose, 500 ml 1.4% sodium bicarbonate, 500 ml 5% dextrose
↓
At end of first hour check input/output chart

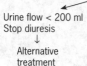

Urine flow < 200 ml
Stop diuresis
↓
Alternative
treatment
needed

Urine flow > 200 ml
Continue fluids to maintain:
• Urine pH 7.5–8.5
• Urine 500 ml/h (i.v. frusemide if needed)
• Normal serum potassium
Check.
• Urine pH half-hourly
• Arterial blood gases 2-hourly
• Serum electrolytes 2-hourly

Figure 11.2
Forced alkaline diuresis.

- *Haemoperfusion* involves the passage of heparinized blood through devices containing absorbent particles such as activated charcoal or resins, to which drugs are absorbed. Its use should be considered in patients severely poisoned with certain drugs (e.g. theophylline, short- and medium-acting barbiturates and glutethimide), who fail to improve despite the use of adequate supportive measures.

Antagonizing the effects of poisons Specific antidotes are available for a small number of drugs; these will be considered under the individual drugs.

Psychiatric assessment All suicide attempts must be taken seriously and an assessment made of suicidal intent (Table 11.2). In some patients, often young females, the act was not premeditated, they have no wish to die and the tablets were taken in response to an acute situation, e.g. an argument with the boyfriend. The risk of suicide is low and formal psychiatric assessment is not always necessary. In the absence of potential medical problems these patients may not necessarily need to be admitted to hospital, provided there is the necessary social and emotional back-up at home. In

Table 11.2 Factors associated with increased risk of suicide and need for psychiatric referral

Sociodemographic
Patients over 45 years
Male
Unmarried
Living alone

Psychiatric
Clinical depression
Psychotic illness of any kind
Family history of suicide
Previous suicide attempts
Addiction to alcohol or drugs
Major unresolved crisis: financial, family, occupational

Persistent suicidal behaviour/thoughts
Patient expresses intention to die
Cogent plan
Lethal means available
Expressions of despair, hopelessness and pessimism about the future

other patients there is clear suicidal intent: the act was planned, a suicide note was written and efforts were made not to be discovered. These patients must be assessed by a psychiatrist before they leave hospital.

SPECIFIC DRUG PROBLEMS

In this section only specific treatment regimens will be discussed. The general principles of management of self-poisoning should always be applied.

Aspirin

Overdosage of aspirin (salicylate) stimulates the respiratory centre, directly increasing the depth and rate of respiration and thereby producing a respiratory alkalosis. Compensatory mechanisms include renal excretion of bicarbonate and potassium, which results in a metabolic acidosis and a fall in arterial pH indicates serious poisoning. Salicylates also interfere with carbohydrate, fat and protein metabolism, as well as with oxidative phosphorylation. This gives rise to increased lactate, pyruvate and ketone bodies, all of which contribute to the acidosis.

Clinical features

Symptoms and signs of aspirin poisoning include tinnitus, nausea and vomiting, overbreathing, hyperpyrexia and sweating with a tachycardia. Alternatively, the patient may appear completely well, even with high blood levels of salicylate. Ingestion of 10–20 g of aspirin by an adult (or one-tenth of this amount for a child) is likely to cause moderate or severe toxicity.

In severe poisoning (blood salicylate levels 800–1000 mg/l; 5.6–7.2 mmol/l) there may be cerebral and pulmonary oedema resulting from increased capillary permeability. Coma and respiratory depression may be seen with severe poisoning, but more frequently are due to the ingestion of a second drug or alcohol.

Management

- Gastric lavage up to 24 hours after ingestion in severe cases
- Activated charcoal in repeated doses (see page 458)
- Correct dehydration and hypokalaemia with intravenous fluids
- Intramuscular vitamin K to correct hypoprothrombinaemia
- Consider forced alkaline diuresis if blood salicylate level >500 mg/l (3.6 mmol/l)
- Haemodialysis may be indicated if the concentration of salicylate exceeds 700 mg/l (5.1 mmol/l).

Paracetamol

Paracetamol in overdose may cause fatal hepatic necrosis and is the commonest form of poisoning encountered in the UK today, being responsible for over 200 deaths per year. Paracetamol is converted to a toxic metabolite, N-acetyl-p-benzoquinoimine, which is normally inactivated by conjugation with reduced glutathione. After a large overdose glutathione is depleted and the toxic metabolite binds covalently with sulphydryl groups on liver cell membranes, causing necrosis. Marked liver cell necrosis can occur with as little as 7.5 g (15 tablets) and death with 15 g. The prothrombin time or international normalized ratio (INR) is the best guide to the severity of the liver damage.

Clinical features

The main danger is liver failure, which usually becomes apparent in 72–96 hours after drug ingestion. Initial symptoms include malaise, nausea and vomiting, with preserved consciousness unless another drug has also been taken. Acute renal failure may occur in the absence of severe liver failure.

Management

Treatment depends on the interval between overdose and presentation and on the plasma concentrations of paracetamol. The investigation and management of paracetamol poisoning are summarized in Emergency Box 11.1 and Figure 11.3. The two antidotes in use for paracetamol poisoning increase the availability of glutathione. Intravenous N-acetylcysteine (NAC) is the

> ### ! Emergency
>
> - Take blood for paracetamol levels, INR and ALT/AST, V+E and glucose
>
> - Gastric lavage or activated charcoal if patients presents early (<1 h)
>
> - Give intravenous NAC if potentially serious overdose taken (>7.5 g)
>   150 mg/kg in 200 ml 5% dextrose over 15 min, then
>   50 mg/kg in 500 ml 5% dextrose over 4 h, then
>   100 mg/kg in 1 litre 5% dextrose over 16 h.
>
> - Make decision to continue treatment based on nomogram (Figure 11.3)
>
> - If patient presents >15 h following ingestion Figure 11.3 is unreliable. Give NAC if a potentially serious overdose was taken. Repeat investigations (PT, AST/ALT) and consider continuing NAC treatment (100 mg/kg in 1 litre 5% dextrose over 16 h repeated until recovery)
>
> - Patients with established liver disease or on enzyme-inducing drugs may be at greater risk of paracetamol-induced liver damage and treatment should be commenced if levels are above the lower (100 mg) line of the nomogram

Emergency Box 11.1
Management of paracetamol poisoning

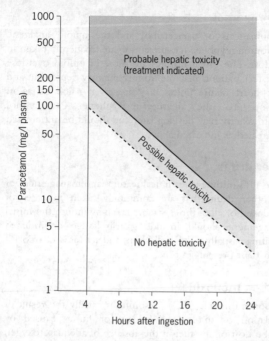

Figure 11.3
Nomogram for treatment of paracetamol poisoning

treatment of choice; there are few side effects other than occasional hypersensitivity reactions. Oral methionine is an alternative, but absorption and efficacy are erratic if the patient is vomiting. Patients who develop liver damage with a raised INR should remain in hospital until the values are returning to normal. Fresh frozen plasma should not normally be given to patients with a raised INR, as the trend in the INR is important in assessing prognosis and in determining the need for possible transplantation. A poor prognosis is indicated by an INR value above 3, raised serum creatinine concentration or a blood pH below 7.3 recorded more than 24 hours after the overdose. If any of these abnormalities is present, advice should be sought from a specialist liver unit. Patients with severe hepatic damage may require liver transplantation.

Co-proxamol

Combinations of paracetamol and the opioid analgesic dextropropoxyphene (co-proxamol) are frequently taken in overdose. The initial features are those of opioid overdose (see later); patients may die from respiratory depression and acute heart failure unless they are given naloxone as an antidote to the dextropropoxyphene. Paracetamol hepatotoxicity may develop later and should be anticipated and treated as indicated above.

Other drugs

Table 11.3 outlines the clinical features and management of the other drugs that are commonly taken in cases of overdose. For all of those that are taken by mouth the initial management should include gastric lavage or induced vomiting (usually only in children) and activated charcoal if the patient presents in time.

Carbon monoxide

Carbon monoxide (CO) poisoning is usually the result of inhalation of smoke, car exhaust or fumes caused by combustion of any fuel in the absence of adequate oxygen and ventilation. CO combines readily with haemoglobin to form carboxyhaemoglobin, thus preventing the formation of oxyhaemoglobin. The clinical features include headache, mental impairment and, in severe cases, coma. In spite of hypoxaemia the skin is pink. Treatment consists of removing the patient from the CO source and giving as high a concentration of inhaled oxygen as possible. Referral for hyperbaric oxygen treatment should be considered if the victim is, or has been, unconscious or has a blood carboxyhaemoglobin concentration of more than 40%.

Alcohol

Acute intoxication with alcohol produces severe depression of consciousness and hypoglycaemia, particularly in children. Treatment usually only consists of gastric lavage with an endotracheal tube in position. Blood glucose is measured and glucose given if indicated.

Table 11.3 Clinical features and specific management for certain drugs taken in over dose

Drug	Clinical features	Management
Tricyclic antidepressants	Tachycardia, hypotension, fixed dilated pupils, convulsions, urinary retention, arrhythmias, decreased conscious level	Treat convulsions with diazepam Arrhythmias may respond to correction of acidosis and hypoxia
Benzodiazepines	Drowsiness, ataxia, dysarthria and coma Potentiate the effect of other CNS depressants taken concomitantly	Flumazenil, a benzodiazepine antagonist given intravenously, is used in cases of severe respiratory depression
Phenothiazines	Hypotension, hypothermia arrhythmias Depression of consciousness and respiration Convulsion and dystonic reactions	Symptomatic treatment of complications, e.g. diazepam for convulsions. Dystonic reactions treated with intravenous benztropine
NSAIDs	Mefenamic acid is the most significant member of this group taken in overdose Convulsions are the most important feature	Convulsions treated with diazepam
β-Blockers	Bradycardia and hypotension. Coma, convulsions and hypoglycaemia with severe overdose	Atropine for hypotension and arrhythmias. In resistant cases intravenous glucagon has a positive inotropic effect

....

DRUG ABUSE

Under the Misuse of Drugs Regulations of 1985, drugs with a high abuse potential, drugs of addiction and other drugs with non-therapeutic psychotropic activity are categorized as controlled drugs. These include opiates, cocaine, barbiturates, lysergide, amphetamines and related drugs. Any patient who is believed to be dependent or addicted to controlled drugs must, by law, be notified to the Home Office.

Opioids

Opioid drugs produce physical dependency, such that an acute withdrawal syndrome develops ('cold turkey') if the drugs are stopped. These severe symptoms – profuse sweating, tachycardia, dilated pupils, leg cramps, diarrhoea and vomiting – may be reduced by giving methadone.

Drug addicts frequently overdose themselves, causing varying degrees of coma, respiratory depression and pinpoint pupils. Treatment is with intravenous naloxone, an opiate antagonist, 0.4–1.2 mg i.v. every 2 minutes until breathing is adequate. The drug is short acting and repeated doses or an infusion may be necessary, with the rate titrated according to the clinical response.

Cannabis

Cannabis is usually smoked and is often taken casually. It is a mild hallucinogen, seldom accompanied by a desire to increase the dose; withdrawal symptoms are uncommon.

Lysergide

Lysergic acid diethylamine (LSD) is a much more potent hallucinogen; its use can lead to severe psychotic states in which life may be at risk. Even in overdose severe physiological reactions do not seem to occur. Adverse reactions are treated with repeated reassurance; a sedative, e.g. diazepam, is sometimes necessary. Phenothiazines may be necessary in severe cases.

Cocaine

Cocaine can be taken by injection, inhalation ('crack') or ingestion. It stimulates the central nervous system, producing euphoria, agitation and tachycardia. Convulsions, pyrexia and cardiorespiratory depression may occur in severe cases of overdose and management is supportive.

Amphetamines

Amphetamines are taken for their stimulatory effect. In overdose there is confusion, delirium, hallucinations and violent behaviour. Cardiac arrhythmias can be a major problem. Treatment is with sedatives, such as diazepam. Forced acid diuresis may be used but is rarely required.

Ecstasy (MDMA, 3,4-methylenedioxymethamphetamine) is a synthetic amphetamine derivative taken orally as tablets or capsules. In Britain it is used almost exclusively as a 'dance drug' and the adverse effects are the result of the drug's pharmacological properties compounded by physical exertion. Serious acute complications are convulsions, hyperpyrexia, coagulopathy, rhabdomyolysis, renal and liver failure and death. Treatment is supportive.

Solvents

The inhalation of organic solvents has become a common problem, particularly in teenagers. The patient presents either in the acute intoxicated state (with euphoria and excitement) or as a chronic abuser with excoriation and rashes over the face and a peripheral neuropathy. Sudden death can occur and is probably the result of cardiac arrhythmias.

Alcohol abuse

Drinking-related problems have increased in recent years. Approximately one in five male admissions to acute medical wards is directly or indirectly the result of alcohol. Over the past 20 years admissions to psychiatric hospitals for the treatment of alcohol-related problems has increased 25-fold.

A number of medical, social and psychiatric problems are related to alcohol abuse (see below) and may be seen in the absence of actual physiological dependence. Alcohol dependence has seven essential elements:

- A compulsive need to drink
- A regular (daily) drinking routine to avoid or relieve withdrawal symptoms

- Drinking takes priority over other activities
- Increased tolerance to alcohol
- Repeated withdrawal symptoms often worse on waking in the morning
- Early morning drinking to avoid withdrawal symptoms (nausea, sweating, agitation)
- Reinstatement after abstinence.

Guidelines for safe limits of drinking are 21 units per week in men and 14 units in women (one unit = a measure of spirits, a glass of wine or half a pint of standard-strength beer). A slightly higher intake is probably unlikely to lead to harm, but more than 36 units per week in men and 24 units in women increases the risk to health. An elevated serum γGT

(γ–Glutamyltranspeptidase) (page 95) and raised red cell mean corpuscular volume (MCV, page 150) are useful screening tests for alcohol abuse and are helpful in monitoring progress. Blood and urine alcohol levels are sometimes measured to demonstrate high intake.

Consequences of alcohol abuse and dependence

Physical complications

These usually occur after a long period of heavy drinking, e.g. 10 years. Problems are generally seen earlier in women than in men. Damage is the result of direct tissue toxicity and the effects of malnutrition and vitamin deficiency which often accompany alcohol abuse.

- *Cardiovascular* A direct toxic effect in the heart leads to a cardiomyopathy and arrhythmias.
- *Neurological* Acute intoxication leads to ataxia, falls and head injury with intracranial bleeds. Long-term complications include polyneuropathy (page 617), myopathy, cerebellar degeneration (page 557), dementia (page 624) and epilepsy.

  Wernicke–Korsakoff syndrome is the result of vitamin B$_1$ deficiency (thiamine) and thus may also be seen in severe starvation and prolonged vomiting. The clinical features include an acute onset of confusion, ataxia, nystagmus and ophthalmoplegia, usually with VIth nerve palsies or defects of conjugate gaze (page 564). Untreated, the patient becomes increasingly drowsy, lapses into a coma and dies. In less acute cases the characteristic features of Korsakoff's syndrome appear. There is a gross defect of short-term memory, associated with confabulation. The diagnosis in these conditions is essentially clinical. Treatment is with parenteral thiamine (100 mg twice daily), which may reverse some of the early changes but the memory impairment is often irreversible. Treatment must be given to all patients in which the diagnosis is even considered.

- *Gastrointestinal effects* These include liver damage (page 125), pancreatitis (page 135), oesophagitis and an increased incidence of oesophageal carcinoma.
- *Haematology* These include thrombocytopenia (alcohol inhibits platelet maturation and release from bone marrow), a raised MCV and anaemia caused by dietary folate deficiency.
- *Psychiatric complications* There is an increased incidence of depression and deliberate self-harm among alcoholics. In these patients attempted suicide must always be taken seriously and psychiatric referral considered (page 460).
- *Social complications* These include marital and sexual difficulties, employment problems, financial difficulties and homelessness.

Alcohol withdrawal

Most heavy drinkers will experience some form of withdrawal symptoms if they attempt to reduce or stop drinking.

- Early mild features occur within 6–12 hours and include tremor, nausea and sweating. Treatment is with a reducing dose of chlormethiazole (see below).
- Late major features usually occur within 2–3 days but may take up to 2 weeks:
  - Generalized tonic–clonic seizures (page 585)
  - Delirium tremens with fever, tremor, tachycardia, agitation and visual halluciantions ('pink elephants'). Treatment must be given urgently (see Emergency Box 11.2)

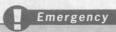

Emergency

- Admit patient to hospital

- Chlormethiazole 9–12 capsules (each capsule contains
  192 mg) for 24 h, then reduced over 5 days, or diazepam
  4–100 mg for 2 days then reduced

- Correct dehydration, electrolyte imbalance

- Treat infection

- B vitamins intravenously

- Intravenous chlormethiazole should be avoided and oral
  treatment should not be carried on long term

Emergency Box 11.2
Management of delirium tremens

Endocrinology

12

Hormones were traditionally thought of as chemical messengers, released from endocrine cells into the circulation and acting at a site distant from their site of secretion. However, the situation is more complex and hormones may act in a variety of ways, such as:

- Neurotransmitters
- A local hormone effect with action on adjacent cells (paracrine action)
- Acting on the cell of origin (autocrine).

Hormones act by binding to specific receptors either on the target cell or within the cell (e.g. thyroid hormones, cortisol). The result is a cascade of intracellular reactions within the target cell which frequently amplifies the original stimulus and leads ultimately to a response by the target cell. Some hormones, e.g. growth hormone and thyroxine, act on most tissues of the body. Others act on only one tissue, e.g. thyroid-stimulating hormone (TSH) and adrenocorticotrophin (ACTH) are secreted by the anterior pituitary and have specific target tissues, namely the thyroid gland and the adrenal cortex.

The hypothalamus and pituitary

The hypothalamus contains many vital centres for functions such as appetite, thirst, thermal regulation and sleep/waking. It also plays a role in circadian rhythm, the menstrual cycle, stress and mood. Releasing factors produced in the hypothalamus reach the pituitary via the portal system, which runs down the pituitary stalk. These releasing factors stimulate or inhibit the production of hormones from distinct cell types (e.g. production of growth hormone by acidophils), each of which secretes a specific hormone in response to unique hypothalamic stimulatory or inhibitory hormones. The anterior pituitary hormones, in turn,

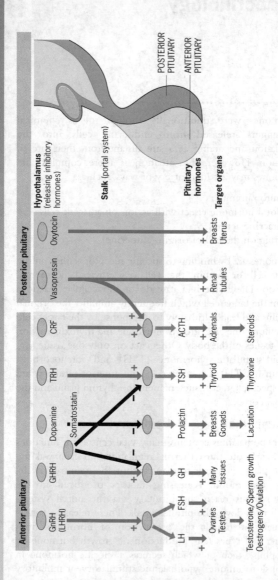

Figure 12.1
Hypothalamic releasing hormones and the pituitary trophic hormones.

stimulate the peripheral glands and tissues. This pattern is illustrated in Figure 12.1 The posterior pituitary acts as a storage organ for antidiuretic hormone (ADH, vasopressin) and oxytocin, which are synthesized in the supraoptic and paraventricular nuclei in the anterior hypothalamus and pass to the posterior pituitary along a single axon in the pituitary stalk. ADH is discussed on page 507; oxytocin produces milk ejection and uterine myometrial contractions.

Control and feedback

Most hormone systems are controlled by some form of feedback; an example is the hypothalamic–pituitary–thyroid axis (Figure 12.2). Thyrotrophin-releasing hormone (TRH), secreted in the hypothalamus, stimulates TSH secretion from the anterior pituitary which, in turn,

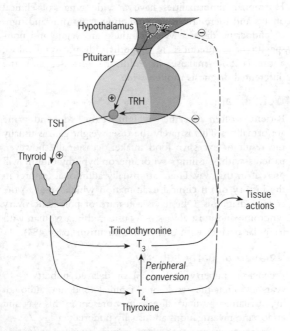

Figure 12.2
The hypothalamic–pituitary–thyroid feedback system. The dotted line indicates probable negative feedback at the hypothalamic level.

stimulates the synthesis and release of thyroid hormones from the thyroid gland. Circulating thyroid hormone feeds back on the pituitary, and possibly the hypothalamus, to suppress the production of TRH and TSH, and hence a fall in thyroid hormone secretion. Conversely, a fall in thyroid hormone secretion (e.g. after thyroidectomy) leads to increased secretion of TRH and TSH.

A patient with a hormone-producing tumour fails to show negative feedback and this is useful in diagnosis, e.g. the dexamethasone suppression test in the diagnosis of Cushing's syndrome.

COMMON PRESENTING SYMPTOMS IN ENDOCRINE DISEASE

Hormonal abnormalities have a wide range of clinical effects and there are many presenting symptoms and signs of endocrine disease. Many of these are vague and non-specific, e.g. tiredness in hypothyroidism, weight loss, anorexia and malaise in Addison's disease, and the differential diagnosis is often wide.

Weight gain

Patients often ascribe weight gain to endocrine abnormalities. This is rarely the case: weight gain is usually the result of excessive food intake; occasionally, however, patients with Cushing's syndrome or hypothyroidism will present in this way. There are usually additional features in the history or on clinical examination which point to the correct diagnosis. Obesity is a feature of polycystic ovary syndrome and must always be considered in a woman with irregular periods with or without hirsutism (page 484).

Delayed or early puberty

Precocious puberty (<9 years) or delayed puberty (>15 years) is often the result of a familial tendency, although hypothalamic–pituitary disease may present in this way, and endocrine investigations are usually undertaken.

Other symptoms that often require specific endocrine investigations include hirsutism (page 484), menstrual irregularities with infrequent or absent periods (page 482), galactorrhoea and infertility. Carpal tunnel syndrome (page 616) is usually idiopathic, but may be a presenting feature of acromegaly or hypothyroidism.

Pituitary tumours

Benign pituitary tumours are the most common form of pituitary disease. Symptoms may arise as a result of excess hormone secretion, inadequate hormone production or from pressure and local infiltration.

Overproduction

Overproduction of pituitary hormones may cause the following:

- Growth hormone (GH) excess, resulting in acromegaly or gigantism (usually acidophil adenomas)
- Prolactin excess (chromophobe adenomas)
- Cushing's disease, resulting from excess ACTH production (basophil adenomas or hyperplasia).

Tumours producing luteinizing hormone (LH), follicle-stimulating hormone (FSH) or TSH are very rare.

Underproduction

This is the result of disease at either a hypothalamic or a pituitary level, and it results in the clinical features of hypopituitarism (page 477).

Local effects

Local infiltration of or pressure on surrounding structures (Figure 12.3), may result in:

- Visual loss with field defects. This is typically a bitemporal hemianopia caused by pressure on the optic chiasm (page 560).
- Headache produced by tumour involvement of the meninges and bony structures
- Obesity and altered appetite and thirst. This is due to involvement of the hypothalamus. In children, hypothalamic involvement may lead to early puberty (precocious puberty)
- Hydrocephalus caused by interruption of CSF flow
- Cranial nerve lesions by infiltration of the cavernous sinus (see Table 14.1).

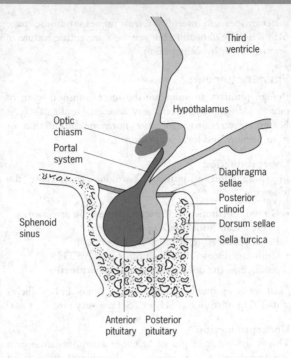

Figure 12.3
A sagittal section of the pituitary fossa, showing the important anatomical relationships.

Hypopituitarism

Deficiency of hypothalamic-releasing hormones or pituitary hormones may be either selective or multiple. Multiple deficiencies usually result from tumour growth or other destructive lesions, and there is usually a progressive loss of function, with LH and FSH being affected first and TSH and ACTH last. Rather than prolactin deficiency, hyperprolactinaemia occurs relatively early because of loss of tonic inhibitory control by dopamine (see Figure 12.1). Panhypopituitarism is a deficiency of all anterior pituitary hormones and is most commonly caused by tumours, surgery or radiotherapy. Vasopressin and oxytocin secretion will only be affected if the hypothalamus is involved by either hypothalamic tumour or by extension of a pituitary lesion.

Aetiology

The causes of hypopituitarism are listed in Table 12.1

Table 12.1 Causes of hypopituitarism

Neoplastic	Primary tumours Secondary deposits Craniopharyngioma	Traumatic	Skull fracture Surgery
Infective	Meningitis Encephalitis Syphilis	Infiltrations	Sarcoidosis Haemochromatosis
Vascular	Pituitary apoplexy Sheehan's syndrome	Others	Radiation damage Chemotherapy 'Empty sella' syndrome
Immunological	Pituitary antibodies	Functional	Anorexia Starvation Emotional deprivation
Congenital	Kallman's syndrome		

Clinical features

These depend on the extent of hypothalamic–pituitary deficiencies. Gonadotrophin deficiency results in loss of libido, amenorrhoea (absent menstruation) and impotence, whereas hyperprolactinaemia results in galactorrhoea and hypogonadism. Growth hormone deficiency is usually silent except in children, although it may impair wellbeing in adults. Secondary hypothyroidism and adrenal failure lead to tiredness, slowness of thought and action, and mild hypotension. Long-standing hypopituitarism may give the classic picture of pallor with hairlessness (alabaster skin). Particular syndromes related to hypopituitarism are:

- *Kallman's syndrome*: isolated gonadotrophin deficiency with anosmia, colour blindness, midline facial deformities and renal abnormalities
- *Sheehan's syndrome*: this situation, now rare, is pituitary infarction following severe postpartum haemorrhage
- *Pituitary apoplexy*: infarction or haemorrhage into a pituitary tumour which may result in life-threatening hypopituitarism. Additional features include severe headaches, visual loss and cranial nerve palsy

• *'Empty sella' syndrome*: the sella turcica appears radiologically devoid of pituitary tissue; the pituitary is actually placed eccentrically and function is usually normal.

Investigation

Each axis of the hypothalamic–pituitary system may require separate investigation. The presence of normal gonadal function (ovulatory menstruation or normal libido/erections) suggests that multiple defects of the anterior pituitary are unlikely. Tests range from measurement of basal hormone levels to stimulatory tests of the pituitary and tests of feedback for the hypothalamus .

Management

Steroid and thyroid hormones are essential for life and are given as oral replacement drugs (e.g. 15–40 mg hydrocortisone daily in divided doses, 100–150 μg thyroxine daily) with the aim of restoring clinical and biochemical normality. Androgens and oestrogens are replaced for symptomatic control. If fertility is desired, LH and FSH analogues may be used. GH therapy should be given to the growing child under appropriate specialist supervision and it may also produce substantial benefits to the GH-deficient adult in terms of work capacity and psychological wellbeing.

Two important warnings are necessary:

• Thyroid replacement should not commence until normal glucocorticoid function has been demonstrated or replacement steroid therapy initiated, as an adrenal 'crisis' may otherwise be precipitated.
• Glucocorticoid deficiency may mask impaired urine concentrating ability. Diabetes insipidus is apparent after steroid replacement, the steroids being necessary for excretion of a water load.

MALE REPRODUCTION AND SEX

Luteinizing hormone-releasing hormone (LHRH, also called gonadotrophin-releasing hormone, GnRH) is synthesized in the hypothalamus. It is released episodically into the pituitary portal circulation (during and after puberty) and stimulates LH and FSH secretion from the anterior pituitary gland. LH and FSH stimulate the production of testosterone and sperm respectively from the testes.

Normal puberty, delayed and precocious puberty.

Disorders of sexual differentiation.

Male hypogonadism

Male hypogonadism is a descriptive term for the clinical features associated with androgen deficiency. The presentation depends on the age of onset of hypogonadism (Table 12.2). In prepubertal onset the patient presents with delayed puberty and eunuchoid body proportions resulting from the continued growth of long bones, which occurs because of delayed fusion of the epiphyses.

Table 12.2 Consequences of androgen deficiency in the male

Prepubertal onset with eunuchoidism
Increased height and arm span
Lack of adult hair distribution
High-pitched voice
Small penis, testes and scrotum
Decreased muscle mass

Hypogonadism beginning after puberty
Decreased prostate size
Diminished rate of growth of beard and body hair
Fine feminine skin
Decreased potency and libido

A large number of diseases can lead to destruction or malfunction of the hypothalamic–pituitary–testicular axis (Table 12.3). Klinefelter's syndrome is the most common cause of male hypogonadism, with an incidence of 1 in 1000 live births. It is the result of the presence of an extra X chromosome (47, XXY). Accelerated atrophy of the germ cells gives rise to sterility and small firm testes. The clinical picture varies: in the most severely affected there is complete failure of sexual maturation, eunuchoid body proportions, gynaecomastia and mental handicap.

Table 12.3 Causes of male hypogonadism

Hypothalamic–pituitary disorder	Hypopituitarism
	Selective gonadotrophic
	  deficiency (Kallman's syndrome)
	Severe systemic illness
	Severe malnourishment
	Hyperprolactinaemia (interferes
	  with pulsatile secretion of LH
	  and FSH)

Primary gonadal disease	
Congenital	Klinefelter's syndrome, anorchia, Leydig cell agenesis, failure of testicular descent
Acquired	Trauma, torsion, chemotherapy, radiation
Target tissues	Androgen receptor deficiency

Investigations

Measurement of basal serum testosterone, LH and FSH will confirm the diagnosis and allow the distinction between primary gonadal (testicular) failure and hypothalamic–pituitary disease. Intesticular failure testosterone levels will be low but LH/FSH levels high, as a result of loss of the negative feedback of testosterone on the hypothalamus–pituitary. Further investigations, e.g. serum prolactin, chromosomal analysis, pituitary MRI scan and pituitary function tests, will depend on the site of the defect.

Management

The cause can rarely be reversed and the mainstay of treatment is androgen replacement. Although hypogonado-trophic patients have the potential for fertility, LH and FSH or pulsatile GnRH are only used (instead of testosterone) when fertility is desired, as these regimens are expensive and complex.

Loss of libido and impotence

Erectile impotence is defined as failure to initiate an erection or to maintain an erection until ejaculation. Erection is the result of increased vascularity of the penis controlled via the sacral parasympathetic outflow; it may be impaired by vascular disease, autonomic neuropathy and nerve damage after pelvic surgery. The nervous pathways for ejaculation are centred on the lumbar sympathetics, and abnormalities may occur with autonomic neuropathy and traumatic nerve damage. Psychological factors, endocrine factors (causes of hypogonadism described above), alcohol and drugs, e.g. cannabis, β-blockers and diuretics, may cause abnormalities at either stage. A careful history and examination will identify the cause in many patients. The presence of nocturnal emissions and morning erections is suggestive of psychogenic impotence.

Apart from cessation of the offending drug, methods of treatment include intracavernosal injections of alprostadil, papaverine or phentolamine, penile implants and vacuum expanders. Recently, sildenafil citrate, a phosphodiesterase inhibitor which increases penile blood flow, has been introduced.

Many cases are the result of psychological factors and the patient may respond to psychosexual counselling.

Gynaecomastia

The development of benign breast tissue in the male is the result of an increase in the oestrogen:androgen ratio (Table 12.4). Gynaecomastia is common in early puberty as a result of relative oestrogen excess, and usually resolves spontaneously. Unexplained gynaecomastia occurs, especially in elderly people, and is a diagnosis of exclusion after thorough examination and investigation. The treatment is either of the underlying cause or by removal of the drug if possible. Occasionally surgery is needed.

Table 12.4 Causes of gynaecomastia

Physiological	Neonatal, resulting from the influence of maternal hormones Pubertal Old age
Deficient testosterone secretion	Any cause of hypogonadism (see Table 12.3)
Oestrogen-producing tumours	Of the testis or adrenal gland
HCG-producing tumours	Of the testis or the lung
Drugs	Oestrogens, digitalis, cannabis, heroin, spironolactone, cyproterone, cimetidine
Other	Hyperthyroidism, liver disease

HCG, human chorionic gonadotrophin.

FEMALE REPRODUCTION AND SEX

In the adult female higher brain centres impose a menstrual cycle of 28 days upon the activity of hypothalamic GnRH. Pulses of GnRH stimulate the release of pituitary LH and FSH. LH stimulates ovarian androgen production and FSH stimulates follicular development and aromatase activity (an enzyme required to convert ovarian androgens to oestrogens). Oestrogens are necessary for normal pubertal development and maintenance of the menstrual cycle; they also have effects on a variety of tissues.

The menopause

The menopause, or cessation of periods, naturally occurs about the age of 45–55 years. During the late 40s, first FSH and then LH concentrations begin to rise, probably as a result of diminishing follicle supply. Oestrogen levels fall and the cycle becomes disrupted. Menopause may also occur surgically, with radiotherapy to the ovaries and with ovarian disease (e.g. premature menopause in the 20s and 30s). Symptoms of the menopause are hot flushes, vaginal dryness and breast atrophy. There may also be vague symptoms of depression, loss of libido and weight gain. There is loss of bone density (osteoporosis, page 239) and the premenopausal protection against ischaemic heart disease disappears. Most of these effects may be reduced by hormone replacement therapy (HRT), which is now given long term to most women with menopausal symptoms; some authorities would recommend giving HRT to all women to protect against osteoporosis and ischaemic heart disease. HRT is always given to women with premature ovarian failure. Oestrogens, when given alone, increase the risk of endometrial cancer and so combination treatment with progestogens is given to women with an intact uterus.

Female hypogonadism and amenorrhoea

Amenorrhoea is the absence of menstruation. It is often physiological, e.g. during pregnancy and lactation, and after the menopause. Primary amenorrhoea is failure to start spontaneous menstruation by the age of 16 years. Secondary amenorrhoea is the absence of menstruation for 3 months in a woman who has previously had menstrual cycles. In the female, hypogonadism almost always presents as amenorrhoea or oligomenorrhoea (irregular periods with long cycles). The other features of oestrogen deficiency include atrophy of the breasts and vagina, loss of pubic hair and osteoporosis.

Aetiology

The causes of amenorrhoea are listed in Table 12.5. Polycystic ovary syndrome is the most common cause of oligomenorrhoea and amenorrhoea in clinical practice, though one should always consider pregnancy as a possible cause. Severe weight loss (e.g. anorexia nervosa) has long been associated with amenorrhoea, but it is now recognized that less severe forms of weight loss, produced by dieting and exercise, are a common cause of amenorrhoea caused by abnormal secretion of GnRH.

Table 12.5 Pathological causes of amenorrhoea

Hypothalamic	*GnRH deficiency (isolated or as part of Kallman's syndrome) Weight loss, physical exercise, stress Post oral contraceptive therapy
Pituitary	Hyperprolactinaemia Hypopituitarism
Gonadal	Polycystic ovary syndrome Premature ovarian failure – autoimmune basis *Defective ovarian development (dysgenesis) Androgen-secreting ovarian tumours Radiotherapy
Other diseases	Thyroid dysfunction, Cushing's syndrome Adrenal tumours, severe illness
Uterine/vaginal abnormality	*Imperforate hymen or absent uterus

* Presents as primary amenorrhoea.

Investigations

The cause of amenorrhoea may be apparent after a full history and examination. Basal levels of serum FSH, LH, oestrogen and prolactin will allow a distinction between primary gonadal and hypothalamic–pituitary causes. Further investigations, e.g. ultrasonography of the ovaries, laparoscopy and ovarian biopsy, pituitary MRI and measurement of serum testosterone, will depend on the probable site of the defect and the findings on clinical examination.

Management

Treatment is of the cause where possible, e.g. increase weight, treat hypothyroidism and hyperprolactinaemia. In patients where the underlying defect cannot be corrected, cyclical oestrogens are given to reverse the symptoms of oestrogen deficiency and prevent early osteoporosis. Patients with isolated GnRH deficiency or hypopituitarism are treated with human FSH/LH. The management of polycystic ovaries is discussed on page 486. The treatment, however is different in those patients who want to become pregnant.

Hirsutism and polycystic ovary syndrome

Hirsutism is an excess growth of hair in a male pattern: beard area, abdominal wall, thigh and around the nipples. There is, however, considerable variation in normal hair growth between individuals, families and races, being more extensive in the Mediterranean and some Asian Indian subcontinent populations.

It has been traditional to divide patients with hirsutism into those with no elevation of serum androgen levels and no other clinical features (usually labelled 'idiopathic hirsutism') and those with an identifiable endocrine imbalance (most commonly polycystic ovary syndrome – PCOS – or rarely other causes). However, in recent years it has become apparent that most patients with 'idiopathic hirsutism' have some radiological or biochemical evidence of PCOS on more detailed investigation, and indeed several studies have demonstrated evidence of mild PCOS in up to 20% of the normal female population. Therefore, in routine clinical practice the majority of patients with objective signs of androgen-dependent hirsutism will have PCOS, and investigation is mainly required to exclude rarer and more serious causes (Table 12.6) of virilization (male secondary sexual characteristics).

PCOS, originally known in its severe form as the Stein–Leventhal syndrome, is characterized by multiple small cysts within the ovary and by excess androgen

Table 12.6 Causes of hirsutism

Familial and racial	
Ovarian	Polycystic ovary syndrome
	Androgen-secreting tumours
Adrenal	Androgen-secreting tumours
	Congenital adrenal hyperplasia
Androgenic drugs	Androgens, phenytoin, minoxidil, cyclosporin
Idiopathic	Target organ hypersensitivity

production from the ovaries and, to a lesser extent, from the adrenals, although whether the basic defect is in the ovary, adrenal or pituitary remains unknown. The ovarian 'cysts' represent arrested follicular development. Recent studies have shown an association of PCOS with anovulation and insulin resistance, which may also be associated with hypertension and hyperlipidaemia. The precise mechanisms that link the aetiology of polycystic ovaries, hyperandrogenism, anovulation and insulin resistance remain to be elucidated, but may prove important in the causation of macrovascular disease in women.

Clinical features

Typically, PCOS presents with amenorrhoea/oligomenorrhoea, hirsutism and acne, usually beginning shortly after menarche. It is sometimes associated with marked obesity, but the weight may be normal. Mild virilization may occur in severe cases. A short history, accompanying virilization, and severe menstrual disturbance are suggestive of significant androgen secretion with a more serious underlying cause, e.g. adrenal tumour.

Investigations

The diagnosis of PCOS is made on a clinical basis supported by ultrasound and biochemical tests.

- Serum testosterone concentrations are increased.
- Serum LH concentrations are increased or normal.
- Serum FSH concentrations are normal.
- Ovarian ultrasound shows a thickened capsule with multiple cysts.

Other investigations in a patient presenting with hirsutism include measurement of serum androgens and CT/MRI of the adrenal glands.

Management

The management is to identify and treat the underlying cause. Excess hair can be removed or disguised by shaving, bleaching and waxing. Other treatments for hirsuitism are the antiandrogen cyproterone acetate, and oestrogens that reduce free androgens by increasing levels of the sex hormone-binding globulin.

For PCOS, patients who require induction of ovulation are treated with the antioestrogen clomiphene. For those not concerned with fertility, menstrual irregularity can be managed with oral contraceptives. Symptoms of hyperandrogenism can be managed by antiandrogens such as cyproterone acetate.

Hyperprolactinaemia

Unlike other pituitary hormones, prolactin release is tonically inhibited by dopamine from the hypothalamus via the pituitary stalk. There is a physiological increase in prolactin during pregnancy and postpartum breastfeeding.

Aetiology

The most important pathological cause of high prolactin levels is a prolactin-secreting pituitary adenoma. Other pituitary or hypothalamic tumours may also cause hyperprolactinaemia by interfering with dopamine inhibition of prolactin release. Other causes include primary hypothyroidism (high TRH levels stimulate prolactin) and drugs metoclopramide and phenothiazines (caused by inhibition of dopamine), oestrogens and cimetidine.

Clinical features

The cardinal feature is galactorrhoea. Other features such as oligo- or amenorrhoea, subfertility and impotence occur as a result of inhibition of GnRH by high levels of prolactin. If there is a pituitary tumour there may be headache and visual field defects.

Investigations

- Serum prolactin level. At least three measurements should be taken. Further tests are appropriate after physiological and drug causes have been excluded.
- Visual fields should be checked (page 560).
- Pituitary function should be checked if a pituitary tumour is suspected.
- Thyroid function tests, as hypothyroidism is a cause of hyperprolactinaemia.
- Magnetic resonance imaging of the pituitary.

Management

Causative drugs should be withdrawn if possible and hypothyroidism treated. In the case of a prolactinoma, the dopamine agonist bromocriptine will reduce plasma prolactin concentrations and produce some shrinkage in tumour size. Definitive therapy is controversial and depends on the size of the tumour, the patient's wish for fertility and the facilities available. Transsphenoidal surgery, combined with postoperative radiotherapy for large tumours, often restores normoprolactinaemia but there is a high late recurrence rate (50% at 5 years). Small tumours (microadenomas) in asymptomatic patients may only need observation.

THE GROWTH AXIS

GH is secreted from the anterior pituitary and its tissue effects are mediated by insulin-like growth factor (IGF-1) synthesized in the liver and other tissues. Deficiency of GH produces short stature in children but in adults it is often clinically silent, although recent evidence suggests that it may result in significant impairment in wellbeing and work capacity. Excessive GH production leads to gigantism in children (if acquired before epiphyseal fusion) and acromegaly in adults.

Acromegaly

Acromegaly is rare and caused by a benign pituitary adenoma in almost all cases. Hyperplasia resulting from an excess of GH-releasing hormone (GHRH) is rare. Males and females are affected equally and the incidence is highest in middle age.

Clinical features

Symptoms and signs are shown in Figure 12.4. One-third of patients present with changes in appearance and 10% with visual field defects or headaches.

Investigations

- Glucose tolerance test is diagnostic. In a positive test there is failure of the normal suppression of serum GH below 1 mU/l in response to a glucose load. Some show a paradoxical rise. Twenty-five per cent of individuals with acromegaly have a diabetic glucose tolerance test.
- Serum GH levels are usually elevated, but levels fluctuate and a normal level does not exclude the diagnosis.

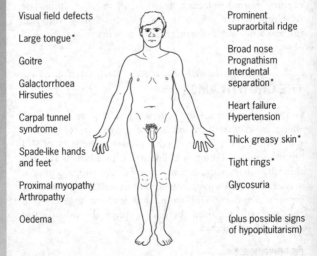

Visual field defects

Large tongue*

Goitre

Galactorrhoea
Hirsuties

Carpal tunnel
syndrome

Spade-like hands
and feet

Proximal myopathy
Arthropathy

Oedema

Prominent
supraorbital ridge

Broad nose
Prognathism
Interdental
separation*

Heart failure
Hypertension

Thick greasy skin*

Tight rings*

Glycosuria

(plus possible signs
of hypopituitarism)

Figure 12.4
The symptoms and signs of acromegaly. *These indicate signs of greater discriminant value.

- IGF-1 levels are almost always raised in acromegaly, and fluctuate less than those of GH.
- MRI scan of the pituitary will almost always reveal the adenoma.
- Visual field defects are common and should be plotted by perimetry.
- Pituitary function testing usually shows evidence of hypopituitarism.
- Hyperprolactinaemia occurs in 30%.

Management

Treatment is indicated in all except elderly people or those with minimal abnormalities, because untreated acromegaly is associated with markedly reduced survival. Most deaths result from heart failure, coronary artery disease and hypertension-related causes. The aim of therapy should be to reduce mean GH level to below 5 mU/l, which has been shown to reduce mortality to normal levels. The preferred treatment is controversial and complete cure, if possible, is often slow. The choice lies between the following:

- Surgery: this is the treatment of choice in suitable cases and may be transsphenoidal, or transfrontal if the tumour is large. Surgery is often combined with radiotherapy because excision is rarely complete with large tumours (macroadenomas, i.e. >1 cm in diameter).
- External beam radiotherapy is normally used after pituitary surgery fails to normalize GH levels, rather than as primary therapy. It may take 1–10 years to be effective when used alone.
- Drugs: subcutaneous octreotide, a somatostatin analogue, or lanreotide, a longer-acting preparation, are now the treatments of choice in resistant cases. They are given to shrink tumours before definitive treatment or to control symptoms. Bromocriptine is usually reserved for elderly and frail people.

THE THYROID AXIS

The thyroid gland secretes predominantly thyroxine (T_4) and only a small amount of the biologically active hormone triiodothyronine (T_3). These hormones control the metabolic rate of many tissues. Most circulating T_3 is produced by peripheral conversion of T_4. Over 99% of T_4 and T_3 circulate bound to plasma proteins, mainly thyroxine-binding globulin (TBG). The feedback pathway that controls the secretion of TSH is discussed on pages 473–474. Measurement of plasma TSH is the first-line investigation in patients with suspected thyroid gland dysfunction.

Hypothyroidism

Underactivity of the thyroid gland may be primary, from disease of the thyroid gland, or, much less commonly, secondary to hypothalamic–pituitary disease.

Aetiology

Atrophic (autoimmune) hypothyroidism This is the most common cause of hypothyroidism and is associated with microsomal antibodies and lymphoid infiltration of the gland, with eventual fibrosis and atrophy. It is six times more common in females and the incidence increases with age. It is associated with other autoimmune conditions, such as pernicious anaemia.

Hashimoto's thyroiditis This autoimmune thyroiditis, also associated with thyroid microsomal antibodies, produces atrophic changes with regeneration leading to goitre formation. It is more common in females and in late middle age. Patients may be hypothyroid, euthyroid, or go through an initial toxic phase.

Iatrogenic Forty per cent are hypothyroid by 25 years following radioactive iodine or surgery for hyperthyroidism.

Iodine deficiency This still exists in some areas, particularly mountainous areas (Alps, Himalayas, South America). Goitre, occasionally massive, is common. The patient may be euthyroid or hypothyroid, depending on the severity of the iodine deficiency.

Dyshormonogenesis This rare condition is caused by genetic defects in the synthesis of thyroid hormones.

Clinical features

Symptoms and signs of hypothyroidism are illustrated in Figure 12.5. Features are often difficult to distinguish in elderly people and young women. Hypothyroidism should

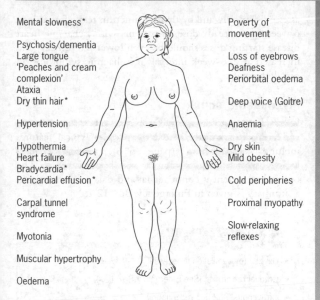

Mental slowness*

Psychosis/dementia
Large tongue
'Peaches and cream
complexion'
Ataxia
Dry thin hair*

Hypertension

Hypothermia
Heart failure
Bradycardia*
Pericardial effusion*

Carpal tunnel
syndrome

Myotonia

Muscular hypertrophy

Oedema

Poverty of
movement

Loss of eyebrows
Deafness
Periorbital oedema

Deep voice (Goitre)

Anaemia

Dry skin
Mild obesity

Cold peripheries

Proximal myopathy

Slow-relaxing
reflexes

Figure 12.5
The symptoms and signs of hypothyroidism. *These indicates signs of
greater discriminant value.

be excluded in all patients with oligomenorrhoea/amenor-
rhoea, menorrhagia, infertility and hyperprolactinaemia.

Investigations

Measurement of serum TSH is the investigation of choice.
A high TSH confirms primary hypothyroidism.

- Serum free T_4 levels are low.
- Thyroid antibodies and other organ-specific antibodies
  may be present in the serum.
- Other features include anaemia (normocytic or
  macrocytic), hypercholesterolaemia and hyponatraemia
  (increased antidiuretic hormone and impaired clearance
  of free water).

Management

Replacement therapy with thyroxine (100–200 μg/day) is
required for life. The starting dose is 100 μg/day (50 μg/day
in elderly people) and the adequacy of replacement is

assessed clinically and by thyroid function tests after at least 6 weeks on a steady dose. In patients with ischaemic heart disease starting doses should be even lower (25 μg/day) and increased at 2–6-week intervals if ischaemic symptoms do not deteriorate.

Myxoedema coma

Severe hypothyroidism may rarely present with confusion and coma, particularly in elderly people. Typical features include hypothermia (page 516), cardiac failure, hypoventilation, hypoglycaemia and hyponatraemia. The optimal treatment is controversial and data are lacking, but a summary is given in Emergency Box 12.1.

 Emergency

- Oxygen (by ventilation if necessary)

- Gradual rewarming (See Emergency Box 12.4)

- Intravenous T$_3$ 2.5–5 μg 8 hourly

- Intravenous hydrocortisone 100 mg 8 hourly (in case hypothyroidism is a manifestation of hypopituitarism)

- Intravenous dextrose to prevent hypoglycaemia

Emergency Box 12.1
Management of myxoedema coma

Myxoedema madness

Depression is common but occasionally, with severe hypothyroidism in elderly people, the patient may become frankly demented or psychotic, sometimes with striking delusions. This may occur shortly after starting thyroxine replacement.

Hyperthyroidism

Hyperthyroidism (thyroid overactivity, thyrotoxicosis) is common, affecting 2–5% of all women at some time, mainly between the ages of 20 and 40 years. Three intrinsic thyroid disorders account for the vast majority of cases of hyperthyroidism: Graves' disease, toxic adenoma and toxic multinodular goitre. Rarer causes include de Quervain's thyroiditis, thyroiditis factitia (surreptitious T_4 consumption), drugs (amiodarone), metastatic differentiated thyroid carcinoma and TSH-secreting tumours (e.g. of the pituitary).

Graves' disease Graves' disease is the most common cause of hyperthyroidism and is the result of IgG antibodies binding to the TSH receptor and stimulating thyroid hormone production. It is associated with typical eye changes (see below), vitiligo, pretibial myxoedema and, rarely, lymphadenopathy and splenomegaly. It is also associated with other autoimmune diseases, such as pernicious anaemia and myasthenia gravis.

Toxic multinodular goitre Many patients with toxic multinodular goitre have been euthyroid for several years before the development of nodular autonomy. Toxic multinodular goitre commonly occurs in older women, and drug therapy is rarely successful in inducing a prolonged remission.

Solitary toxic nodule (Plummer's disease) This is responsible for about 5% of cases. Prolonged remission is again rarely induced by drug therapy.

de Quervain's thyroiditis Transient hyperthyroidism sometimes results from acute inflammation of the gland, probably as a result of viral infection. It is usually accompanied by fever, malaise and pain in the neck. Treatment is with aspirin, reserving prednisolone for severely symptomatic cases.

Clinical features

Typical symptoms and signs of hyperthyroidism are shown in Figure 12.6.

Clinical features vary with age and the underlying aetiology. Eye signs (see below), pretibial myxoedema (raised, purple-red symmetrical skin lesions over anterolateral aspects of the shins) and thyroid acropachy (clubbing, swollen fingers and periosteal new bone formation) occur only in Graves' disease. Elderly patients may present with atrial fibrillation and/or heart failure, or with a clinical picture resembling hypothyroidism ('apathetic thyrotoxicosis').

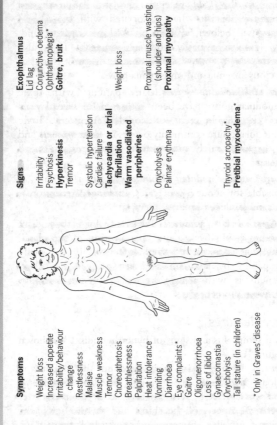

Symptoms

Weight loss
Increased appetite
Irritability/behaviour
 change
Restlessness
Malaise
Muscle weakness
Tremor
Choreoathetosis
Breathlessness
Palpitation
Heat intolerance
Vomiting
Diarrhoea
Eye complaints*
Goitre
Oligomenorrhoea
Loss of libido
Gynaecomastia
Onycholysis
Tall stature (in children)

*Only in Graves' disease

Signs

Irritability
Psychosis
Hyperkinesis
Tremor

Systolic hypertension
Cardiac failure
**Tachycardia or atrial
 fibrillation**
**Warm vasodilated
 peripheries**

Onycholysis
Palmar erythema

Thyroid acropachy*
Pretibial myxoedema*

Exophthalmus
Lid lag
Conjunctive oedema
Ophthalmoplegia*
Goitre, bruit

Weight loss

Proximal muscle wasting
 (shoulder and hips)
Proximal myopathy

Figure 12.6
The symptoms and signs of hyperthyroidism. The bold type indicates signs of greater discriminatory value.

494

Investigations

- Serum TSH is suppressed.
- Serum T_4 and T_3 are elevated. Occasionally T_3 alone is elevated (T_3 toxicosis).
- Serum microsomal and thyroglobulin antibodies are present in most cases of Graves' disease. TSH receptor antibodies are not measured routinely.
- Thyroid ultrasound will help differentiate Grave's disease from adenoma.

Management

- Antithyroid drugs: carbimazole (10–20 mg 8 hourly) blocks thyroid hormone biosynthesis and also has immunosuppressive effects which will affect the Grave's disease process. As clinical benefit may not be apparent for 10–20 days, β-blockers may be used to provide rapid symptomatic control because many manifestations are mediated via the sympathetic system. Carbimazole is then reduced according to clinical state over the next 12–18 months. Some physicians prefer the 'block and replace regimen', where by full doses of carbimazole 30–45 mg/day are given for 18 months to suppress the thyroid completely, while replacing thyroid activity with thyroxine. Claimed advantages are avoidance of under- or over-treatment and better use of the immunosuppressive action. Fifty per cent of patients with Graves' disease will relapse on discontinuation of drug treatment, mostly within the following 2 years.

  The most severe side effect of carbimazole is agranulocytosis. All patients starting treatment must be warned to stop and seek an urgent blood count if they develop a sore throat or unexplained fever.
- Radioactive iodine: ^{131}I accumulates in the gland and destroys it by local irradiation. The indications for radioactive iodine are similar to those for surgery, and include recurrence after drug treatment, poor compliance, or side effects with drugs. It is more commonly used in older patients. It is effective in 75% of patients in 4–12 weeks. If hyperthyroidism persists a further dose of ^{131}I can be given, although this increases the rate of subsequent hypothyroidism

- Surgery: subtotal thyroidectomy should only be performed in patients who have been rendered euthyroid. Antithyroid drugs are stopped 10–14 days before the operation and replaced with oral potassium iodide, which inhibits thyroid hormone release and reduces the vascularity of the gland. Indications for surgery include those for ^{131}I and large goitres. Complications of surgery include transient hypocalcaemia, hypothyroidism, hypoparathyroidism, recurrent laryngeal nerve palsy and recurrent hyperthyroidism

Thyroid crisis

Thyroid crisis or storm is a rare life-threatening condition in which there is a rapid deterioration of thyrotoxicosis with hyperpyrexia, tachycardia, extreme restlessness and eventually delirium, coma and death. It is most commonly precipitated by infection, stress, and surgery or radioactive iodine therapy in an unprepared patient. Management (Emergency Box 12.2) includes the administration of large doses of carbimazole and propranolol, iodine to block acutely the release of thyroid hormone from the gland, and dexamethasone which inhibits peripheral conversion of T_4 to T_3.

! Emergency

- Take blood for full blood count, glucose, serum urea and eletrolytes, and serum thyroxine

- Propranolol 5 mg i.v. four times daily or 80 mg orally twice daily

- Carbimazole 20 mg orally three times daily

- Potassium iodide orally 15 mg four times daily

- Dexamethasone 2 mg i.v. four times daily

- Supportive treatment, including oxygen, i.v. fluids and management of hyperpyrexia

- Search for and treat precipitating cause

Emergency Box 12.2
Management of thyroid crisis

Thyroid eye disease

Lid retraction (white of sclera visible above the cornea as the patient looks forwards) and lid lag are a result of increased catecholamine sensitivity of the levator palpebrae superioris and may occur in any form of hyperthyroidism. Exophthalmos (protruding eyeballs) and ophthalmoplegia (limitation of eye movements) only occur in patients with Graves' disease (ophthalmic Graves' disease).

Aetiology

It is currently believed that the exophthalmos of Graves' disease, which may be unilateral or bilateral, is the result of specific antibodies causing retro-orbital inflammation, with swelling and oedema of the extraocular muscles leading to limitation of movement. TSH antibodies are found in the serum although their role in pathogenesis is not clear.

Clinical features

The clinical appearances are characteristic. Exophthalmos and ophthalmoplegia are direct effects of the inflammation, whereas conjunctival oedema (chemosis), lid lag and corneal scarring are secondary to the proptosis and lack of eye cover. Eye manifestations do not parallel the clinical course of Graves' disease and may appear before the onset of hyperthyroidism. CT and MRI of the orbits will exclude other causes of proptosis, e.g. retro-orbital tumour, and show enlarged muscles and oedema.

Management

Thyroid status should be normalized and hypothyroidism avoided because this may exacerbate the eye problem. Smoking increases the severity of ophthalmopathy and patients should be advised to stop. Specific treatment includes methylcellulose eye drops or, if more severe, high-dose systemic steroids to reduce inflammation. Lateral tarsorraphy will protect the cornea if the lids cannot be closed. Occasionally irradiation of the orbits or surgical decompression of the orbit(s) is required.

Goitre (thyroid enlargement)

Goitre is more common in women than in men and may be physiological or pathological in origin (Table 12.7). The

Table 12.7 Causes of goitre

Physiological: puberty, pregnancy
Multinodular goitre
Autoimmune: Graves' disease, Hashimoto's disease
Thyroiditis: acute (de Quervain's thyroiditis), chronic fibrotic (Riedel's thyroiditis)
Iodine deficiency (endemic goitre)
Dyshormonogenesis
Diffuse goitre
Benign cysts, lymphoma, carcinoma

presence of a goitre gives no indication about the thyroid status of the patient.

Clinical features

It is usually noticed as a cosmetic defect, although discomfort and pain in the neck can occur, and occasionally oesophageal or tracheal compression produces dysphagia or difficulty in breathing. The gland may be diffusely enlarged, multinodular or possess a solitary nodule. A bruit may be present and occasionally there is lymphadenopathy.

Investigations

- Thyroid function tests: TSH plus T_4 or T_3.
- Radiography of the chest and thoracic inlet where appropriate to detect tracheal compression.
- Fine needle aspiration for cytology should be performed for solitary nodules or a dominant nodule in a multinodular goitre because there is a 5% chance of malignancy.
- Other tests are not usually required. Thyroid ultrasonography can delineate nodules and demonstrate whether they are solid or cystic. Thyroid scan (^{125}I or ^{131}I) distinguishes between a functioning ('hot') or non-functioning ('cold') nodule. Hot nodules are rarely malignant, whereas cold nodules are malignant in up to 10% of cases.

Management

Treatment is usually not required, apart from inducing euthyroidism if necessary. Surgical intervention may be required for cosmetic reasons, pressure effects, or if there is a possibility of malignancy.

Thyroid carcinoma

Thyroid cancer is relatively uncommon, being responsible for 400 deaths annually in the UK. Characteristics are listed in Table 12.8. Most differentiated thyroid cancers present as asymptomatic thyroid nodules, but the first sign of disease is occasionally lymph-node metastases or, in rare cases, lung or bone metastases. Features that suggest carcinoma in a patient presenting with a thyroid nodule are a history of progressive increase in size, a hard and irregular nodule, and the presence of enlarged lymph nodes on examination. Fine-needle aspiration cytology is the best test for distinguishing between benign and malignant thyroid nodules. Treatment of follicular and papillary cancers is surgical, with total thyroidectomy. Ablative radioactive iodine is subsequently given which will be taken up by remaining thyroid tissue or metastatic lesions. Treatment of anaplastic carcinoma is largely palliative.

The glucocorticoid axis

The adrenal gland consists of an outer cortex producing steroids (cortisol, aldosterone and androgens) and an inner medulla secreting catecholamines. Aldosterone secretion is under the control of the renin–angiotensin system (see later). Corticotrophin-releasing factor (CRF) from the hypothalamus stimulates ACTH (from the anterior pituitary), which stimulates cortisol production by the adrenal cortex. The cortisol secreted feeds back on the hypothalamus and pituitary to inhibit further CRF/ACTH release. CRF release, and hence cortisol release, is in response to a circadian rhythm, stress and other factors. Random 'one-off' cortisol measurements may therefore be misleading in the diagnosis of hypoadrenalism or Cushing's syndrome. Cortisol has many effects, particularly on carbohydrate metabolism. It leads to increased protein catabolism, increased deposition of fat and glycogen, sodium retention, increased renal potassium loss and a diminished host response to infection.

Addison's disease – primary hypoadrenalism

This is an uncommon condition in which there is destruction of the entire adrenal cortex.

Table 12.8 Characteristics of thyroid cancer

Cell type	Frequency (%)	Behaviour	Spread	Prognosis
Papillary	70	Young people, slow growing	Local	Good
Follicular	20	More common in females	Lung/bone	Good if resected
Anaplastic	<5	Aggressive	Local	Very poor
Lymphoma	2	Variable		Variable*
Medullary cell	5	Often familial and part of MEN syndrome	Local/metastases	Poor

* Sometimes responsive to radiotherapy.

Aetiology

More than 90% of cases result from destruction of the adrenal cortex by organ-specific autoantibodies. This is associated with other autoimmune conditions, e.g. Hashimoto's thyroiditis, Graves' disease, pernicious anaemia and insulin-dependent diabetes mellitus. Rarer causes are adrenal gland tuberculosis, surgical removal, haemorrhage (in meningococcal septicaemia), malignant infiltration and secondary adrenocortical failure as a result of pituitary disease (page 476).

Clinical features

Adrenal insufficiency has an insidious presentation with lethargy, depression, anorexia and weight loss. It may also present as an emergency (Addisonian crisis), with vomiting, abdominal pain, profound weakness and hypovolaemic shock. The important signs are hypotension (which may only be postural) caused by salt and water loss, and hyperpigmentation (buccal mucosa, pressure points, skin creases and recent scars) resulting from stimulation of melanocytes by excess ACTH. There may be vitiligo and loss of body hair in women because of the dependence on adrenal androgens.

Investigations

- Serum urea and electrolytes may be normal but classically there is hyponatraemia, hyperkalaemia, a raised urea and hypoglycaemia.
- Blood count shows a neutrophil leucocytosis and eosinophilia.
- Adrenal antibodies are detected in most cases of autoimmune adrenalitis.
- Radiographs of the chest and abdomen may show evidence of TB, with calcified adrenals.
- The diagnosis is usually made using the short tetracosactrin (Synacthen or synthetic ACTH) test (Table 12.9). Acutely ill patients with Addisonian crisis need immediate treatment before full investigation (Emergency Box 12.3).

Management

This is with lifelong steroid replacement taken as tablets.

Table 12.9 Tetracosactrin (Synacthen) tests

Short test
1. Take blood for measurement of plasma cortisol
2. Administer tetracosactrin 250 µg i.m.
3. Take blood for measurement of cortisol at 30 and 60 minutes
4. Interpretation: adrenal failure is excluded if the basal plasma cortisol exceeds 170 nmol/l and rises by at least 330 nmol/l to 690 nmol/l. An inadequate rise in plasma cortisol is due either to primary adrenal failure or to secondary adrenocortical failure. A long test is then performed to differentiate between these.

Long test
1. Take blood for measurement of plasma cortisol
2. Administer tetracosactrin 1 mg i.m.
3. Take blood for cortisol at 1, 4, 8 and 24 hours
4. Interpretation: patients with normal adrenal glands reach a plasma cortisol concentration of over 1000 nmol/l by 4 hours. In patients with Addison's disease the cortisol response is impaired throughout, and in secondary adrenal insufficiency a delayed but normal response is seen.

Emergency

Take blood for plasma cortisol (will be inappropriately low) and ACTH (will be high because of loss of negative feedback) *before administration of hydrocortisone*. Take blood for full blood count, urea and electrolytes, glucose and blood cultures.

Immediate treatment
• Hydrocortisone 100 mg intravenously
• 1 litre of 0.9% saline over 30–60 minutes
• 50 ml of 50% dextrose if hypoglycaemic

Subsequent treatment
• Hydrocortisone 100 mg intramuscular 6 hourly until BP stable and vomiting ceased
• 0.9% saline 2–4 litres intravenously in 12–24 hours; monitor by JVP or CVP
• Expect recovery, with normal BP, blood glucose and serum sodium, within 12–24 hours
• When stable, convert to maintenance treatment (see below) continued lifelong
• Search for and treat precipitating cause, e.g. infection

Emergency Box 12.3
Management of Addisonian crisis

- Hydrocortisone. The usual dose is 20 mg on waking and 10 mg in the evening, which mimics the normal diurnal rhythm. The dose is best monitored by measuring a series of cortisol levels throughout the day.
- Fluorocortisone, a synthetic mineralocorticoid, 0.05–0.4 mg daily. The dose is adequate when there is no postural drop in blood pressure and plasma renin levels are suppressed to within the normal range.

In a normal individual stress of any type, e.g. infection, trauma and surgery, causes an immediate and marked increase in ACTH and hence in cortisol. This is a necessary response and therefore it is very important in patients on steroid replacement that the dose is increased when they are placed in any of these situations. The usual dose is 100 mg hydrocortisone intramuscularly for minor surgery and, for major surgery, 100 mg hydrocortisone 6 hourly until oral medication is resumed. Patients who are being treated with steroids for a variety of inflammatory conditions, e.g. inflammatory bowel disease, asthma or rheumatological conditions, are also at risk of adrenal suppression perioperatively. Therefore, a similar regimen is given to patients who are currently being treated with steroids, or who have been treated in the previous 12 months. All patients on steroids must carry a 'steroid card' and a MedicAlert bracelet must be worn in case of accidents.

Secondary hypoadrenalism

This may arise from hypothalamic–pituitary disease or from long-term steroid therapy leading to hypothalamic–pituitary–adrenal suppression. The clinical features are the same as those of Addison's disease but there is no pigmentation because ACTH levels are low and, in pituitary disease, there are usually features of failure of other pituitary hormones. A long tetracosactrin (Synacthen) test (see Table 12.9) will differentiate between primary and secondary adrenal failure. Treatment is with hydrocortisone; fludrocortisone is unnecessary. If adrenal failure is secondary to long-term steroid therapy, the adrenals will recover if steroids are withdrawn very slowly.

Cushing's syndrome

Cushing's syndrome is caused by persistently and inappropriately elevated glucocorticoid levels. Most cases result from administration of steroids for the treatment of medical conditions, e.g. asthma. Spontaneous Cushing's syndrome is rare (Table 12.10). Cushing's disease must be distinguished from Cushing's syndrome. The latter is a general term which refers to the abnormalities resulting from a chronic excess of glucocorticoids whatever the cause, whereas Cushing's disease specifically refers to excess glucocorticoids resulting from inappropriate ACTH secretion from the pituitary (usually a microadenoma, less often corticotroph hyperplasia). Alcohol excess mimics Cushing's syndrome clinically and biochemically (pseudo-Cushing's syndrome). The pathogenesis is incompletely understood but the features resolve when alcohol is stopped.

Table 12.10 Aetiology of spontaneous Cushing's syndrome

	% of cases
ACTH-dependent causes	
Pituitary disease (Cushing's disease)	60–70
Ectopic ACTH-producing tumours (small cell lung cancer, carcinoid tumours)	15
Non-ACTH-dependent causes	
Adrenal adenomas	9
Adrenal carcinomas	7
Rare causes, e.g. adrenal hyperplasia	

Clinical features

Patients are obese: fat distribution is typically central, affecting the trunk, abdomen and neck (buffalo hump). They have a plethoric complexion with a moon face. Many of the features are the result of the protein-catabolic effects of cortisol: the skin is thin and bruises easily, and there are purple striae on the abdomen, breasts and thighs (Figure 12.7). Pigmentation occurs with ACTH-dependent cases. Patients with ectopic production of ACTH tend to have rapidly progressive symptoms and signs, and may have evidence of the primary tumour.

Symptoms

Weight gain (central)
Change of appearance
Depression
Psychosis
Insomnia
Amenorrhoea/
  oligomenorrhoea
Poor libido
Thin skin/easy bruising
Hair growth/acne
Muscular weakness
Growth arrest in children
Back pain
Polyuria/polydipsia

Old photographs may
  be useful
Symptoms of
  hypopituitarism are rare

Signs

Depression/psychosis
Acne, hirsuties
Thin skin
Bruising
Hypertension
Rib fractures
Osteoporosis

Pathological fractures

Poor wound healing

Proximal muscle wasting
Proximal myopathy

Oedema

Frontal balding (female)

Moon face
Plethora
'Buffalo-hump'
Kyphosis

Centripetal obesity
Pigmentation

Striae (purple)

Skin infections

Glycosuria

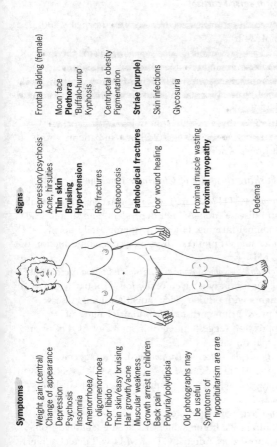

Figure 12.7
The symptoms and signs of Cushing's syndrome. The bold type indicates signs of greater discriminatory value.

Investigations

In a patient with suspected Cushing's syndrome the purpose of investigation is (1) to confirm the presence of cortisol excess, and then (2) to determine the cause.

Confirm raised cortisol

- Raised 24-hour urinary free cortisol (normal <700 nmol/24 h).
- The *low-dose dexamethasone suppression test* is the most reliable screening test. Dexamethasone (a potent synthetic glucocorticoid) 0.5 mg 6 hourly is given orally for 48 hours. Normal individuals suppress serum cortisol by 48 hours.
- Circadian rhythm studies show loss of the normal circadian fall of cortisol at 24 hours in patients with Cushing's syndrome.

Establishing the cause of Cushing's syndrome

- *Plasma ACTH levels* are low or undetectable in adrenal gland disease (non-ACTH dependent) and should lead to adrenal imaging. High or inappropriately normal values suggest pituitary disease or ectopic production of ACTH.
- *High-dose dexamethasone suppression test*: dexamethasone 2.0 mg 6 hourly is given orally for 48 hours. Most patients with pituitary-dependent Cushing's disease suppress serum cortisol by 48 hours. Failure of suppression suggests an ectopic source of ACTH or an adrenal tumour.
- *Corticotrophin-releasing hormone test*. An exaggerated plasma ACTH response to exogenous CRF (bolus given intravenously) suggests pituitary-dependent Cushing's disease.
- *Other tests* will depend on the probable cause of Cushing's syndrome, which has been established from the above tests. Adrenal CT or MRI will detect adrenal adenomas and carcinomas. Pituitary MRI and CT will detect some, but not all, pituitary adenomas. Chest radiography, bronchoscopy and CT of the body may localize ectopic ACTH-producing tumours. Selective venous sampling for ACTH will localize pituitary

tumours and an otherwise occult ectopic ACTH–producing tumour.
- *Radiolabelled octreotide* (^{111}In octreotide) shows promise in locating ectopic ACTH sites.

Management

- Surgical removal is indicated for most pituitary (usually a transsphenoidal approach) and adrenal tumours and may be appropriate for many cases of ectopic ACTH-producing tumours.
- Drugs which inhibit cortisol synthesis (metyrapone, ketoconazole or aminoglutethimide) may be useful in cases not amenable to surgery.
- External-beam irradiation of the pituitary produces a very slow response and is restricted to cases where surgery is unsuccessful, contraindicated or unacceptable to the patient.

Iatrogenic Cushing's syndrome responds to a reduction in steroid dosage when possible. Immunosuppressant drugs such as azathioprine may be used in conjunction with steroids to enable lower doses to be used to control the underlying disease.

Incidental adrenal tumours

With the advent of improved abdominal imaging, unsuspected adrenal masses have been discovered in about 1% of scans. These include primary tumours, metastases and cysts. If found, functional tests to exclude secretory activity should be performed; if none is found then most authorities recommend surgical removal of large (>4–5 cm) and functional tumours but observation of smaller hormonally inactive lesions.

THE THIRST AXIS

The secretion of antidiuretic hormone (ADH, vasopressin) from the posterior pituitary gland is determined principally by the plasma osmolality. ADH secretion is suppressed at levels below 280 mmol/kg, thus allowing maximal water diuresis. Secretion increases to a maximum at a plasma osmolality of 295 mmol/kg. Large falls in blood pressure or volume also stimulate vasopressin secretion. The major hormonal action is on the collecting tubule of the kidney to cause water reabsorption. At high concentrations vasopressin also causes vasoconstriction.

Syndrome of inappropriate ADH secretion (SIADH)

There is continued ADH secretion in spite of plasma hypotonicity and a normal or expanded plasma volume.

Aetiology

SIADH is caused by ectopic production of ADH, e.g. small cell lung cancer or disordered hypothalamic–pituitary secretion (Table 12.11).

Table 12.11 Causes of SIADH

Cancer	Many tumours, of which the most common is small cell cancer of the lung
Brain	Meningitis, cerebral abscess, head injury, tumour
Lung	Pneumonia, tuberculosis, lung abscess
Metabolic	Porphyria, alcohol withdrawal
Drugs	Opiates, chlorpropramide, carbamazepine, vincristine

Clinical features

There is nausea, irritability and headache with mild hyponatraemia (115–125 mmol/l). Fits and coma may occur with severe hyponatraemia (<115 mmol/l).

Investigations

SIADH must be differentiated from other causes of dilutional hyponatraemia (page 259). The criteria for diagnosis are:

- Low serum sodium (<125 mmol/l)
- Low plasma osmolality
- Urine osmolality 'inappropriately' higher than plasma osmolality
- Continued urinary sodium excretion (>30 mmol/l)
- Absence of hypotension and hypovolaemia
- Normal renal, adrenal and thyroid function.

Management

Mild asymptomatic cases need no treatment other than that of the underlying cause. For symptomatic cases the options are:

- Water restriction: 500–1000 ml in 24 hours
- Dimethylchlorotetracycline inhibits the action of vasopressin on the kidney and may be useful if water restriction is poorly tolerated or ineffective
- Hypertonic saline (300 mmol/l i.v. slowly), with frusemide to prevent circulatory overload, may be necessary in severe cases.

Diabetes insipidus

Impaired vasopressin secretion (cranial diabetes insipidus, CDI) or renal resistance to its action (nephrogenic diabetes insipidus, NDI) leads to polyuria (dilute urine in excess of 3 l/day), nocturia and compensatory polydipsia. It must be distinguished from other primary polydipsia, which is a psychiatric disturbance characterized by excessive intake of water, and other causes of polyuria and polydipsia, e.g. hyperglycaemia.

Aetiology

The causes are listed in Table 12.12.

Clinical features

There is polyuria (as much as 15 litres urine a day) and polydipsia. Patients depend on a normal thirst mechanism and access to water to maintain normonatraemia.

Investigations

- Urine volume must be measured to confirm polyuria.
- Plasma biochemistry shows high or high–normal sodium concentration and osmolality. Blood glucose, serum potassium and calcium should be measured to exclude common causes of polyuria.
- Urine osmolality is inappropriately low for the high plasma osmolality.
- A water deprivation test with exogenous desmopressin (a synthetic vasopressin analogue) is the usual investigation for polyuric patients with normal blood

Table 12.12 Causes of diabetes insipidus

Cranial diabetes insipidus	Nephrogenic diabetes insipidus
Familial	Familial
Idiopathic*	Renal tubular acidosis
Head injury*	Metabolic
	Hypercalcaemia
Surgery: transfrontal, transsphenoidal*	Hypokalaemia*
	Prolonged polyuria of any
Hypothalamic – pituitary tumours	cause
Granulomas: Sarcodosis, histiocytosis	Drugs*
	Lithium chloride
Infections: meningitis, encephalitis	Dimethylchlorotetracycline
	Glibenclamide
Vascular: hamorrhage, thrombosis	

* Indicate the most common causes. Diabetes insipidus after surgery may only be transient.

glucose and serum electrolytes. It confirms the diagnosis of DI and will usually distinguish between CDI, NDI and primary polydipsia (Table 12.13). Water is restricted for 8 hours, during which time blood and urine osmolality are measured hourly. Patients are weighed hourly and the test stopped if body weight drops by 5%, as this indicates significant dehydration. In equivocal cases the measurement of plasma vasopressin during water deprivation provides a definitive diagnosis, but this test is not routinely available.

Table 12.13 Response to fluid deprivation and desmopressin in polyuric patients

Urine osmolality (mmol/kg)		Diagnosis
After 8 h fluid deprivation	After desmopressin	
< 300	> 800	CDI
< 300	< 300	NDI
> 800	> 800	Primary polydipsia

- MRI of the pituitary and hypothalamus is performed in cases of CDI.

Management

Treatment of the underlying condition seldom improves established CDI. In mild cases (3–4 litres urine per day) no specific treatment is necessary. Desmopressin, administered orally, nasally or intramuscularly, is useful for more severe cases. Treatment of the cause will usually improve NDI.

ENDOCRINOLOGY OF BLOOD PRESSURE CONTROL

Blood pressure is determined by cardiac output and peripheral resistance and thus an increase in blood pressure may be due to an increase in one or both of these. In approximately 90% of cases no cause can be found (page 385) and patients are said to have essential hypertension. In the remaining minority an underlying cause can be identified, and these include endocrine causes (Table 12.14). Young patients (<35 years), those with abnormal baseline screening test (page 386) or patients with hypertension resistant to treatment should be screened for secondary causes.

Table 12.14 Endocrine causes of hypertension

Excessive production of	
Renin	Renal artery stenosis Renin-secreting tumours
Aldosterone	Adrenal adenoma Adrenal hyperplasia
Mineralocorticoids	Cushing's syndrome (cortisol is a weak mineralocorticoid)
Catecholamines	Phaeochromocytoma
Growth hormone	Acromegaly
Oral contraceptive pill (mechanism unclear)	

The renin–angiotensin system

The renin–angiotensin–aldosterone system is illustrated in Figure 12.8. *Angiotensin*, an α_2-globulin of hepatic origin, circulates in plasma. The enzyme *renin*, is secreted by the kidney in response to decreased renal perfusion pressure or flow; it cleaves the decapeptide *angiotensin I* from angiotensinogen. Angiotensin I is inactive but is further cleaved by converting enzyme (present in lung and vascular endothelium) in to the active peptide, *angiotensin II*, which has two major actions:

- It causes powerful vasoconstriction (within seconds).
- It stimulates the adrenal zona glomerulosa to increase aldosterone production

Aldosterone causes sodium retention and urinary potassium loss (hours to days). This combination of changes leads to an increase in blood pressure and the stimulus to renin production is reduced. Sodium deprivation or urinary loss also increases renin production, whereas dietary sodium excess will suppress production.

Primary hyperaldosteronism

This is a rare condition (<1% of all hypertension) where high aldosterone levels exist independent of the renin–angiotensin system. It is caused by an adrenal adenoma secreting aldosterone (Conn's syndrome, 60% of cases) or by bilateral adrenal hyperplasia.

Clinical features

The major function of aldosterone is to cause an exchange transport of sodium and potassium in the distal renal tubule, that is, absorption of sodium (and hence water) and excretion of potassium. Therefore, hyperaldosteronism causes hypertension, resulting from expansion of intravascular volume, and hypokalaemia, which is rarely low enough to produce symptoms.

Investigations

- Urea and electrolytes show a low serum potassium and normal or high sodium.

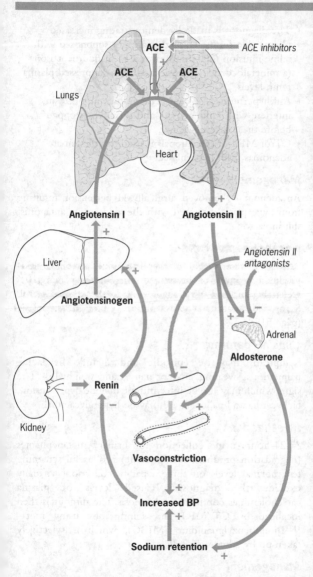

Figure 12.8
The renin–aldosterone system. ACE, angiotensin converting enzyme. Angiotensin II antagonists act on the adrenals and blood vessels.

- The diagnosis is made by demonstrating increased plasma aldosterone levels that are not suppressed with saline infusion (300 mmol over 4 h) or fludrocortisone (a mineralocorticoid), associated with suppressed plasma renin levels.
- Antihypertensives, except bethanidine and prazosin, interfere with renin activity and should be stopped before these investigations.
- CT or MRI of the adrenals is used to differentiate adenomas from hyperplasia.

Management

An adenoma is removed surgically. Hypertension resulting from hyperplasia is treated with the aldosterone antagonist spironolactone.

Phaeochromocytoma

This is a rare (0.1% of hypertension) catecholamine-producing tumour of the sympathetic nervous system; 10% are malignant and 10% occur outside the adrenal gland. Some are associated with multiple endocrine neoplasia (page 515).

Clinical features

Symptoms may be episodic and include headache, palpitations, sweating, anxiety, nausea and weight loss. The signs, which may also be intermittent, include hypertension, tachycardia and pallor. There may be hyperglycaemia.

Investigations

A 24-hours urine collection for urinary metanephrines (degradation products of adrenaline) is a useful screening test; normal levels on three separate collections virtually exclude the diagnosis. Raised levels of plasma catecholamines confirm the diagnosis. The tumour is then localized by CT/MRI and scintigraphy using meta-[131I]iodobenzylguanidine (MIBG), which is selectively taken up by adrenergic cells.

Management

The treatment of choice is surgical excision of the tumour under α- and β-blockade using phenoxybenzamine and propranolol, which is started before the operation. These drugs can also be used long term where operation is not possible.

Multiple endocrine neoplasia

This is the name given to the synchronous or metachronous (i.e. occurring at different times) occurrence of tumours involving a number of endocrine glands (Table 12.15). Multiple endocrine neoplasia (MEN) is subdivided into type 1, type 2A and type 2B. They are inherited in an autosomal dominant manner. MEN type 1 is due to a mutation in the menin gene on chromosome 11; the normal protein product of this gene may act as a tumour suppressor. The genetic abnormality in MEN2 lies within the RET proto-oncogene on chromosome 1. Management involves surgical excision of the tumours if possible and biochemical screening of first- and second-degree relatives. In a patient known to have MEN constant surveillance is

Table 12.15 Multiple endocrine neoplasia (MEN) syndrome

Organ	Frequency	Tumours/clinical manifestations
Type 1		
Functioning adenomas in		
Parathyroid	95%	Hypercalcaemia
Pituitary	70%	Prolactinoma, acromegaly, Cushing's disease
Pancreatic islets	50%	Gastrinoma, Insulinoma, VIPoma, glucagonoma
Adrenal	40%	Non-functional adenomas
Thyroid	20%	Adenomas – multiple or single
Type 2A		
Medullary thyroid carcinoma	Most	Thyroid mass, diarrhoea, raised plasma calcitonin
Adrenal	Most	Phaeochromocytoma, Cushing's syndrome
Parathyroid hyperplasia	60%	Hypercalcaemia
Type 2B		
Like type 2A (but parathyroid disease does not occur) with a typical phaeotypic appearance: slim body habitus, cutaneous ganglioneuromas around the lips, tongue, eyelids, and throughout the gastrointestinal tract especially the large bowel.		

VIP, vasoactive intestinal polypeptide.

required for additional features of the syndrome, which may develop many years after the initial presentation.

DISORDERS OF TEMPERATURE REGULATION

Normal body temperature is 36.5–37.5°C and is controlled by temperature-sensitive cells within the hypothalamus which control heat generation and loss. Fever during an infection is due to cytokines, particularly interleukin-1, released from inflammatory cells acting in the hypothalamus affecting the thermoregulatory set point.

Hypothermia

Hypothermia is defined as a drop in core (i.e. rectal) temperature to below 35°C. It is frequently fatal when the temperature falls below 32°C.

Aetiology

Very young and elderly individuals are particularly prone to hypothermia, the latter having a reduced ability to feel the cold. Hypothyroidism, hypnotics, alcohol or intercurrent illness may contribute. In healthy individuals, prolonged exposure to extremes of temperature or prolonged immersion in cold water are the most common underlying causes.

Clinical features

Mild hypothermia (32–35°C) causes shivering and a feeling of intense cold. More severe hypothermia leads progressively to altered consciousness and coma. This is usually associated with a fall in pulse rate and blood pressure, muscle stiffness and depressed reflexes. As coma ensues the pupillary and other brain-stem reflexes are lost. Ventricular arrhythmias or asystole are the usual causes of death.

Diagnosis

Measurement of core temperature with a low-reading thermometer makes the diagnosis. Alteration in consciousness usually indicates a core temperature of below 32°C this is a medical emergency. With severe hypothermia there are ECG changes, including an increase in the PR interval, widening of the QRS complex and 'J' waves (deflections at the junction of the QRS complex and ST segment).

! Emergency

- Measure arterial blood gases, urea and electrolytes, blood glucose

- Search for and treat infection

- Intubate and ventilate patients who are comatose or in respiratory failure

- Warmed (37°C) intravenous fluids to achieve urine output 30–40 ml/h

- External warming if core temperature >32°C
    place patient in a warm room (27°–29°C)
    'space' blankets
    warm bath water

- Internal rewarming if core temperature <32°C
    Humidifed and warmed air
    Extracorporeal shunt (haemodialysis, arteriovenous or venovenous) rewarming
    Cardiopulmonary bypass – treatment of choice for arrested hypothermic patients

- Monitor core temperature, urine output and central venous pressure

---

Emergency Box 12.4
Management of hypothermia

Management

The principles of treatment are to rewarm the patient gradually while correcting metabolic abnormalities (if severe) and treating cardiac arrythmias (Emergency Box 12.4). Hypothyroidism should always be looked for and, if suspected, should be treated with intravenous triiodothyronine. Hypothermia may protect organs from ischaemia in patients with prolonged hypothermia-induced cardiopulmonary arrest. Therefore, it is usually recommended that resuscitation efforts are continued (maybe for some hours) until arrest persists after rewarming.

Hyperthermia (hyperpyrexia)

Hyperpyrexia is a body temperature above 41°C. Causes include:

- Injury to the hypothalamus (trauma, surgery, infection)
- Malignant hyperpyrexia – rare autosomal dominant condition in which skeletal muscle generates heat in presence of certain anaesthetic drugs, e.g. suxamethonium
- Ingestion of 3,4-methylenedioxymetamphetamine (Ecstasy).
- Neuroleptic malignant syndrome: idiosyncratic reaction to therapeutic dose of neuroleptic medication, e.g. phenothiazines.

Treatment includes stopping the offending drug, cooling, and the administration of dantrolene sodium.

Diabetes mellitus and other disorders of metabolism

13

....

DIABETES MELLITUS

Insulin is the key hormone that facilitates the storage of nutrients in the form of glycogen in liver and muscle, and triglyceride in fat. During a meal it is released from the beta (β) cells of the pancreatic islets.

The normal venous *whole blood glucose* concentration is between 3.5 and 8.0 mmol/l. It should be noted that whole blood values are about 10–15% lower than *plasma values*, and *capillary values* are about 7% higher than plasma values.

Diabetes mellitus is a common group of metabolic disorders that are characterized by chronic hyperglycaemia resulting from relative insulin deficiency, insulin resistance or both. Diabetes is usually primary but may be secondary to other conditions, which include pancreatic (e.g. total pancreatectomy, chronic pancreatitis, haemochromatosis) and endocrine diseases (e.g. acromegaly and Cushing's disease). It may also be drug induced, most commonly by thiazide diuretics and corticosteroids.

Primary diabetes is divided into insulin–dependent diabetes mellitus (type 1 diabetes, IDDM) and non–insulin dependent diabetes (type 2 diabetes, NIDDM). In clinical terms these represent two ends of a spectrum (Table 13.1).

Aetiology and pathogenesis

Non-insulin dependent diabetes mellitus Single gene mutations that cause NIDDM have been identified and include abnormalities of genes coding for glucokinase, hepatocyte nuclear factors 1α and 4α, and the insulin receptor. It is thought that some of these mutations affect β-cell response to glucose. However, the mutations detected to date are likely to contribute to only a minority of cases of NIDDM, and the genetic defects responsible for most cases have yet to be identified. Environmental factors, notably

Table 13.1 The spectrum of diabetes: a comparison of insulin-dependent diabetes mellitus and non-insulin-dependent diabetes

	Type 1	Type 2

Epidemiology	Patients are
	  Younger (usually
	  juvenile onset)
	  Usually lean
	  European extraction
	  (usually)
	  Seasonal incidence
	  (↑ spring & autumn)
		Affects 2% of UK population
		Patients are
		  Older (usually present
		  after age 40)
		  Often overweight
		  All racial groups

Inheritance	HLA-DR3 or DR4
	  in >90%
	30–35% concordance
	  in identical twins
		No HLA links
		90% concordance in
		  identical twins

Pathogenesis	Autoimmune β-cell destruction	No evidence of immune disturbance
Clinical picture	Complete insulin deficiency May develop ketoacidosis Always need insulin	Partial insulin deficiency, insulin resistance May develop non-ketotic hyperosmolar state Sometimes need insulin

central obesity, appear to trigger the disease in genetically susceptible individuals. The β-cell mass is reduced to about 50% of normal in NIDDM. Hyperglycaemia is the result of reduced insulin secretion (inappropriately low for the glucose level) and peripheral insulin resistance.

Insulin-dependent diabetes mellitus IDDM is thought to be a polygenic disorder and the genes causing diabetes to be transmitted along with particular HLA types (Table 13.1). An autoimmune aetiology is suggested by:

- Antibodies directed against insulin and several islet cell antigens (e.g. glutamic acid decarboxylase) predating clinical onset by many years
- Infiltration of pancreatic islets by mononuclear cells resembles that in other autoimmune diseases, e.g. thyroiditis.
- Association with other organ-specific autoimmune diseases, e.g. autoimmune thyroid disease, Addison's disease and pernicious anaemia.

Clinical features

- *Acute presentation*: Young people present with a brief history (2–4 weeks) of thirst, polyuria, weight loss and lethargy. Polyuria is the result of an osmotic diuresis that results when blood glucose levels exceed the renal tubular reabsorptive capacity (the renal threshold). Fluid and electrolyte losses stimulate thirst. Weight loss is caused by fluid depletion and breakdown of fat and muscle as a result of insulin deficiency. Ketoacidosis (see later) is the presenting feature if these early symptoms are not recognized and treated.
- *Subacute presentation*: Older patients may present with the same symptoms, although less marked and extending over several months. They may also complain of lack of energy, visual problems and pruritus vulvae or balanitis due to *Candida* infection.
- *With complications* (see later)
- *In asymptomatic individuals* diagnosed at routine medical examinations, e.g. for insurance purposes.

Investigations

The criteria for the diagnosis of diabetes mellitus have recently been changed.

The diagnosis is made by demonstrating:

- Fasting venous blood glucose ≥6.2 mmol/l or,
- Random blood glucose ≥10 mmol/l.

A glucose tolerance test (Table 13.2) is only used for borderline cases when the blood glucose is outside the normal range but the criteria above are not satisfied. Glycosuria does not necessarily indicate diabetes and may be the result of a low renal threshold for glucose excretion.

Other routine investigations include Stix testing the urine for proteinuria (page 272), full blood count, serum urea and electrolytes, and a fasting blood sample for cholesterol and triglyceride levels.

Management

Management involves:

- Achieving good glycaemic control. In young patients with IDDM the aim is to maintain blood glucose

Table 13.2 The oral glucose tolerance test

	Fasting blood glucose (mmol/l)	2-hour blood glucose (mmol/l)
Normal	≤5.6	≤5.6
Diabetes mellitus	≥6.2	≥10
Impaired glucose tolerance (IGT)	≤5.6	5.6–10
Impaired fasting glucose (IFG)	5.6–6.2	<10

After an overnight fast 75 g of glucose is taken in 250–350 ml of water. Blood samples are taken before, and 2 hours after the glucose has been given. Individuals with IGT and IFG have an increased risk of cardiovascular disease compared to the normal population and some will go on to develop diabetes.

concentrations as near normal as possible to minimize long-term complications
- Advice regarding regular physical activity and reduction of body weight in the obese, both of which improve glycaemic control in NIDDM
- Aggressive treatment of hypertension and hyperlipidaemia
- Physical examination at diagnosis, and at least yearly thereafter for evidence of diabetic complications.

Management of the diabetic involves a multidisciplinary approach involving, among others, the hospital doctor, the general practitioner, community nurse and dietitian.

Principles of treatment All patients with diabetes require diet therapy. Insulin is always indicated in a patient who presents in ketoacidosis and is usually indicated in those under 40 years of age. Insulin is also indicated in other patients who do not achieve satisfactory control with oral hypoglycaemics.

- *Diet.* In older patients the first approach is by diet alone. The diet itself is no different from the normal healthy diet recommended for the rest of the population. Fat should be reduced to 30–35% of total energy intake and consist mainly of unsaturated fats. Protein should be 10–15% and carbohydrate 50% of total energy intake. Patients should eat complex carbohydrates (e.g. potato, pasta), which are absorbed relatively slowly from the gastrointestinal tract, thus preventing the rapid fluctuations in blood glucose that occur when simple sugars, such as sucrose or glucose, are eaten. The nutrient load should be spread throughout the day (three main meals with snacks in between times and at bedtime), which reduces swings in blood glucose.

- *Oral hypoglycaemics.* These are used in association with dietary treatment when this alone has failed to control hyperglycaemia

  – *Sulphonylureas* increase β-cell insulin release and reduce peripheral resistance to insulin action. Glibenclamide (2.5–20 mg daily in one or two divided doses) is the most popular choice, but is best avoided in elderly people and in those with renal failure because of its relatively long duration of action (12–20 hours) and renal excretion. Tolbutamide, which is shorter acting and metabolized by the liver, is a better choice in these patient groups. The most common side effect of this group of drugs is hypoglycaemia, which may be prolonged.

  – *Biguanides.* Metformin, the only available biguanide, reduces hepatic glucose production and increases insulin sensitivity. It is used in combination with sulphonylureas when a single agent has failed to control diabetes. It is also used as the first-line agent in obese diabetic individuals because, unlike with sulphonylureas, appetite is not increased. Side effects include anorexia and diarrhoea. Lactic acidosis has occurred in patients with severe hepatic or renal disease, in whom its use is contraindicated.

  – *α-Glucosidase inhibitors.* Acarbose inhibits intestinal α-glucosidases, thus impairing carbohydrate digestion and slowing glucose absorption. Postprandial glucose peaks are reduced. Gastrointestinal side effects, e.g. flatulence, bloating and diarrhoea, are common and limit the dose and acceptability of this treatment.

- *Insulin.* Insulin of three species is available: human, porcine and bovine. Most patients receive human insulin, which is manufactured biosynthetically using recombinant DNA technology.

There are two main types of insulin:

1. Insulins prepared in a clear solution (soluble or crystalline). These insulins start working within 30–60 minutes and last for 4–6 hours. They are the only insulins to be used in emergencies such as ketoacidosis, or for surgical operations.
2. Insulins premixed with retarding agents (either protamine or zinc) that precipitate crystals of varying size according to the conditions employed. These insulins are intermediate (12–24 hours) or long acting (more than 24 hours). The protamine insulins are also known as isophane or NPH insulins, and the zinc insulins as lente insulins.

Insulin lispro (Humalog) is similar to human regular insulin except that two amino acids, lysine and proline, are reversed in order. As a result, molecules of lispro bind only weakly to each other (in contrast to regular insulin) and the onset of action is quicker (within 15 minutes), with a shorter duration of action (2–4 hours) than regular insulin. The exact role of lispro is not fully defined, but potential advantages include administration immediately before or even during meals, reduced postprandial blood glucose and reduced frequency of night-time lows.

In young patients a reasonable starting regimen is subcutaneous injection of an intermediate-acting insulin, 8–10 units administered half an hour before breakfast and before the evening meal. In many patients who present acutely with diabetes there is some recovery of endogenous insulin secretion soon after diagnosis ('the honeymoon period') and the insulin dose may need to be reduced. Requirements rise thereafter and a multiple injection regimen (often using a 'pen injector' device), which may improve control and allows greater meal flexibility, is then appropriate for most younger patients. An example of this is soluble insulin administered before each meal and a long-acting insulin given at bedtime. An alternative is to use a small pump strapped to the waist which delivers a continuous subcutaneous insulin infusion (CSII). Mealtime doses are delivered when the patient presses a button on the side of the pump. This should only be used under the guidance of specialized centres.

In many patients with NIDDM who eventually require insulin, a twice-daily regimen of premixed soluble and isophane insulin (e.g. Mixtard) is suitable.

Measuring control

Patients may feel very well and be asymptomatic even if their blood glucose is consistently above the normal range. Self-monitoring at home is therefore necessary because of the immediate risks of hyper- and hypoglycaemia, and because it has been shown that persistently good control (i.e. near normoglycaemia) reduces the risk of progression to retinopathy, nephropathy and neuropathy in IDDM.

Home testing

- Most patients, especially those on insulin, are taught to monitor control by testing finger-prick blood samples with enzyme-impregnated reagent strips, which change colour according to the capillary blood glucose level. Patients are asked to take regular profiles (e.g. four times daily samples on 2 days each week) and to note these in a diary or record book.
- Urine testing for glucose (using Stix) is a crude measure of glycaemic control because glycosuria only appears above the renal threshold for glucose (which varies between a blood glucose of 7 and 13 mmol/l) and because urine glucose lags behind blood glucose. It is usually reserved for the elderly patient in whom tight control is unnecessary.
- Urine ketones, also measured with Stix (Ketostix), are useful if the patient is unwell because ketonuria indicates potentially serious metabolic derangement.

Hospital testing
Single random blood glucose measurements, obtained at clinic visits, are of limited value.

- Glycosylated haemoglobin (HbA1c) is produced by the attachment of glucose to Hb and measurement of this Hb fraction (normally 4–8%) is a useful measure of the average glucose concentration over the life of the Hb molecule (approximately 6 weeks)

- Glycosylated plasma proteins (fructosamine) are less reliable than HbA1c but may be useful in certain situations, e.g. thalassaemia where haemoglobin is abnormal.

··

DIABETIC METABOLIC EMERGENCIES

Hypoglycaemia (blood glucose <2.2 mmol/l)

This is the most common complication of insulin treatment and may also occur in patients taking sulphonylureas.

Clinical features

Increased sympathetic activity causes hunger, sweating, pallor and tachycardia. Hours later there is personality change, fits, occasionally hemiparesis, and finally coma. In patients with long-standing diabetes and autonomic neuropathy the early 'adrenergic features' may be absent.

Investigations

Immediate diagnosis and treatment are essential. A blood glucose confirms the diagnosis but treatment should begin immediately (while waiting for the result) if hypoglycaemia is suspected on clinical grounds.

Management

A rapidly absorbed carbohydrate, e.g. sugary water, should be given orally if possible. In unconscious patients, treatment is with intravenous glucose (50 ml of 50% dextrose into a large vein though a large gauge needle) or intramuscular glucagon (1 mg), which acts rapidly by mobilizing hepatic glycogen and is particularly useful where intravenous access is difficult. Oral glucose is given to replenish glycogen reserves once the patient revives.

Diabetic ketoacidosis

Diabetic ketoacidosis results from insulin deficiency and is the result of previously undiagnosed diabetes, the stress of intercurrent illness (e.g. infection or surgery) or the interruption of insulin therapy. A common error is for insulin to be reduced or stopped if the patient is ill and feels unable to eat. Insulin should never be stopped and most patients in fact need a larger dose when ill.

Pathogenesis

Ketoacidosis is a state of uncontrolled catabolism associated with insulin deficiency. In the absence of insulin there is an unrestrained increase in hepatic gluconeogenesis. High circulating glucose levels result in an osmotic diuresis by the kidneys and consequent dehydration. In addition, peripheral lipolysis leads to an increase in circulating free fatty acids, which are converted within the liver to acidic ketones, leading to a metabolic acidosis. These processes are accelerated by the 'stress hormones' – catecholamines, glucagon and cortisol – which are secreted in response to dehydration and intercurrent illness.

Clinical features

There is profound dehydration secondary to water and electrolyte loss from the kidney. The eyes are sunken, tissue turgor is reduced, the tongue is dry and, in severe cases, the blood pressure is low. Kussmaul's respiration (deep rapid breathing) may be present, as a sign of respiratory compensation for metabolic acidosis, and the breath smells of ketones. Some disturbance of consciousness is common, but only 5% present in coma. Body temperature is often subnormal despite intercurrent infection.

Investigations

The diagnosis is based on the demonstration of hyperglycaemia in combination with acidosis and ketosis.

- Blood glucose is elevated, usually >20 mmol/l.
- Plasma ketones are easily detected by centrifuging a blood sample and testing the plasma obtained with a dipstick that measures ketones, which will usually show ++ or +++.
- Urine Stix testing shows heavy glycosuria and ketonuria.
- Arterial blood gases show a metabolic acidosis.
- Serum urea and electrolytes. Urea and creatinine are often raised as a result of dehydration. The total body potassium is low as a result of osmotic diuresis, but the serum potassium concentration is often raised because of

the absence of the action of insulin, which allows potassium to shift out of cells. Serum bicarbonate is low.
- Full blood count may show an elevated white cell count even in the absence of infection.
- Further investigations are directed towards identifying a precipitating cause: blood cultures, chest radiograph and urine microscopy and culture to look for evidence of infection, and an ECG to look for evidence of myocardial infarction.

Management

Admission to the intensive care unit is recommended in the seriously ill. The aims of treatment are to replace fluid and electrolyte loss (Table 13.3), replace insulin, and restore acid–base balance over a period of about 24 hours. Therapy of diabetic ketoacidosis shifts potassium into cells, which may lead to profound hypokalaemia and death if not treated prospectively. A treatment regimen for a patient with severe ketoacidosis is set out below (Emergency Box 13.1). When the patient has recovered it is necessary to educate them to prevent recurrence.

Table 13.3 Average loss of fluid and electrolytes in an adult with ketoacidosis

Water	6 litres
Sodium	500 mmol
Potassium	400 mml

Non-ketotic hyperosmolar state   HONK

This condition, in which severe hyperglycaemia develops without significant ketosis, is the metabolic emergency characteristic of uncontrolled NIDDM.

Clinical features

Endogenous insulin levels are reduced but are still sufficient to inhibit hepatic ketogenesis, whereas glucose production is unrestrained. Patients present with profound dehydration (secondary to an osmotic diuresis) and a decreased level of consciousness, which is directly related to the elevation of

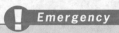 **Emergency**

Early management

Intravenous fluids
- 0.9% saline: 1 litre in 30 min, then 1 litre in 1 hour, then 1 litre in 2 hours, then 1 litre in 4 hours, then 1 litre in 6 hours
- Initial rapid replacement with 1 litre colloid is indicated for severe hypovolaemia with systolic BP <80 mmHg
- Administer 0.45% saline if serum sodium >150 mmol/l

Potassium
- Add 20 mmol KCl to each litre of saline
- Temporarily delay if serum potassium >5 mmol/l
- Increase to 30–40 mmol if serum potassium is low, e.g. <3.5 mmol/l

Insulin
6 units of soluble insulin bolus intravenous injection and then intravenous infusion 6 units hourly thereafter by infusion pump. Aim to reduce blood glucose by 5 mmol/h. Alternatively insulin is given by intramuscular injection 20 units stat and then 6 units hourly

Bicarbonate
Intravenous bicarbonate 1.26%, 500 ml plus 10 mmol/l KCl if blood pH <7.0

Subsequent management

Intravenous fluids
Change intravenous fluids to 5% dextrose, 1 litre 6 hourly plus 20 mmol KCl, when blood glucose falls to 10–12 mmol/l

Potassium
Continue intravenous potassium at 10–40 mmol/l (added to saline or dextrose, drip) until ketoacidosis is cleared (blood pH >7.35, serum ketones negative)

Insulin
Blood glucose must not be allowed to fall below 12 mmol/l in the first 24 h or until ketoacidosis has resolved. Once blood glucose falls to 10–12 mmol/l change infusion fluid to 5% dextrose. Continue insulin at 3 units hourly and

continued

Emergency Box 13.1
Management of diabetic ketoacidosis

	adjust dose depending on blood glucose. When ketoacidosis has cleared switch to 4 times daily soluble subcutaneous insulin and stop intravenous infusion if patient eating
Monitoring	• Hourly blood glucose • 2 hourly serum electrolytes • 4 hourly blood gases and serum ketones • Hourly pulse, BP, temperature and respiratory rate; pulse and BP more frequently in the hypotensive patient
Special measures	Treat infection with broad-spectrum antibiotics. A urinary catheter is passed if oliguria persists 2 hours after rehydration begins. In elderly or seriously ill individuals a central venous pressure line (page 639) may be necessary to monitor fluid replacement accurately. Consider s.c. heparin in the elderly, obese or comatose patient. Coma necessitates standard care of the unconscious patient (page 572) and placement of a nasogastric tube to prevent aspiration and the rare but fatal complication of acute gastric dilatation

Emergency Box 13.1 *Cont'd*

Table 13.4 The main biochemical differences between diabetic ketoacidosis and non-ketotic hyperosmolar coma

Examples of blood values	Severe ketoacidosis	Non-ketotic hyperosmolar coma
Na^+ (mmol/l)	140	155
K^+ (mmol/l)	5	5
Cl^- (mmol/l)	100	110
HCO_3 (mmol/l)	5	30
Urea (mmol/l)	8	15
Glucose (mmol/l)	30	50
Serum osmolality (mosmol/kg)*	328	385
Arterial pH	7.0	7.35

* See page 250 for definition and discussion of plasma osmolality.

plasma osmolality. The main biochemical differences between ketoacidosis and hyperosmolar coma are illustrated in Table 13.4.

Management

Investigations and treatment are the same as for ketoacidosis, with some exceptions. Half physiological saline (0.45%) is given if the serum sodium is more than 170 mmol/l and a lower rate of insulin infusion (3 U/h) is often sufficient as these patients are extremely sensitive to insulin. The hyperosmolar state predisposes to thrombosis, and prophylactic subcutaneous heparin is given.

Prognosis

Mortality rate is around 20–30%, mainly because of the advanced age of the patients and the frequency of intercurrent illness. Unlike ketoacidosis, non-ketotic hyperglycaemia is not an absolute indication for subsequent insulin therapy, and survivors may do well on diet and oral agents.

Lactic acidosis

Lactic acidosis is a rare complication in patients taking metformin. Patients present with severe metabolic acidosis without significant hyperglycaemia or ketosis. Treatment is rehydration with intravenous saline. Intravenous bicarbonate is used only in severe acidosis (pH ≤7).

....

COMPLICATIONS OF DIABETES

Patients with diabetes have a reduced life expectancy. Insulin-treated patients diagnosed before the age of 20 have only a 60–70% chance of living past the age of 50, the excess deaths being mainly the result of diabetic nephropathy. Heart disease, peripheral vascular disease and stroke are the major causes of death in patients over the age of 50.

Vascular

Macrovascular complications

Diabetes is a risk factor for atherosclerosis and this is additive with other risk factors for large vessel disease, e.g.

smoking, hypertension and hyperlipidaemia. Atherosclerosis results in stroke, ischaemic heart disease and peripheral vascular disease.

Microvascular complications

Small vessels throughout the body are affected, but the disease process is of particular danger in three sites: the retina, the renal glomerulus and the nerve sheath. Diabetic retinopathy, nephropathy and neuropathy tend to manifest 10–20 years after diagnosis in young patients. They present earlier in older patients, probably because they have had unrecognized diabetes for months or even years before diagnosis.

Diabetic eye disease

About one-third of young diabetics develop visual problems and in the UK 5% have in the past become blind after 30 years of diabetes. However, the prevalence is now falling.

Retinopathy

Background retinopathy is the earliest feature of retinopathy. Capillary microaneurysms appear on ophthalmoscopy as tiny red dots, haemorrhages are seen as larger red spots (blot haemorrhages), and capillary leaks of fluid rich in lipid and protein give rise to hard exudates (yellow-white discrete patches). There is no specific treatment for background retinopathy, but patients should undergo regular eye examination by an ophthalmologist to look for any deterioration. Background retinopathy does not itself constitute a threat to vision, but may progress to two other distinct forms of retinopathy: maculopathy or proliferative retinopathy. Both are the consequence of damage to retinal blood vessels and resultant retinal ischaemia.

Maculopathy Macular oedema is the first feature of maculopathy and will result in permanent damage if not treated early. It cannot be detected by standard ophthalmoscopy and the only sign may be deteriorating visual acuity detected by Snellen chart testing. At a later stage there are perimacular haemorrhages and hard exudates.

Pre-proliferative retinopathy is characterized by 'cottonwool spots', which are indistinct pale lesions and represent oedema from retinal infarcts. Venous beading and/or venous loops are other pre-proliferative changes.

Proliferative retinopathy Hypoxia is thought to be the signal for new vessel formation. These are fragile and bleed easily, resulting in loss of vision because of vitreous haemorrhage. Fibrous tissue associated with new vessels may shrink and cause retinal detachment.

Maculopathy and proliferative retinopathy are treated by laser photocoagulation of the retina. Effective early therapy of proliferative retinopathy reduces the risk of visual loss by about 50%.

Other eye complications

- Blurred vision (caused by reversible osmotic changes in the lens in patients with acute hyperglycaemia)
- Cataracts
- Glaucoma
- External ocular palsies.

The diabetic kidney

The kidney may be damaged by diabetes as a result of:

- Glomerular disease
- Ischaemic renal lesions
- Ascending urinary tract infection.

Diabetic glomerulosclerosis Nephropathy secondary to glomerular disease affects 25–30% of patients diagnosed under the age of 30 years. On histological investigation there is thickening of the glomerular basement membrane and later glomerulosclerosis, which may be a diffuse or nodular form (Kimmelstiel–Wilson lesion). The earliest evidence of glomerular damage is 'microalbuminuria' (defined as an increase above the normal range in urinary albumin excretion but undetectable by conventional dipsticks) which in turn may, after some years, progress to intermittent albuminuria followed by persistent proteinuria, sometimes with a frank nephrotic syndrome. At the stage of persistent proteinuria the plasma creatinine is normal but the average patient is only some 5–10 years from end-stage renal failure.

The urine of all patients should be checked regularly by dipsticks for the presence of protein. Most centres also screen for microalbuminuria, because meticulous glycaemic control and treatment with angiotensin-converting enzyme (ACE) inhibitors at this stage (even in the absence of hypertension) may delay the onset of frank proteinuria. Aggressive control of blood pressure is the most important factor to reduce disease progression in those with established proteinuria, and ACE inhibitors are the treatment of choice. Many will develop end-stage renal failure and need dialysis and eventually renal transplantation.

Ischaemic lesions Arteriolar lesions with hypertrophy and hyalinization of the vessels affect both afferent and efferent arterioles. The appearances are similar to those of hypertensive disease but are not necessarily related to the blood pressure in patients with diabetes.

Infective lesions Urinary tract infections are common (page 284). A rare complication is renal papillary necrosis, in which renal papillae are shed in the urine and may cause ureteral obstruction.

Diabetic neuropathy (Table 13.5)

Diabetic neuropathy is thought to result from nerve ischaemia or the accumulation of fructose and sorbitol (metabolized from glucose in peripheral nerves), which disrupts the structure and function of the nerve.

Table 13.5 Diabetic neuropathies

Progressive	Symmetrical sensory polyneuropathy (distal)
	Autonomic neuropathy
Reversible	Acute painful neuropathy
	Mononeuropathy and mononeuritis multiplex
	Cranial nerve lesions
	Isolated peripheral nerve lesions
	Diabetic amyotrophy

Symmetrical sensory neuropathy This is the most common form of neuropathy and first affects the most distal parts of the longest nerves, i.e. the toes and the soles of the feet. Symptoms consist of numbness, tingling and pain, which is typically worse at night. Involvement of the hands is less common and results in a 'stocking and glove' sensory loss. Complications include unrecognized trauma, beginning as blistering caused by an ill-fitting shoe or a hot-water bottle, and leading to ulceration. Abnormal mechanical stress and repeated minor trauma, usually prevented by pain, may lead to the development of a neuropathic arthropathy (Charcot's joints) in the ankle and knee, where the joint is grossly deformed and swollen.

Autonomic neuropathy may present with impotence (page 480), postural hypotension, diarrhoea, and nausea and vomiting as a consequence of gastroparesis. In addition, bladder involvement may result in a neuropathic bladder with painless urinary retention.

Acute painful neuropathy The patient describes burning or crawling pains in the lower limbs. These symptoms are typically worse at night, and pressure from bedclothes may be intolerable. There is usually a good response to improved glycaemic control.

Diabetic mononeuropathy Individual nerves are affected. In some instances this relates to local pressure, e.g. carpal tunnel syndrome. In others it results from a localized nerve infarction: commonly the IIIrd and VIth cranial nerves are affected, resulting in diplopia (page 564). More than one nerve may be affected: mononeuritis multiplex.

Diabetic amyotrophy (proximal motor neuropathy) This presents with painful wasting, usually asymmetrical, of the quadriceps muscles. The wasting may be very marked and knee reflexes are diminished or absent.

Infections

Poorly controlled diabetes impairs the function of polymorphonuclear leukocytes and confers an increased risk of infection, particularly of the urinary tract and skin, e.g. cellulitis, boils and abscesses. Tuberculosis and mucocutaneous candidiasis are more common in diabetic individuals. Infections may lead to loss of glycaemic control and are a common cause of ketoacidosis. Insulin–treated patients may need to increase their insulin therapy even if they feel nauseated and unable to eat. Non–insulin treated patients may need insulin for the same reasons.

The skin

Lipohypertrophy is where fat lumps develop at frequently used insulin injection sites, and may be avoided by varying the injection site from day to day. Necrobiosis lipoidica diabeticorum is an unusual complication of diabetes characterized by erythematous plaques, often over the shins, which gradually develop a brown waxy discoloration. Other skin lesions are vitiligo (symmetrical white patches seen in organ-specific autoimmune diseases) and granuloma annulare, which presents as flesh-coloured rings and nodules, principally over the extensor surfaces of the fingers.

SPECIAL SITUATIONS

Surgery

Smooth control of diabetes minimizes the risk of infection and balances the catabolic response to anaesthesia and surgery. If possible, diabetic patients should be admitted 1 or 2 days before surgery and glucose control optimized. They should be first on the operating list and a blood glucose of 6–11 mmol/l maintained during the perioperative period.

IDDM

- Stop long-acting insulins the day before surgery; substitute with soluble insulin.
- Start glucose/potassium/insulin infusion (GKI, 500 ml 10% dextrose + 15 U soluble insulin + 10 mmol KCl over 5 hours) on the morning of surgery and continue until first meal.
- Check blood glucose levels hourly and serum potassium 4–6 hourly.
- Increase or decrease insulin in GKI by 5 U if blood glucose >11 or <6 mmol/l respectively.

NIDDM

- Omit oral hypoglycaemics on day of surgery.
- Check blood glucose 2 hourly.
- Start GKI infusion in patients with high blood glucose on morning of surgery.
- Restart oral hypoglycaemics with first meal.

Pregnancy and diabetes

Poorly controlled diabetes is associated with congenital malformations, macrosomia (large babies), hydramnios, pre-eclampsia and intrauterine death. In the neonatal period there is an increased risk of hyaline membrane disease and neonatal hypoglycaemia (unlike insulin, maternal glucose crosses the placenta and causes hypersecretion of insulin from the fetal islets, which continues when the umbilical cord is cut). Meticulous control of blood glucose levels achieves results comparable to those with non-diabetic pregnancies.

Gestational diabetes is diabetes that develops in the course of pregnancy and remits following delivery. Treatment is with diet in the first instance, but most patients require insulin cover during pregnancy. It is likely to recur in subsequent pregnancies, and non-insulin dependent diabetes may develop later in life.

Brittle diabetes

There is no precise definition for this term, which is used to describe patients with recurrent ketoacidosis and/or recurrent hypoglycaemic coma. Of these, the largest group is made up of those who experience recurrent severe hypoglycaemia.

Hypoglycaemia

The causes and mechanism of hypoglycaemia are listed in Table 13.6. Insulin or sulphonylurea therapy for diabetes accounts for the vast majority of cases of severe hypoglycaemia encountered in an accident and emergency department.

Insulinomas

These are rare pancreatic islet cell tumours (usually benign) that secrete insulin. They may be part of the multiple endocrine neoplasia syndrome (page 515).

Clinical features

The classic presentation is with fasting hypoglycaemia. Hypoglycaemia produces symptoms as a result of neuroglycopenia and stimulation of the sympathetic nervous system. These include sweating, palpitations, diplopia and weakness, progressing to confusion, abnormal behaviour, fits and coma.

Investigations

The diagnosis is made by demonstrating hypoglycaemia in association with inappropriate and excessive insulin secretion:

Table 13.6 Causes of hypoglycaemia

Cause	Mechanism of hypoglycaemia
Drug induced: insulin, sulphonylureas, quinine, pentamidine and salicylates in overdose	Variety of mechanisms
Islet cell tumour of the pancreas (insulinoma)	Inappropriately high circulating insulin levels
Non-pancreatic tumours, e.g. sarcoma, hepatoma	Secretion of IGF-1 by some tumours
Endocrine causes: Addison's disease	Impaired counterregulation to the action of insulin
Fulminant liver failure	Failure of hepatic gluconeogenesis
End-stage renal failure	Failure of renal cortical gluconeogenesis
Excess alcohol	Enhanced insulin response to carbohydrate Inhibition of hepatic gluconeogenesis by alcohol
After gastric surgery	Rapid gastric emptying, mismatch of food and insulin
Factitious hypoglycaemia	Surreptitious self-administration of insulin or sulphonylureas, often in a non-diabetic

IGF-1, insulin-like growth factor: produced by the liver, primarily a growth factor in physiological concentrations.

- Measurement of overnight fasting glucose and plasma insulin levels on three occasions
- Performing a prolonged 72-hour supervised fast if overnight testing is inconclusive and symptoms persist.

Further investigations are used to localize the tumour before surgery. Most tumours express somatostatin receptors on their surface, and an octreotide scan (page 139) is now the primary investigation. High-resolution CT scanning and endoscopic ultrasound may also be helpful.

Treatment

The treatment of choice is surgical excision of the tumour. Diazoxide, which inhibits insulin release from islet cells, is useful when the tumour is malignant, in patients in whom a tumour is very small and cannot be located, or in elderly patients with mild symptoms. Symptoms may also remit using octreotide, a long-acting analogue of somatostatin.

DISORDERS OF LIPID METABOLISM

Fats are transported in the bloodstream as lipoprotein particles composed of lipids (principally triglycerides, cholesterol and cholesterol esters), phospholipids and proteins, called apoproteins. These proteins exert a stabilizing function and allow the particles to be recognized by receptors in the liver and peripheral tissues.

There are five principal types of lipoprotein particles:

- *Chylomicrons* are synthesized in the small intestine and serve to transport exogenous dietary fat (mainly triglycerides, small amounts of cholesterol) to the liver and peripheral tissues.
- *Very-low-density lipoproteins (VLDLs)* are synthesized and secreted by the liver and transport endogenous triglycerides (formed in the liver from plasma free fatty acids) to the periphery. In fat and muscle, triglycerides are removed from chylomicrons and VLDLs by the tissue enzyme lipoprotein lipase and the essential cofactor apoprotein C-II.
- *Intermediate-density lipoproteins (IDLs)*, derived from the peripheral breakdown of VLDLs, are transported back to the liver and metabolized to yield the cholesterol-rich particles – low-density lipoproteins (LDLs).
- *Low-density lipoproteins (LDLs)* deliver most cholesterol to the periphery and liver with subsequent binding to LDL receptors in these tissues.
- *High-density lipoproteins (HDLs)* transport cholesterol from peripheral tissues to the liver. HDL particles carry 20–30% of the total quantity of cholesterol in the blood.

The major clinical significance of hypercholesterolaemia (both total plasma and LDL concentration) is as a risk factor for atheroma and hence ischaemic heart disease. The risk is greatest in those with other risk factors, e.g. smoking. There is a weak independent link between raised concentrations of (triglyceride-rich) VLDL particles and cardiovascular risk. In addition, severe hypertriglyceridaemia may induce acute pancreatitis. In contrast, HDL particles, which transport cholesterol away from the periphery, appear to protect against atheroma.

Measurement of plasma lipids

Most patients with hyperlipidaemia are asymptomatic, with no clinical signs, and they are discovered through routine screening. A single fasting blood sample is necessary for the measurement of total plasma cholesterol, total triglyceride and HDL cholesterol levels. Specific diagnosis of the defect (see below) requires the measurement of individual lipoproteins by electrophoresis, but this is not usually necessary. If a lipid disorder has been detected it is vital to carry out a clinical history, examination and simple special investigations (i.e. blood glucose, urea and electrolytes, liver biochemistry and thyroid function tests) to detect the causes of secondary hyperlipidaemia (Table 13.7).

Table 13.7 Causes of secondary hyperlipidaemia

Poorly controlled diabetes mellitus

Alcohol

Obesity

Hypothyroidism

Renal impairment

Nephrotic syndrome

Dysglobulinaemia

Hepatic dysfunction

Drugs: oral contraceptives in susceptible individuals, thiazide diuretics, corticosteroids

The primary hyperlipidaemias

Hypertriglyceridaemia alone

- Polygenic hypertriglyceridaemia accounts for most cases, in which there are many genes both acting together and interacting with environmental factors to produce a modest elevation in serum triglyceride levels.

- Familial hypertriglyceridaemia is inherited in an autosomal dominant fashion. The exact defect is not known and the only clinical feature is a history of pancreatitis or retinal vein thrombosis in some individuals.
- Lipoprotein lipase deficiency and apoprotein C-II deficiency are rare diseases which usually present in childhood with severe hypertriglyceridaemia complicated by pancreatitis, retinal vein thrombosis and eruptive xanthomas – crops of small yellow lipid deposits in the skin.

Hypercholesterolaemia alone

- Familial hypercholesterolaemia is the result of underproduction of the LDL cholesterol receptor in the liver, which results in high plasma concentrations of LDL cholesterol. Heterozygotes may be asymptomatic or develop coronary artery disease in their 40s. Typical clinical features include tendon xanthomas (lipid nodules in the tendons, especially the extensor tendons of hands and the Achilles tendon) and xanthelasmas. Homozygotes have a total absence of LDL receptors in the liver. They have grossly elevated plasma cholesterol levels (>16 mmol/l) and, without treatment, die in their teens from coronary artery disease.
- Polygenic hypercholesterolaemia accounts for those patients with a modest elevation in cholesterol who do not have familial hypercholesterolaemia. The precise nature of the polygenic variation in plasma cholesterol remains unknown.

Combined hyperlipidaemia (hypercholesterolaemia and hyperlipidaemia)

Polygenic combined hyperlipidaemia and familial combined hyperlipidaemia account for the vast majority of patients in this group. A small minority is the result of the rare condition remnant hyperlipidaemia.

Management of hyperlipidaemia

The aim of treatment is to reduce serum cholesterol to at least <6.5 mmol/l, which is the upper limit of the normal range. A serum triglyceride concentration below 2.0

mmol/l is normal; in the range 2.0–6.0 mmol/l no specific intervention will be needed. However, if there are other cardiovascular risk factors, particularly hypercholesterolaemia, the aim should be to reduce serum triglycerides into the normal range.

Guidelines to therapy

The initial treatment in all cases of hyperlipidaemia is dietary modification, but additional measures are usually necessary. Patients with familial hypercholesterolaemia will probably need drug treatment. Secondary hyperlipidaemia should be managed by treatment of the underlying condition wherever possible.

Lipid-lowering diet

- Dairy products and meat are the principal sources of fat in the diet. Chicken and poultry should be substituted for red meats and the food grilled rather than fried. Low-fat cheeses and skimmed milk should be substituted for the full-fat varieties.
- Polyunsaturated fats, e.g. corn and soya oil, should be used instead of saturated fats.
- Reduction of cholesterol intake from liver, offal and fish roe.
- Increased intake of soluble fibres, e.g. pulses and legumes, which reduce circulating cholesterol.
- Avoid excess alcohol and obesity, both causes of secondary hyperlipidaemias.

Lipid-lowering drugs

- Statins
  e.g. pravastatin, simvastatin, inhibit the enzyme hydroxymethylglutaryl-coenzyme A (HMG CoA) reductase, thereby limiting the synthesis of cholesterol in the liver. They principally reduce LDL cholesterol.
- Fibric acid derivatives
  e.g. clofibrate, bezafibrate, lower total serum cholesterol, LDL cholesterol and tryglyceride concentrations,

though the exact mechanism of action is unknown.

- Bile acid-binding resins e.g. cholestyramine, colestipol, bind and prevent reabsorption of bile acids. They reduce LDL cholesterol but raise levels of triglycerides.

- Nicotinic acid This agent reduces total and LDL cholesterol levels and can reduce triglyceride levels.

Whom to treat

Primary prevention In patients without clinically apparent vascular disease the need to measure blood cholesterol levels and treat if abnormal is determined by the patient's coronary heart disease risk factors. Specific guidelines to aid determination of an individual's risk, and thus the need for treatment, are widely available.

Secondary prevention Patients with clinical evidence of cardiovascular disease, e.g. those with a previous myocardial infarction, previous coronary revascularization, or those with angina, are at high risk of progressive heart disease. These patients should have their blood lipids measured and treatment with a stain instituted if the LDL cholesterol is above 3.3 mmol/l or total cholesterol more than 4.8 mmol/l.

Table 13.8 summarizes the drugs used in the management of hyperlipidaemia. They may be used singly or in combination.

Table 13.8 Drugs used in the management of hyperlipidaemias (listed in the order in which they are usually selected for treatment)

Hypertriglyceridaemia	Hypercholesterolaemia	Combined
Fibric acid derivatives	HMG-CoA reductase inhibitors	Fibric acid derivatives
Nicotinic acid	Fibric acid derivatives	Nicotinic acid
Fish oil capsules (ω-3 marine triglycerides)	Bile acid-binding resins	

THE PORPHYRIAS

The porphyrias are a rare group of inherited heterogeneous disorders resulting from abnormalities of a number of enzymes involved in the biosynthesis of haem. This leads to an overproduction of the intermediate compounds called porphyrins (Figure 13.1).

In porphyrias the excess production of porphyrins occurs within the liver (hepatic porphyria) or in the bone marrow (erythropoietic porphyria), but porphyrias can also be classified in terms of clinical presentation as acute or non-acute (Table 13.9). Acute porphyrias usually produce neuropsychiatric problems and are associated with excess production and urinary excretion of δ-aminolaevulinic acid (δALA) and porphobilinogen. These metabolites are not increased in the non-acute porphyrias.

Acute intermittent porphyria

This is an autosomal dominant disorder caused by a defect at the level of porphobilinogen deaminase. Presentation is in early adult life, and women are affected more than men.

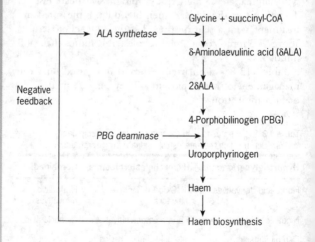

Figure 13.1
Pathways in porphyrin metabolism.

Table 13.9 The classification of porphyrias

	Hepatic	Erythropoietic
Acute	Acute intermittent porphyria	
	Variegate porphyria	
	Hereditary coproporphyria	
Non-acute	Porphyria cutanea tarda	Congenital porphyria
		Erythropoietic protoporphyria

Clinical features

Abdominal pain, vomiting and constipation are the most common presenting features, occurring in 90% of patients (mimicking an acute abdomen, especially as there may be fever and leucocytosis). Additional features include polyneuropathy (especially motor), hypertension, tachycardia and neuropsychiatric disorder (fits, depression, anxiety and frank psychosis). The urine may turn red or brown on standing. Attacks may be precipitated by alcohol and a variety of drugs, especially those such as barbiturates, which are enzyme-inducing drugs and increase δALA synthetase activity.

Investigations

During an attack there may be a neutrophil leucocytosis, abnormal liver biochemistry and a raised urea.

The diagnosis is made during an attack by demonstrating increased urinary excretion of porphobilinogen. Erythrocyte porphobilinogen deaminase may be measured between attacks or, in some cases, urinary porphobilinogen remains high.

Management

This is largely supportive. A high carbohydrate intake must be maintained because this depresses δALA synthetase activity, as does an intravenous haematin infusion which is used in some cases.

Other porphyrias

Variegate porphyria and hereditary coproporphyria present with features similar to those of acute intermittent porphyria, together with the cutaneous features of porphyria cutanea tarda. Porphyria cutanea tarda has a genetic predisposition and presents with a bullous eruption on exposure to light. The eruption heals with scarring. Most patients give a history of alcohol abuse.

The erythropoietic porphyrias are very rare and present with photosensitive skin lesions.

Amyloidosis

This is a heterogeneous group of disorders characterized by extracellular deposition of an insoluble fibrillar protein called amyloid. Amyloidosis is acquired or hereditary, and may be localized or systemic. Clinical features are the result of amyloid deposits affecting the normal structure and function of the affected tissue. The diagnosis of amyloidosis is usually made with Congo red staining of a biopsy of affected tissues. In systemic amyloid a simple rectal biopsy may be used for histological diagnosis. Amyloid deposits stain red and show green fluorescence in polarized light. The features of some systemic amyloid types are shown in Table 13.10.

Table 13.10 Classification of the more common types of amyloid and amyloidosis

Type	Fibril protein precursor	Clinical syndrome
AL	Monoclonal immunoglobulin light chains	Associated with myeloma, Waldenström's macroglobulinaemia and non-Hodgkin's lymphoma. Presents with cardiac failure, nephrotic syndrome, carpal tunnel syndrome and macroglossia (large tongue)
ATTR (familial)	Abnormal transthyretin (plasma carrier protein)	Neuropathy and cardiomyopathy
AA	Protein A, a precursor of serum amyloid A (an acute phase reactant)	Occurs with chronic infections (e.g. TB), inflammation (e.g. rheumatoid arthritis) and malignancy (e.g. Hodgkin's disease). Presents with proteinuria and hepatosplenomegaly

Localized amyloid deposits occur in the brain of patients with Alzheimer's disease and in the joints of patients on long-term dialysis.

Inborn errors of metabolism

Most of the inborn errors of metabolism are rare and tend to present early in childhood.

COMMON NEUROLOGICAL SYMPTOMS

Headache

Headache is a common complaint and does not usually indicate serious disease. In most patients presenting with headache there are no abnormal physical signs, so the diagnosis may depend entirely upon an accurate history. The causes of headache can be broadly divided depending on their onset and subsequent course (Table 14.1). The underlying causes of acute or subacute onset of headache are all potentially serious and require urgent investigation and assessment. The exception is headache due to drugs or migraine (page 607) which, although not serious, may be disabling for the patient. The following points in the clinical history and examination may also help to differentiate between patients who have a serious underlying disease and

Table 14.1 Causes of headache

Acute severe (onset in minute or hours)
Subarachnoid haemorrhage
Meningitis
Head injury
Migraine
Drugs, e.g., glyceryl trinitrate
Alcohol

Subacute onset (onset in days to weeks)
Intracranial mass lesion
Encephalitis
Meningitis
Giant cell arteritis
Malignant hypertension

Recurrent/chronic
Migraine
Tension headache
Sinusitis
Migrainous neuralgia

those who do not. Headache described by the patient as the 'worst ever' is typical of a subarachnoid haemorrhage (page 582). Progressively worsening headaches, or chronic headaches that change in character, may be caused by raised intracranial pressure and require further investigation. Other features which suggest raised intracranial pressure include headache waking the patient from sleep and headache associated with nausea and vomiting (which may also occur with migraine). Ataxia, neurological deficit, papilloedema and altered mental status also indicate a potentially serious underlying cause. Neck stiffness and a positive Kerning's sign indicate meningeal irritation, which usually occurs because of bacterial or viral meningitis, or subarachnoid haemorrhage. Fever may also occur with these conditions. Temporal arteritis (page 608) causes headache in the elderly and requires urgent treatment with steroids to prevent blindness.

Dizziness, faints and 'funny turns'

Episodes of transient disturbance of consciousness are common clinical problems (Table 14.2). Differentiation of seizures from other disorders often depends entirely on the medical history. An eye witness account is invaluable.

Table 14.2 Common causes of attacks of altered consciousness and falls in adults

Syncope
  'Simple faint'
  Cough
  Effort
  Micturition
  Carotid sinus

Cardiac arrhythmias

Postural hypotension

Epilepsy

Hypoglycaemia

Transient ischaemic attacks

Psychogenic attacks
  Panic attacks
  Hyperventilation

Narcolepsy and cataplexy

Dizziness and syncope

Syncope is the term used to describe a temporary impairment of consciousness caused by a reduction in cerebral blood flow. *Dizziness* (faintness) is the symptom that precedes syncope, and represents an incomplete form in which cerebral perfusion has not fallen sufficiently to cause loss of consciousness. Dizziness should be differentiated from *vertigo* (page 569), which is an illusion of movement resulting from disease of the inner ear, the eighth cranial nerve, or its central connections.

The most frequent cause of dizziness is vasovagal syncope (a simple faint), which occurs as a result of reflex bradycardia and peripheral and splanchnic vasodilatation. Fear, pain and prolonged standing are the principal causes. Fainting almost never occurs in the recumbent position. Rapid recovery from the attack and the absence of jerking movements or incontinence of urine suggest a faint as opposed to a fit. Syncope may occur after micturition in men (particularly at night), and when the venous return to the heart is obstructed by breath-holding and severe coughing. Carotid sinus syncope is thought to be the result of excessive sensitivity of the sinus to external pressure. It may occur in elderly patients who lose consciousness on touching the neck. Postural hypotension occurs on standing in those with impaired autonomic reflexes, e.g. elderly people, in autonomic neuropathy and with some drugs (phenothiazines, tricyclic antidepressants).

Narcolepsy is a rare disorder characterized by periods of irresistible sleep in inappropriate circumstances. Cataplexy is a related condition in which sudden loss of tone develops in the lower limbs, with preservation of consciousness. Attacks are set off by sudden surprise or emotion.

Weakness and sensory loss

Skeletal muscle contraction is controlled by the motor axis of the central nervous system, and muscle weakness may be due to a defect or damage in one or more components of this system, i.e. the upper motor neuron, the lower motor neuron and peripheral nerve, the neuromuscular junction and muscle fibers. Lesions that affect the upper motor neuron and peripheral nerve will also often involve the sensory system because of the proximity of sensory to motor nerves in these areas. It is important to determine whether there is true weakness rather than 'tiredness' or 'slowness', as in Parkinson's disease.

The corticospinal tracts

The upper motor neuron The corticospinal tracts originate from neurons of the motor cortex and terminate on the motor nuclei of the cranial nerves and the anterior horn cells. The clinically important pathways cross over in the medulla and pass to the contralateral halves of the spinal cord as the crossed lateral corticospinal tracts (Figure 14.1), which then synapse with the anterior horn cells. This is known as the pyramidal system, disease of which results in upper motor neuron (UMN) lesions with characteristic clinical features (Table 14.3).

Two main patterns of clinical features occur in UMN disorders: hemiparesis and paraparesis:

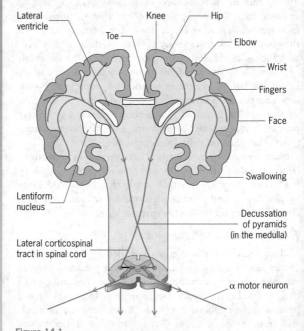

Figure 14.1
The crossed corticospinal ('pyramidal') tracts showing cortical representation of various parts of the body.

Table 14.3 Comparison of the clinical features of upper and lower motor neuron lesions

Upper motor neuron lesion*	Lower motor neuron lesion
Signs are on the opposite side to the lesion	Signs are on the same side as the lesion
No fasciculation	Fasciculation (visible contraction of single motor units)
No muscle wasting	Wasting
Spasticity ± clonus	Hypotonia
Weakness with a characteristic distribution (predominantly extensors in the arms, flexors in the legs)	Weakness
Exaggerated tendon reflexes Extensor plantar response Loss of abdominal reflexes Drift of the outstretched hand (downwards, medially with a tendency to pronate)	Loss of tendon reflexes

* Acute injury to the UMN can, however, be manifested by transient flaccid weakness and hyporeflexia.

- Hemiparesis means weakness of the limbs of one side, and is usually caused by a lesion within the brain or brain stem, e.g. a stroke.
- Paraparesis (weak legs) indicates bilateral damage to the corticospinal tracts and is most often caused by lesions in the spinal cord below T1 (page 610). Tetraparesis (quadriplegic, weakness of the arms and legs) indicates high cervical cord damage, most commonly resulting from trauma.

The lower motor neuron The lower motor neuron (LMN) is the motor pathway from the anterior horn cell or cranial nerve via a peripheral nerve to the motor end-plate. Physical signs (Table 14.3) follow rapidly if the LMN is interrupted at any point in its course. Muscle disease may give a similar clinical picture, but reflexes are usually preserved.

LMN lesions are most commonly caused by the following:

- Anterior horn cell lesions, e.g. motor neuron disease, poliomyelitis
- Spinal root lesions, e.g. cervical and lumbar disc lesions
- Peripheral nerve lesions, e.g. trauma, compression or polyneuropathy.

The commonest disease of the neuromuscular junction is myasthenia gravis, which characteristically produces weakness of skeletal muscle and is rarely associated with wasting. Myopathies are discussed on page 619.

Numbness

The sensory system

The peripheral nerves carry all the modalities of sensation from nerve endings to the dorsal root ganglia and thence to the cord. These then ascend to the thalamus and cerebral cortex in two principal pathways (Figure 14.2):

- Posterior columns, which carry sensory modalities for vibration, joint position sense, two-point discrimination and light touch. These fibres ascend uncrossed to the gracile and cuneate nuclei in the medulla. Axons from the second order neurons cross the midline to form the medial lemniscus and pass to the thalamus.
- Spinothalamic tracts, which carry sensations of pain and temperature. These fibres synapse in the dorsal horn of the cord, cross the midline and ascend as the spinothalamic tracts to the thalamus.

Paraesthesiae (pins and needles), numbness and pain are the principal symptoms of lesions of the sensory pathways below the level of the thalamus. The quality and distribution of the symptoms may suggest the site of the lesion.

Peripheral nerve lesions Symptoms are felt in the distribution of the affected peripheral nerve, e.g. the ulnar or median nerve.

Spinal root lesions Symptoms are referred to the dermatome supplied by that root, often with a tingling discomfort in that dermatome (Figure 14.3). This is in contrast to lesions of sensory tracts within the central nervous system, which characteristically present as general defects in an extremity rather than specific dermatome defects.

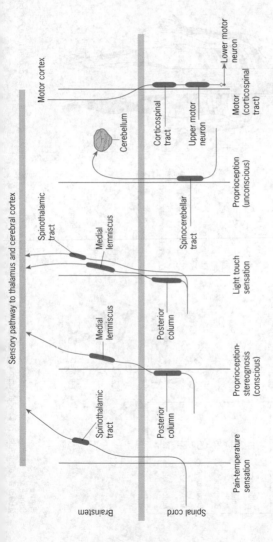

Figure 14.2
A schematic outline of the major motor and sensory pathways.

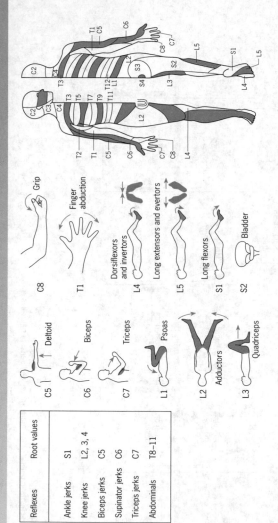

Reflexes	Root values
Ankle jerks	S1
Knee jerks	L2, 3, 4
Biceps jerks	C5
Supinator jerks	C6
Triceps jerks	C7
Abdominals	T8–11

Figure 14.3
Simple scheme depicting motor and sensory innervation of arms and legs and root values for reflexes. (Part of figure adapted from Parsons, M. (1993) A Colour Atlas of Clinical Neurology. London, Mosby Wolfe.)

Spinal cord lesions Symptoms (e.g. loss of sensation) are usually evident below the level of the lesion. A lesion of the pain–temperature pathway (spinothalamic tract), whether within the brain stem or the spinal cord, will result in loss of pain–temperature sensation contralaterally, below the level of the lesion. A lesion at the spinal level of the pathway for proprioception will result in loss of these senses ipsilaterally below the level of the lesion. Dissociated sensory loss suggests a spinal cord lesion, for instance loss of pain–temperature sensation in the right leg and loss of proprioception in the left leg.

Pontine lesions The pons lies above the decussation of the posterior columns. As the medial lemniscus and spinothalamic tracts are close together, pontine lesions result in the loss of all forms of sensation on the side opposite the lesion.

Thalamic lesions A thalamic lesion is a rare cause of complete contralateral sensory loss. Spontaneous pain may also occur, most commonly as the result of a thalamic infarct.

Cortical lesions Sensory loss, neglect of one side of the body and subtle disorders of sensation may occur with lesions of the parietal cortex. Pain is not a feature of cortical lesions.

Coordination of movement

The extrapyramidal system (page 590) and the cerebellum coordinate movement. Disorders of these systems will not produce muscular weakness but may produce incoordination.

The cerebellum

Each lateral lobe of the cerebellum is responsible for coordinating movement of the ipsilateral limb. The midline vermis is concerned with maintenance of axial (midline) balance and posture. Causes of cerebellar disease are listed in Table 14.4.

A lesion within one cerebellar lobe causes one or all of the following:

- An ataxic gait with a broad base; the patient falters to the side of the lesion

Table 14.4 Some causes of cerebellar disease

Multiple sclerosis

Space-occupying lesion
  Primary tumour, e.g. medulloblastoma
  Secondary tumour
  Abscess
  Haemorrhage

Chronic alcohol abuse

Anticonvulsant drugs

Non-metastatic manifestation of malignancy

- An 'intention tremor' (compare Parkinson's disease) with past-pointing
- Clumsy rapid alternating movements, e.g. tapping one hand on the back of the other (dysdiadochokinesis)
- Horizontal nystagmus with the fast component towards the side of the lesion (page 569)
- Dysarthria, usually with bilateral lesions. The speech has a halting jerking quality – 'scanning speech'
- Titubation (rhythmic tremor of the head), hypotonia and depressed reflexes. There is no muscle weakness.

Lesions of the cerebellar vermis cause a characteristic ataxia of the trunk, so that the patient has difficulty sitting up or standing.

THE CRANIAL NERVES

The 12 cranial nerves and their nuclei are distributed approximately equally between the three brain-stem segments (Figure 14.4). The exceptions are the first and second cranial nerves (nerves I and II), whose neurons project to the cerebral cortex. In addition, the sensory nucleus of nerve V extends from the midbrain to the spinal cord, and the nuclei of nerves VII and VIII lie not only in the pons but also in the medulla.

The olfactory nerve (first cranial nerve)

The olfactory nerve subserves the sense of smell. The most common cause of anosmia (loss of the sense of smell) is

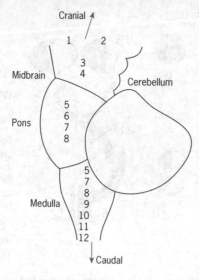

Figure 14.4
The location of the cranial nerves and their nuclei within the midbrain, pons and medulla as seen laterally.

simply nasal congestion. Neurological causes include tumours on the floor of the anterior fossa and head injury.

The optic nerve (second cranial nerve) and the visual system

The optic nerves enter the cranial cavity through the optic foramina and unite to form the optic chiasma, beyond which they are continued as the optic tracts. Fibres of the optic tract project to the visual cortex (via the lateral geniculate body) and the third nerve nucleus for pupillary light reflexes (Figures 14.5 and 14.6).

The assessment of optic nerve function includes measurement of visual acuity (using a Snellen test chart), colour vision (using Ishihara colour plates) and the visual fields (by confrontation and perimetry), and examination of the fundi with the ophthalmoscope. In addition the pupillary responses, mediated by both the optic and the oculomotor nerve (third cranial nerve), must be tested.

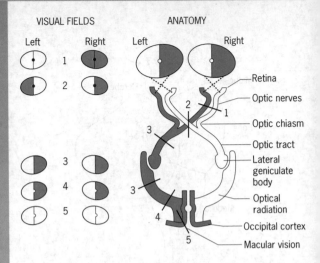

Figure 14.5
Diagram of the visual pathways demonstrating the main field defects. At the optic chiasm, fibres derived from the nasal half of the retina (the temporal visual field) decussate, whereas the fibres from the temporal half of the retina remain uncrossed. Thus the right optic tract is composed of fibres from the right half of each retina which 'see' the left half of both visual fields. Lesion at 1 produces blindness in the right eye with loss of direct light reflex. Lesion at 2 produces bitemporal hemianopia. Lesion at 3 produces homonymous hemianopia with macular involvement. Lesion at 4 produces homonymous hemianopia with macular sparing and a lesion at 5 produces a macular defect. (Adapted from Swash (1989) Hutchison's Clinical Methods, 19th edn. London, Baillière Tindall.)

Visual field defects

There are three main types of visual field defects (Figure 14.5):

- Monocular, caused by damage to the eye or nerve
- Bitemporal, resulting from lesions at the chiasma
- Homonymous hemianopia, caused by lesions in the tract, radiation, or a lesion in the visual cortex.

Optic nerve lesions Unilateral visual loss, starting as a central or paracentral scotoma (an area of depressed vision within the visual field), is characteristic of optic nerve lesions. Complete destruction of one optic nerve results in blindness in that eye and loss of the pupillary light reflex

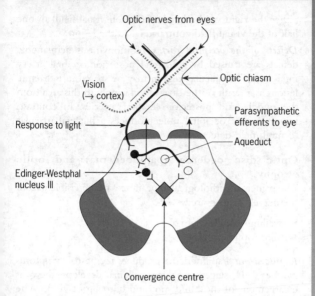

Figure 14.6
Midbrain control of response to light, accommodation and convergence. Afferent impulses in the optic nerve are distributed bilaterally; thus when a light is shone in one eye both pupils will constrict (direct and consensual reflex). The reflex arc for the pupillary response to light is complete within the brain stem and thus the pupils of a patient rendered blind by damage to the occipital lobe will still react when illuminated.

Labels in figure: Optic nerves from eyes; Optic chiasm; Vision (→ cortex); Parasympathetic efferents to eye; Response to light; Aqueduct; Edinger-Westphal nucleus III; Convergence centre

(direct and consensual). Optic nerve lesions result from demyelination (e.g. multiple sclerosis), nerve compression and occlusion of the retinal artery (e.g. in giant cell arteritis). Other causes include trauma, papilloedema, severe anaemia and drugs or toxins, e.g. ethambutol, quinine, tobacco and methyl alcohol.

Defects of the optic chiasm The most common cause of bitemporal hemianopia (i.e. blindness in the outer half of each visual field) is a pituitary adenoma, which compresses the decussating fibres from the nasal half of each eye. Other causes are craniopharyngioma and secondary neoplasm.

Defects of the optic tract and radiation Damage to the tracts or radiation, usually by tumour or a vascular accident, produces a homonymous hemianopia (blindness affecting either the right or the left half of each visual field) in one half of the visual field contralateral to the lesion.

Defects of the occipital cortex Homonymous hemianopic defects are caused by unilateral posterior cerebral artery infarction. The macular region may be spared in ischaemic lesions as a result of the dual blood supply to this area from the middle and posterior cerebral arteries. In contrast, injury to one occipital pole produces a bilateral macular (central) field defect.

Optic disc oedema (papilloedema) and optic atrophy

The principal pathological appearances of the visible part of the nerve, the disc, are:

- Swelling (papilloedema)
- Pallor (optic atrophy).

Papilloedema Papilloedema produces few visual symptoms in the early stages. As disc oedema develops there is enlargement of the blind spot and blurring of vision. The exception is optic neuritis, in which there is early and severe visual loss. The common causes of papilloedema are:

- Raised intracranial pressure, e.g. from a tumour, an abscess or meningitis
- Retinal vein obstruction (thrombosis or compression)
- Optic neuritis (inflammation of the optic nerve, often caused by demyelination)
- Accelerated hypertension.

Optic atrophy Optic atrophy is the end result of many processes that damage the nerve (see Optic nerve lesions, above). The degree of visual loss depends upon the underlying cause.

The pupils

The pupils constrict in response to bright light and convergence (when the centre of focus shifts from a distant to a near object). The parasympathetic efferents that control the constrictor muscle of the pupil arise in the Edinger–Westphal nucleus in the midbrain, and run with the oculomotor (third) nerve to the eye. The Edinger–Westphal nucleus receives afferents from the optic nerve (for the light reflex) and from the convergence centre in the midbrain (Figure 14.6).

Sympathetic fibres which arise in the hypothalamus produce pupillary dilatation. They run from the hypothalamus through the brain stem and cervical cord and emerge from the spinal cord at T1. They then ascend in the neck as the cervical sympathetic chain, and travel with the carotid artery into the head.

The main causes of persistent pupillary dilatation are:

- A third cranial nerve palsy (see later)
- Antimuscarinic eye drops (instilled to facilitate examination of the fundus)
- The myotonic pupil (Holmes Adie pupil): this is a dilated pupil seen most commonly in young women. There is absent (or very delayed) reaction to light and convergence. It is of no pathological significance and may be associated with absent tendon reflexes.

The main causes of persistent pupillary constriction are:

- Parasympatheticomimetic eye drops used in the treatment of glaucoma
- Horner's syndrome, resulting from the interruption of sympathetic fibres to one eye. There is unilateral pupillary constriction, slight ptosis (sympathetic fibres innervate the levator palpebrae superioris), enophthalmos (backward displacement of the eyeball in the orbit) and loss of sweating on the ipsilateral side of the face. A lesion affecting any part of the sympathetic pathway to the eye results in a Horner's syndrome. Causes include diseases of the cervical cord, e.g. syringomyelia, involvement of the T1 root by apical lung cancer (Pancoast's tumour), and lesions in the neck, such as trauma, surgical resection or malignant lymph nodes
- The Argyll Robertson pupil: this is the pupillary abnormality seen mainly in neurosyphilis and diabetes mellitus (page 603). There is a small irregular pupil which is fixed to light but which constricts on convergence
- Opiate addiction

Cranial nerves III–XII

The cranial nerves III–XII may be damaged by lesions in the brain stem or during their intracranial and extracranial course. The causes are listed in Table 14.5. The site of a lesion may be suggested if clinical examination shows the involvement of other cranial nerves at that site, e.g. a seventh-nerve palsy, together with cerebellar signs and involvement of the fifth, sixth and eighth cranial nerves, suggests a lesion of the cerebellopontine angle, commonly a meningioma or acoustic neuroma. In contrast, an isolated seventh-nerve palsy in a patient with a parotid tumour suggests involvement during its extracranial course in the parotid.

The ocular movements and the third, fourth and sixth cranial nerves

These three cranial nerves supply the six external ocular muscles which move the eye in the orbit (Figure 14.7). The abducens nerve (sixth cranial nerve) supplies the lateral rectus muscle and the trochlear (fourth cranial nerve) supplies the superior oblique muscle. All the other extraocular muscles, the sphincter pupillae (parasympathetic fibres) and the levator palpebrae superioris are supplied by the oculomotor nerve (third cranial nerve). Normally the brain stem (with input from the cortex, cerebellum and vestibular nucleus) coordinates the functions of these three cranial nerves, so that eye movement is symmetrical (conjugate gaze). Thus *infranuclear (lower motor neuron)* lesions of the third, fourth and sixth cranial nerves lead to paralysis of individual muscles or muscle groups. *Supranuclear (upper motor neuron)* lesions, e.g. brain-stem involvement by multiple sclerosis, lead to paralysis of conjugate movements of the eyes.

A lesion of the oculomotor nerve causes unilateral complete ptosis, the eye faces 'down and out', and the pupil is dilated and fixed to light and accommodation. This is the picture of a complete third-nerve palsy, of which the most common cause is a 'berry' aneurysm arising in the posterior communicating artery which runs alongside the nerve. Frequently the lesion is partial, particularly in diabetes mellitus, when parasympathetic fibres are spared and the pupil reacts normally. Less common causes are listed in Table 14.5.

In a sixth-nerve lesion the eye cannot be abducted beyond the midline. The unopposed pull of the medial

Table 14.5 Some structural causes of lesions of cranial nerves III–XII

Nerve	Brain stem (UMNL)	Intracranial course (LMNL)	Extracranial course (LMNL)
III IV	Infarction Tumour MS	Posterior communicating artery aneurysm (III) 'Coning' of the temporal lobe (III) Cavernous sinus lesions, e.g. internal carotid artery aneurysm	Orbital trauma
V VI VII VIII	Infarction Tumour MS MND	Cerebellopontine angle tumours Cavernous sinus lesions (V and VI) Petrous temporal bone lesions (VII and VIII)	Neoplastic infiltration of skull base Parotid gland tumour (VII)
IX X XI XII	Infarction Tumour MS MND Syringobulbia	Infiltrating nasopharyngeal carcinoma Skull-base trauma	Tumours and trauma in the neck

MS, multiple sclerosis; MND, motor neuron disease; UMNL, upper motor neuron lesion; LMNL, lower motor neuron lesion.
The nerves may also be involved by any of the causes of mononeuritis multiplex (page 617). Diabetes mellitus particularly affects the third and sixth nerves.

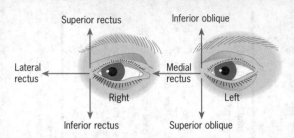

Figure 14.7
The action of the external ocular muscles. (Adapted from Swash (1989)
Hutchison's Clinical Methods. London, Bailliere Tindall.)

rectus muscle causes the eye to turn inward, thereby
producing a squint (squint, or *strabismus*, is the appearance
of the eyes when the visual axes do not meet at the point
of fixation). The patient complains of diplopia or double
vision, which worsens when they attempt to gaze to the
side of the lesion.

Isolated lesions of the trochlear nerve are rare. The patient
complains of diplopia when attempting to look down and
away from the affected side.

Disordered ocular movements may also result from
disease of the ocular muscles (e.g. muscular dystrophy,
dystrophia myotonica) or of the neuromuscular junction
(e.g. myasthenia gravis). In these conditions all the muscles
tend to be affected equally, presenting a generalized
restriction of eye movements.

The trigeminal nerve (fifth cranial nerve)

The trigeminal nerve, through its three divisions, supplies
sensation to the face and scalp as far back as the vertex
(Figure 14.8). It also supplies the mucous membranes of the
sinuses, the nose, mouth, tongue and teeth. The motor root
travels with the mandibular division and supplies the
muscles of mastication.

Diminution of the corneal reflex is often the first sign of
a fifth-nerve lesion. A complete fifth-nerve lesion on one
side causes unilateral sensory loss on the face, tongue and
buccal mucosa. The jaw deviates to the side of the lesion
when the mouth is opened. A brisk jaw jerk is seen with

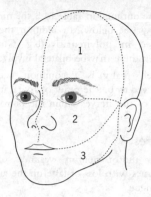

Figure 14.8
Cutaneous distribution of the trigeminal nerve. 1, ophthalmic or first division; 2, maxillary or second division; 3, mandibular or third division.

upper motor neuron lesions, i.e. above the motor nucleus in the pons.

The facial nerve (seventh cranial nerve)

The facial nerve is largely motor in function, supplying the muscles of facial expression. It has, in addition, two major branches: the chorda tympani, which carries taste from the anterior two-thirds of the tongue, and the nerve to the stapedius muscle (this has a damping effect to protect the ear from loud noise). These two branches arise from the facial nerve during its intracranial course through the facial canal of the petrous temporal bone. Therefore, damage to the facial nerve in the temporal bone (e.g. Bell's palsy, trauma, herpes zoster, middle-ear infection) may be associated with undue sensitivity to sounds (hyperacusis) and loss of taste to the anterior two-thirds of the tongue.

Lower motor neuron (LMN) lesions

A unilateral LMN lesion causes weakness of all the muscles of facial expression on the same side as the lesion. The face, especially the angle of the mouth, falls and dribbling occurs from the corner of the mouth. There is weakness of frontalis, the eye will not close and the exposed cornea is at risk of ulceration. The structural causes of a lower motor neuron lesion are outlined in Table 14.5, the most common being Bell's palsy (see below). In addition, the nerve may also be affected in polyneuritis (e.g. Guillain–Barré syndrome), when there may be bilateral involvement.

Bell's palsy Bell's palsy is a common, acute, isolated facial palsy believed to be the result of a viral infection that causes swelling of the nerve within the petrous temporal bone.

Clinical features

There is lower motor neuron weakness of the facial muscles, sometimes with loss of taste on the anterior two-thirds of the tongue.

Investigations

The diagnosis is clinical.

Management

The eyelid must be closed to protect the cornea from ulceration (either adhesive tape or surgery in prolonged cases). Oral prednisolone reduces the proportion of patients with a severe deficit if given at the onset of symptoms.

Prognosis

Most patients recover completely, although 15% are left with a severe permanent weakness.

Ramsay Hunt syndrome This is herpes zoster (shingles) of the geniculate ganglion (the sensory ganglion for taste fibres) situated in the facial canal. There is an LMN facial palsy, with herpetic vesicles in the external auditory meatus and sometimes in the soft palate. Deafness may occur as a result of involvement of the eighth nerve in the facial canal. Treatment is with aciclovir.

Upper motor neuron (UMN) lesions

An upper motor neuron lesion causes weakness of the lower part of the face on the side opposite the lesion. Upper facial muscles are spared because of the bilateral cortical innervation of neurons supplying the upper face. Wrinkling of the forehead (frontalis muscle) and eye closure are normal. The most common cause is a stroke, when there is an associated hemiparesis.

The vestibulocochlear nerve (eighth cranial nerve)

The eighth cranial nerve has two components: cochlear and vestibular, subserving hearing and equilibrium, respectively. The clinical features of a cochlear nerve lesion are sensorineural deafness and tinnitus. The causes of a cochlear nerve lesion are outlined in Table 14.5; however, deafness is very rare in pontine lesions. Sensorineural deafness may also be the result of disease of the cochlea itself: Ménière's disease (see below), drugs (e.g. gentamicin) and presbyacusis (deafness of old age).

The main symptom of a vestibular nerve lesion is vertigo, which may be accompanied by vomiting. Nystagmus is the principal physical sign, often with ataxia (loss of balance).

Vertigo

Vertigo is the definite illusion of movement – a sensation as if the external world were revolving around the patient. It results from disease of the inner ear, the eighth nerve or its central connections (Table 14.6).

Table 14.6 Principal causes of vertigo

Labyrinth	Ménière's disease, vestibular neuronitis, benign positional vertigo
Eighth nerve	Cerebellopontine angle lesions, drugs (e.g. gentamicin)
Brain stem	Tumours, ischaemia/infarction, multiple sclerosis, migraine
Cerebellum	Acute cerebellar lesions

Nystagmus

Nystagmus is a rhythmic oscillation of the eyes, which must be sustained for more than a few beats to be significant. It is a sign of disease of either the ocular or the vestibular system and its connections. Nystagmus is described as either pendular or jerk.

Pendular nystagmus A pendular movement of the eye occurs; there is no rapid phase. It occurs where there is poor visual fixation (i.e. long-standing severe visual impairment) or a congenital lesion.

Jerk nystagmus Jerk nystagmus has a fast and a slow component to the rhythmic movement.

- Horizontal or rotary nystagmus may be either peripheral (middle ear) or central (brain stem and cerebellum) in origin. In peripheral lesions it is usually transient (minutes or hours); in central lesions it is long lasting (weeks, months or more).
- Vertical nystagmus is caused only by central lesions.

Ménière's disease

Ménière's disease is a disorder of the inner ear in which there is dilatation of the membranous labyrinth because of the accumulation of endolymph. The aetiology is unknown and symptoms rarely start before middle age. It is characterized by recurrent attacks, lasting minutes to hours, of vertigo, tinnitus and deafness. Vomiting and nystagmus may accompany an attack. Ultimately deafness develops and the vertigo ceases. Betahistine, a histamine analogue, is useful in some cases. Recurrent severe attacks may require surgery (ultrasonic destruction of the labyrinth or vestibular nerve section).

Vestibular neuronitis

Vestibular neuronitis is believed to be caused by a viral infection affecting the labyrinth. There is a sudden onset of severe vertigo, nystagmus and vomiting, but no deafness. The attack lasts several days or weeks, and treatment is symptomatic with vestibular sedatives (e.g. prochlor-perazine).

Benign positional vertigo

Vertigo occurs with turning and moving. It may follow vestibular neuronitis, head injury or ear infection, and usually lasts for some months; treatment is with vestibular sedatives.

Glossopharyngeal, vagus, accessory and hypoglossal nerves (ninth to 12th cranial nerves)

The lower four cranial nerves (ninth to 12th) which lie in the medulla (the 'bulb') are usually affected together; isolated lesions are rare. A *bulbar palsy* is a weakness of the lower motor neuron type of the muscles supplied by these cranial nerves. There is dysarthria, dysphagia and nasal regurgitation. The tongue is weak, wasted and fasciculating. The most common causes of a bulbar palsy are motor neuron disease (page 614), syringobulbia (page 612) and Guillain–Barré syndrome (page 618). Poliomyelitis is now a rare cause in developed countries. *Pseudobulbar palsy* is an upper motor neuron weakness of the same muscle groups. There is also dysarthria, dysphagia and nasal regurgitation, but the tongue is small and spastic and there is no fasciculation. The jaw jerk is exaggerated and the patient is emotionally labile. In many patients there is a partial palsy with only some of these features. The most common cause of pseudobulbar palsy is a stroke, but it may also occur in motor neuron disease and multiple sclerosis.

....

UNCONSCIOUSNESS AND COMA

The central reticular formation, which extends from the brain stem to the thalamus, influences the state of arousal. It consists of clusters of interconnected neurons throughout the brain stem, with projections to the spinal cord, the hypothalamus, the cerebellum and the cerebral cortex.

Coma is a state of unconsciousness from which the patient cannot be roused. A *stuporous* patient is sleepy but will respond to vigorous stimulation. The Glasgow Coma Scale (Table 14.7) is a simple grading system used to assess the level of consciousness. It is easy to perform and provides an objective assessment of the patient. Serial measurements are particularly useful to monitor the conscious level and thus detect a deterioration which may indicate the need for further investigation or treatment.

Aetiology

Altered consciousness is produced by three types of processes:

- Diffuse metabolic, toxic or neurological disturbance.
- Brain-stem lesions which damage the reticular formation.
- Cortical and cerebellar lesions. These will only cause coma if there is raised intracranial pressure and secondary brain-stem compression, i.e. an indirect effect.

Table 14.7 Glasgow Coma Scale

Category	Score
Eye opening	
Spontaneous	4
To speech	3
To pain	2
None	1
Best verbal response	
Oriented	5
Confused	4
Inappropriate	3
Incomprehensible	2
None	1
Best motor response	
Obeying commands	5
Localizing	4
Flexing	3
Extending	2
None	1

The scores in each category are added up to give an overall score, which may vary from 3 (in the deeply comatose patient) to 14.

The principal causes of coma and stupor are shown in Table 14.8. A common cause of coma is self-poisoning (page 455).

Assessment

Immediate assessment, which takes only seconds, is essential:

- Emergency resuscitation (page 457).
- Clear the airway and intubate if ventilation is inadequate.
- Check the pulse; if absent and rescucitation is appropriate, perform cardiopulmonary resuscitation.
- Check for head injury and, if present, anticipate deterioration.

In all patients presenting in coma a history should be obtained from any witnesses and relatives (e.g. speed of onset of coma, diabetes, drug or alcohol abuse, past medical history, medication and drug abuse).

Further assessment The depth of coma should be noted (Table 14.7) and a full general examination carried out.

Table 14.8 Causes of coma and stupor

Toxins	Drug overdose, alcohol, anaesthetic gases, carbon monoxide poisoning
Metabolic	Hypo- or hyperglycaemia Severe hypo- or hypercalcaemia Severe hypo- or hypernatraemia Hypoxic/ischaemic brain injury Hypoadrenalism Hypothyroidism Renal failure Hepatic failure Respiratory failure with CO_2 retention
Diffuse neurological disease	Subarachnoid haemorrhage Hypertensive encephalopathy Encephalitis, cerebral malaria
Brain-stem lesions	Tumour Haemorrhage/infarction Demyelination, e.g. multiple sclerosis Trauma Wernicke–Korsakoff syndrome
Cortical/cerebellar lesions	Tumour Haemorrhage/infarction Abscess Encephalitis

Clues to the cause of coma should be looked for, for example the smell of alcohol or ketones (in diabetic ketoacidosis) on the breath, needle-track marks in a drug abuser, or a Medic-Alert bracelet, as carried by some diabetic people and patients on steroid replacement therapy. The neurological examination must include:

- The head and neck: the patient should be examined for evidence of trauma and neck stiffness (indicating meningitis or subarachnoid haemorrhage)
- The pupils: the size of the pupils and their reaction to light must be recorded:
  – A *fixed dilated pupil* indicates herniation of the temporal lobe ('coning') through the tentorial hiatus and compression of the third cranial nerve (page 565). This indicates the need for urgent neurosurgical intervention.
  – *Bilateral fixed dilated pupils* are a cardinal sign of brain death. They also occur in deep coma of any cause, but

particularly coma caused by barbiturate intoxication or hypothermia.

– *Pinpoint pupils* are seen with opiate overdose or with pontine lesions that interrupt the sympathetic pathways to the dilator muscle of the pupil.

– *Midpoint pupils* that react to light are characteristic in coma of metabolic origin and coma caused by most CNS-depressant drugs.

• The fundi: these should be examined for papilloedema, which indicates raised intracranial pressure.

• Eye movements: cerebral hemisphere lesions may produce conjugate deviation of the eyes towards the side of the lesion ('the eyes look *towards the normal limbs*'). In a pontine brain-stem lesion, sustained conjugate lateral gaze occurs away from the site of the lesion (*towards the paralysed limbs*).

Passive head rotation normally causes conjugate ocular deviation in the direction opposite to the induced head movement (doll's head reflex). This reflex is lost in very deep coma and is absent in brain-stem lesions.

• Motor responses: asymmetry of spontaneous limb movements, tone and reflexes indicates a unilateral cerebral hemisphere or brain-stem lesion. The plantar responses are often both extensor in coma of any cause.

Investigations

In many cases the cause of coma will be evident from the history, and examination and appropriate investigations should then be carried out. However, if the cause is still unclear further investigations will be necessary.

Blood and urine tests

• Serum and urine for drug analysis, e.g. salicylates
• Serum for urea and electrolytes, liver biochemistry and calcium
• Blood glucose
• Arterial blood gases
• Thyroid function tests and serum cortisol
• Blood cultures.

Radiology CT of the head may indicate an otherwise unsuspected mass lesion or intracranial haemorrhage.

CSF Examination Lumbar puncture (page 652) is performed if subarachnoid haemorrhage or meningoencephalitis is suspected and only if a mass lesion is excluded on CT.

Management

The immediate management consists of treatment of the cause, careful nursing, meticulous attention to the airway and frequent observation to detect any change in vital function.

Prognosis

The outlook depends upon the cause of coma. A cause must be established before decisions are made about withdrawing supportive care.

Brain death

Brain death means the irreversible loss of the capacity for consciousness, combined with the irreversible loss of the capacity to breathe. Two independent senior medical opinions are required for the diagnosis to be made. The three main criteria for diagnosis are as follows:

• Irremedial structural brain damage. A disorder that can cause brain-stem death, e.g. intracranial haemorrhage, must have been diagnosed with certainty. Patients with hypothermia, significant electrolyte imbalance or drug overdose are excluded, but may be reassessed when these are corrected.
• Absent motor responses to any stimulus. Spinal reflexes may be present.
• Absent brain-stem function, demonstrated by:
  – Pupils fixed and unresponsive to light
  – Absent corneal, gag and cough reflexes
  – Absent doll's head reflex (page 574)
  – Absent caloric responses: ice-cold water run into the external auditory meatus causes nystagmus when brain-stem function is normal.
  – Lack of spontaneous respiration.

In suitable cases, and provided the patient was carrying a donor card and/or the consent of relatives has been obtained, the organs of those in whom brain-stem death has been established may be used for transplantation.

CEREBROVASCULAR DISEASE

Stroke

Definitions

Stroke is a focal neurological deficit (e.g. hemiplegia) lasting longer than 24 hours which is the result of a vascular lesion.

A completed stroke is when the neurological deficit has reached its maximum (usually within 6 hours).

Stroke in evolution is when the symptoms and signs are getting worse (usually within 24 hours of onset).

A minor stroke is one in which the patient recovers without a significant neurological deficit, usually within 1 week.

Transient ischaemic attack is a focal deficit lasting less than 24 hours and from which there is complete neurological recovery.

Epidemiology

Stroke is the third most common cause of death in the UK and the most common cause of physical disability in adults. The incidence rises steeply with age; it is uncommon in those under 40 years. It is slightly more common in men.

Pathogenesis

A stroke is caused by cerebral infarction or cerebral haemorrhage. The clinical picture of 'stroke' may also be caused by a space-occupying lesion in the brain, e.g. a tumour or abscess, although the onset of symptoms and signs is usually much slower. In young adults one-fifth of strokes are caused by dissection of a major extracranial or intracranial artery, associated with trauma to, or manipulation of the neck.

Cerebral infarction may be the result of:

- Thrombosis at the site of an atheromatous plaque in a major cerebral vessel
- Emboli arising from atheromatous plaques in the carotid/vertebrobasilar arteries, or from cardiac mural thrombi (e.g. following myocardial infarction), or from the left atrium in atrial fibrillation.

Rarely cerebral infarction is the result of severe hypotension (e.g. systolic blood pressure <75 mmHg), vasculitis, meningovascular syphilis, or emboli from vegetations in infective endocarditis.

Cerebral haemorrhage (15% of strokes) In most cases this is the result of rupture of an intracranial microaneurysm (Charcot–Bouchard aneurysms) in a hypertensive patient.

Risk factors

The major risk factors for thromboembolic stroke are those for atheroma, i.e. hypertension, diabetes mellitus, cigarette smoking and hyperlipidaemia. Others are obesity, oestrogen-containing oral contraceptives, alcohol and polycythaemia.

Clinical features

The history and physical examination in all stroke patients must include a search for risk factors (see above) and source of emboli (?atrial fibrillation, valve lesion, carotid bruits in the neck).

In most patients symptoms and signs develop over a few minutes and reach maximum disability within 1–2 hours. It is usually impossible to distinguish clinically between haemorrhage and infarction; cerebral haemorrhage however, tends, to be accompanied by a severe headache and produces a more diffuse neurological deficit.

The neurological deficit produced by the occlusion of a vessel may be predicted by a knowledge of neuroanatomy and vascular supply (Figures 14.1, 14.9, 14.10). In practice it is less clear-cut because of collateral supply to brain areas.

Cerebral hemisphere infarcts The most common stroke is the hemiplegia caused by infarction of the internal capsule (the narrow zone of motor and sensory fibres that converges on the brain stem from the cerebral cortex; Figure 14.1) following occlusion of a branch of the middle cerebral artery. The signs are contralateral to the lesion: hemiplegia (arm > leg), hemisensory loss, upper motor neuron facial weakness and hemianopia. Initially the patient has a hypotonic hemiplegia with decreased reflexes; within days this develops into a spastic hemiplegia with increased reflexes and an extensor plantar response. Weakness may recover gradually over days or months.

(a)

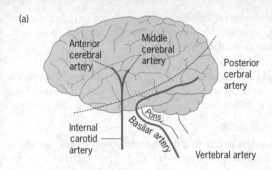

(b)

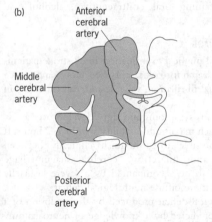

Figure 14.9
The arterial supply to the brain. **(a)** The area above the dotted line is
supplied by the internal carotid artery and the area below the line is supplied
by the vertebral artery. **(b)** A coronal section through the brain. The anterior
cerebral artery suplies the medial surface of the hemisphere and the middle
cerebral artery supplies the lateral surface of the hemisphere, including the
internal capsule.

Occlusion of the main trunk of the middle cerebral artery
produces contralateral hemiplegia, hemisensory loss and
aphasia (if located in the dominant hemisphere). Lacunar
infarcts are small infarcts that produce localized deficits, e.g.
pure motor stroke, pure sensory stroke.

Brain-stem infarction Brain-stem infarction causes complex
patterns of dysfunction depending on the sites involved:

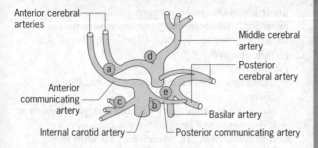

Figure 14.10
The main cerebral arteries showing the Circle of Willis and the most common sites for berry aneurysms. Frequency of occurrence, a–e (decreasing order). a, anterior communicating artery; b, origin of the posterior communicating artery; c, trifurcation of the middle cerebral artery; d, termination of the internal carotid artery; e, basilar artery.

In the figure: Anterior cerebral arteries; Middle cerebral artery; Posterior cerebral artery; Anterior communicating artery; Basilar artery; Internal carotid artery; Posterior communicating artery.

- The lateral medullary syndrome, the most common of the brain-stem vascular syndromes, is caused by occlusion of the posterior inferior cerebellar artery. It presents with sudden vomiting and vertigo, ipsilateral Horner's syndrome, facial numbness, cerebellar signs and palatal paralysis with a diminished gag reflex. On the side opposite the lesion there is loss of pain and temperature.
- Coma as a result of involvement of the reticular formation.
- Pseudobulbar palsy (page 571) may be caused by brain-stem infarction.

Multi-infarct dementia is a syndrome caused by multiple small cortical infarcts, resulting in generalized intellectual loss; there is a stepwise progression with each infarct. The final picture is of dementia, pseudobulbar palsy and a shuffling gait resembling Parkinson's disease.

Investigations

Stroke is usually a straightforward clinical diagnosis. The purpose of the investigation is to differentiate between haemorrhage and infarction, and to identify aetiological or risk factors which can be eliminated or reduced.

- CT or magnetic resonance imaging is indicated in virtually all patients. Imaging will demonstrate the site of the lesion, differentiate between a haemorrhage and infarction, and occasionally may show unexpected mass lesions, e.g. tumour or abscess, leading to the clinical picture of a stroke.

- Further investigations:
  - Blood glucose to identify patients with diabetes mellitus
  - Haemoglobin to identify patients with polycythaemia
  - ESR, which will be raised in the few cases of endocarditis, giant cell arteritis and vasculitis that present with stroke
  - ECG may show evidence of a recent myocardial infarction or atrial fibrillation
  - Syphilis serology will identify the rare cases of meningovascular syphilis.
- Carotid Doppler and duplex scanning are indicated in patients with a cerebral infarct who may be suitable for surgery (see below), to look for carotid atheroma and stenosis.
- Angiography of the carotid territory may be considered in younger patients to define stenotic lesions more accurately before surgery.

Management

Many mild strokes may be managed at home if social circumstances allow.

Immediate therapy is supportive, with maintenance of hydration, frequent turning to avoid pressure sores, and other measures as for the unconscious patient (page 572). An expanding intracerebral haematoma causing deepening coma (with eventual coning) should be considered for urgent neurosurgical removal.

Intravenous administration of the thrombolytic agent, rt-PA (page 184), has been shown in a clinical trial to reduce mortality and neurological deficit when given to patients within 3 hours of the onset of ischaemic stroke. However, in the UK most patients would not reach hospital and have a CT scan within this time frame.

Secondary prevention This involves advice and treatment to reverse risk factors. Control of hypertension is the single most important factor in the prevention of stroke.

- Aspirin (75 mg daily) should be given to all patients with a stroke caused by cerebral infarction. A CT scan should be performed before starting aspirin therapy to exclude haemorrhage.
- Long-term anticoagulation with warfarin is indicated in cerebral infarction when there is atrial fibrillation, with some valvular lesions (uninfected) or dilated cardiomyopathy.
- Internal carotid endarterectomy reduces the risk of recurrent stroke (by 75%) in patients who have had an infarct and who have internal carotid artery stenosis which narrows the arterial lumen by more than 70%. It is considered in patients with a non-disabling stroke who are likely to have some recoverable function.

In all stroke patients rehabilitation plays an important part of management. Physiotherapy is particularly useful in the first few months in reducing spasticity, relieving contractures and teaching patients to use walking aids. Following recovery, the occupational therapist plays a valuable role in assessing the requirement for and arranging the provision of various aids and modifications in the home, such as stair rails, hoists, or wheelchairs etc.

Prognosis

Between 30% and 50% of patients will die in the first month following a stroke, although the prognosis is much worse for bleeds than for infarction. About 10% of patients will suffer a recurrent stroke within 1 year, and of initial survivors only about 30–40% are alive after 3 years. Of the long-term survivors, one-third have a severe disability requiring permanent institutional care.

Transient ischaemic attacks

Transient ischaemic attacks (TIAs) are less common than strokes but are an important predictive factor for stroke and myocardial infarction.

Aetiology

The risk factors and causes of TIAs are the same as those for thromboembolic stroke. Most are the result of emboli (which subsequently lyse) arising from internal carotid artery atheromas.

Clinical features

There is a sudden loss of function in one region of the brain which, by definition, resolves in 24 hours. Symptoms and signs depend on the site of the brain involved (Table 14.9). The history and physical examination must include a search for risk factors and possible sources of emboli.

Table 14.9 Features of TIAs in different arterial territories

Carotid system	Vertebrobasilar system
Amaurosis fugax	Diplopia, vertigo, vomiting
Aphasia	Choking and dysarthria
Hemiparesis	Ataxia
Hemisensory loss	Hemisensory loss
Hemianopic visual loss	Hemianopic visual loss
	Transient global amnesia
	Loss of consciousness (rare)

Amaurosis fugax is a sudden loss of vision in one eye as a result of the passage of emboli through the retinal arteries. Transient global amnesia is a condition in which there are sudden episodes of amnesia associated with confusion, probably caused by ischaemia in the posterior circulation.

The investigation and management of TIAs is similar to that of stroke. Aspirin (75 mg daily) reduces the incidence of subsequent stroke and is given to most patients.

Primary intracranial haemorrhage

Intracerebral haemorrhage

This is discussed under Stroke, above.

Subarachnoid haemorrhage

The term 'subarachnoid haemorrhage' (SAH) describes spontaneous rather than traumatic arterial bleeding into the subarachnoid space.

Incidence

SAH accounts for 10% of cerebrovascular disease and has an annual incidence of 15 per 100 000. The mean age of patients at presentation is 50 years.

Aetiology

SAH is caused by rupture of:

- Saccular ('berry') aneurysms in 70% of cases. These are acquired lesions that are most commonly located at the branching points (Figure 14.10) of the major arteries coursing through the subarachnoid space at the base of the brain (the Circle of Willis).
- Congenital arteriovenous malformations in 10%.

In 20% of cases no lesion can be found.

Clinical features

Most intracranial aneurysms remain asymptomatic until they rupture and cause a subarachnoid haemorrhage. Some, however, become symptomatic because of a mass effect, and the most common symptom is a painful third-nerve palsy. The typical presentation of subarachnoid haemorrhage is the sudden onset of severe headache, often accompanied by nausea and vomiting, and sometimes loss of consciousness. On examination there may be signs of meningeal irritation (neck stiffness and a positive Kernig's sign), focal neurological signs and subhyaloid haemorrhages (between the retina and vitreous membrane) with or without papilloedema. Some patients have experienced small warning headaches a few days before the major bleed.

Investigation

- CT scan shows subarachnoid or intraventricular blood in 95% of cases undergoing scanning within 24 hours of the haemorrhage.
- Lumbar puncture is indicated if there is a strong clinical suspicion of a subarachnoid haemorrhage but the CT scan is normal. Xanthochromia (yellow discoloration caused by the breakdown of blood products) of the supernatant after centrifugation of the CSF is diagnostic of a subarachnoid haemorrhage.

Patients who are potentially fit for surgery should be referred urgently to a neurosurgical unit for cerebral angiography to establish the source and site of bleeding.

Management

Immediate management consists of bed rest and supportive measures with cautious control of hypertension. Oral or intravenous nimodipine (a calcium channel blocker) is given to reduce cerebral artery spasm, an important cause of ischaemia and further neurological deterioration. Surgery (clipping the neck of the aneurysm at craniotomy) is indicated for patients likely to make a reasonable recovery. Endovascular therapy, in which soft metallic coils are placed within the lumen of the aneurysm to promote local thrombus formation, is emerging as a promising alternative to surgical clipping in selected cases.

Prognosis

Approximately 50% of patients die suddenly or soon after the haemorrhage. A further 10–20% die in the early weeks in hospital from further bleeding. The outcome is variable in the survivors; some patients are left with major neurological deficits.

Subdural haematoma

Subdural haematoma (SDH) occurs when blood accumulates in the subdural space following the rupture of a vein running from the hemisphere to the sagittal sinus. It is almost always the result of head injury, often minor, and the latent interval between injury and symptoms may be weeks or months. Elderly patients and alcoholics are particularly susceptible because they are accident prone and their atrophic brains make the connecting veins more susceptible to rupture. The main clinical symptoms are headache, drowsiness and confusion, which may fluctuate. The diagnosis is usually made on CT and treatment is by surgical removal of the haematoma.

Extradural haemorrhage

Extradural haematomas are caused by injuries that fracture the temporal bone and rupture the underlying middle meningeal artery. Clinically there is the picture of a head injury with a brief period of unconsciousness followed by a lucid interval of recovery. This is then followed by rapid deterioration with focal neurological signs and a deterioration in conscious level if surgical drainage is not carried out.

EPILEPSY AND OTHER CAUSES OF RECURRENT LOSS OF CONSCIOUSNESS

Epilepsy

An epileptic seizure is a convulsion or transient abnormal event experienced by the subject as a result of a paroxysmal discharge of cerebral neurons. Epilepsy, by definition, is the continuing tendency to have such seizures.

Epidemiology

Epilepsy is a common condition, with 3% of the UK population having two or more seizures during their lives.

Classification

Epilepsy is classified according to the clinical type of seizure (Table 14.10). They are broadly divided into generalized seizures, in which abnormal electrical activity is widespread in the brain, and partial seizures, in which the electrical abnormality is focal (e.g. temporal lobe), although these may later become generalized.

Table 14.10 The classification of epilepsy

Generalized seizures
Tonic–clonic (grand mal)
Absence seizures (petit mal)
Myoclonic seizures (rare form of epilepsy with involuntary muscle jerks)

Partial seizures
Simple partial seizures (no impairment of consciousness), e.g. Jacksonian seizures
Complex partial seizures (with impairment of consciousness), e.g. temporal lobe epilepsy

- Tonic–clonic: there is a sudden onset of a rigid tonic phase followed by a convulsion (clonic phase) in which the muscles jerk rhythmically. The episode lasts typically for seconds to minutes, may be associated with tongue biting and incontinence, and is followed by a period of drowsiness or coma.
- Typical absences (petit mal): this is usually a disorder of childhood in which the child ceases activity, stares and pales for a few seconds only. It is characterized by 3-Hz spike and wave activity on the electroencephalogram (EEG).

- Jacksonian (motor) seizures: these simple partial seizures originate in the motor cortex and result in jerking movements, typically beginning in the corner of the mouth or thumb and index finger, and spreading to involve the limbs on the opposite side of the epileptic focus. Paralysis of the involved limbs may follow for several hours (Todd's paralysis).
- Temporal lobe seizures: these complex partial seizures are associated with olfactory and visual hallucinations, feelings of unreality (jamais-vu) or undue familiarity (déjà-vu) with the surroundings.

Precipitating factors

Flashing lights or a flickering television screen may provoke an attack in susceptible patients.

Aetiology

No cause for epilepsy is found in over 75% of patients. About 30% of patients have a first-degree relative with epilepsy, although the exact mode of inheritance is unknown. Head injury, brain surgery, cerebral tumours and infarction are common predisposing factors. Inflammatory conditions of the brain, such as encephalitis, chronic meningitis (e.g. TB) and cerebral abscess, may sometimes present initially with seizures. Drug overdose, alcohol withdrawal and metabolic disturbances, e.g. hypoglycaemia, hypoxia, hypocalcaemia and hyponatraemia, are other causes.

Investigations

The diagnosis is often made clinically; a detailed description of the attack from an eye witness is invaluable.

- The electroencephalogram (EEG) is the single most useful test in the diagnosis of epilepsy, but the recording is frequently normal between attacks. During a seizure the EEG is almost always abnormal and is shown typically by a cortical spike focus (e.g. in a temporal lobe) or by generalized spike and wave activity.
- CT or magnetic resonance imaging should be performed in all patients other than children to exclude an underlying lesion. Even in adults, however, the pick-up rate for treatable lesions is very low.

Management

The emergency treatment is to ensure that the patient harms him- or herself as little as possible and that the airway remains patent.

Anticonvulsant drugs are indicated in recurrent seizures; some authorities will treat after a single seizure. Phenytoin, carbamazepine and sodium valproate are generally the most effective drugs prescribed, although phenobarbitone, primidone and clonazepam are also used. Table 14.11 gives a suggested scheme for treatment and lists the idiosyncratic side effects (i.e. non-dose related), which tend to be more common than dose-related effects. Intoxication with all anticonvulsants causes a syndrome of ataxia, nystagmus and dysarthria. Side effects of chronic administration of phenytoin (gum hypertrophy, hypertrichosis, osteomalacia and folate deficiency) are reduced by maintaining serum levels within the therapeutic range. Phenytoin is a potent hepatic enzyme inducer and will reduce the efficacy of the contraceptive pill.

Vigabatrin, lamotrigine and gabapentin are more recently introduced drugs which are generally reserved as second-line agents in those not satisfactorily controlled with other antiepileptics. The question of withdrawal of drug therapy is often raised by patients. Gradual withdrawal of drugs should only be considered when the patient has been seizure-free for at least 2 years. Many patients will have

Table 14.11 A typical scheme for anticonvulsant treatment

Seizure type	Drug	Major side effects of drug treatment
Generalized tonic–clonic seizures	Phenytoin	Rashes, blood dyscrasias, lymphadenopathy
Generalized absence seizures	Sodium valproate	Anorexia, hair loss, liver damage
Partial seizures	Carbamazepine Sodium valproate	Rashes, leukopenia
Second-line drugs	Lamotrigine Vigabatrin Gabapentin	Stevens – Johnson syndrome (toxic necrolysis) Retinal damage

further fits, resulting in a threat to employment and driving (see below).

Neurosurgical treatment (e.g. amputation of the anterior temporal lobe) may be of value in those with poorly controlled epilepsy with a clearly defined focus of abnormal electrical activity.

Advice to patients

Patients should restrict their lives as little as possible but follow simple advice, e.g. avoid swimming alone, avoid dangerous sports, such as rock climbing, leave the door open when taking a bath. In the UK patients with epilepsy (whether on or off treatment) may drive a motor vehicle (but not a heavy goods or public service vehicle), provided that they have had a seizure-free period of 2 years or that seizures have only occurred at night for the last 3 years.

Status epilepticus

Status epilepticus is a medical emergency which exists when seizures follow each other without recovery of consciousness. When grand mal seizures follow one another, there is a significant risk of death from cardiorespiratory failure. Precipitating factors in a known epileptic include intercurrent illness, alcohol abuse, abruptly stopping antiepileptic treatment and poor compliance with therapy; 60% of all episodes occur in patients without any history of epilepsy. The initial treatment of generalized convulsive status epilepticus is with intravenous lorazepam or rectal diazepam. Lorazepam may cause respiratory depression and hypotension, and facilities for resuscitation should be available. If lorazepam fails to control the seizures, an infusion of phenytoin or phenobarbitone should be started. Rapid infusion of phenytoin may cause cardiac dysrhythmias, and full ECG monitoring is necessary during the infusion. Paraldehyde, given rectally or by intramuscular injection, is occasionally used if intravenous access if difficult or where facilities for resuscitation are poor (it causes little respiratory depression). Management of status epilepticus is summarized in Emergency Box 14.1. Once status is controlled, all of these drug treatments must be followed by regular anticonvulsant therapy to present subsequent fits. Intravenous treatment is withdrawn when anticonvulsant therapy is established.

Emergency

General measures
- Secure the airway: remove false teeth and insert oropharyngeal tube
- Administer 60% oxygen
- Secure venous access: many anticonvulsants cause phlebitis, so choose a large vein
- Glucose, 50 ml of 50% i.v. if hypoglycaemia is a possibility
- Thiamine, 250 mg by slow i.v. injection if patient is a chronic alcohol abuser

Control of seizures
- Lorazepam 0.1 mg/kg by slow (2 mg/min) intravenous injection. Give rectal diazepam (10–20 mg) or intramuscular midazolm (0.2 mg/kg) if intravenous access difficult.
- If seizures continue consider i.v. phenytoin; chlormethiazole is sometimes used.
    Phenytoin Loading dose of 15 mg/kg at a rate not exceeding 50 mg/min. Give a further bolus up to a total loading dose of 30 mg/kg if seizures persist. Continue with a maintenance dose of 100 mg i.v. at intervals of 6–8 hours; if seizures continue use:
    Phenobarbitone 15 mg/kg at a rate not exceeding 100 mg/min and repeated at intervals of 6–8 hours if necessary
    Chlormethiazole (0.8%) 40–120 mg/min (5–15 ml) up to a maximum total dose of 320–800 mg to control seizures, followed by a continuous infusion at the lowest dose required to control seizures, usually 4–8 mg/min, occasionally used.
- If seizures continue despite these measures the patient is given a general anaesthetic, such as thiopentone or propofol, and management is continued with full anaesthetic support.

Investigations
Serum anticonvulsant levels, blood glucose, serum electrolytes including calcium and magnesium. Consider brain CT scan, lumbar puncture and blood cultures, depending on clinical circumstances.

Emergency Box 14.1
Management and investigation of status epilepticus

....
EXTRAPYRAMIDAL DISEASE – PARKINSON'S DISEASE AND OTHER MOVEMENT DISORDERS

The extrapyramidal system is a general term for the basal ganglia and their connections with other brain areas, particularly those concerned with movement. The overall function of this system is the initiation and modulation of movement. Clinically, extrapyramidal disorders are broadly classified into the akinetic–rigid syndromes, where there is loss of movement with increase in muscle tone, and dyskinesias, where there are added movements outside voluntary control (Table 14.12). Parkinson's disease is the most common of these movement disorders.

Table 14.12 A classification of movement disorders

Akinetic–rigid syndromes
Idiopathic Parkinson's disease
Drug-induced parkinsonism, e.g. phenothiazines
MPTP-induced parkinsonism
Postencephalitic parkinsonism
'Parkinsonism plus'
Childhood akinetic–rigid syndromes, e.g. Wilson's disease and athetoid
  cerebral palsy

Dyskinesias
Benign essential tremor
Chorea
Hemiballismus
Myoclonus
Tick or habit spasms
Torsion dystonias

MPTP, methylphenyl tetrahydropyridine.

Akinetic rigid syndromes

Idiopathic Parkinson's disease
The clinical features of Parkinson's disease principally result from the depletion of dopamine-containing neurons in the substantia nigra of the basal ganglia and a relative excess of acetylcholine stimulation.

Epidemiology

The disease usually presents in elderly people, the prevalence rising to 1 in 200 in those over 70.

Aetiology

The cause of the disease is unknown. MPTP (methylphenyl tetrahydropyridine, an impurity produced during illegal synthesis of opiates) produces severe and irreversible parkinsonism. Survivors of an encephalitis epidemic (encephalitis lethargica 1918–1930), which was presumed to be a viral disease, developed parkinsonism. There is no evidence, however, that idiopathic Parkinson's disease is caused by an environmental toxin or an infective agent, though interestingly the disease is less prevalent in tobacco smokers than in lifelong abstainers.

Clinical features

There is a combination of tremor, rigidity and akinesia (slow movements), together with changes in posture. The features of Parkinson's disease may be unilateral initially, but the disease subsequently progresses to involve both sides of the body.

- *Tremor.* This is a characteristic 4–7 Hz resting tremor (*cf* cerebellar disease), usually most obvious in the hands ('pill-rolling' of the thumb and fingers), improved by voluntary movement and made worse by anxiety.
- *Rigidity* refers to the increase in tone in the limbs and trunk. The limbs resist passive extension throughout movement (lead-pipe rigidity, or cog-wheel when combined with tremor), in contrast to the hypertonia of an upper motor neuron lesion (page 552), where resistance falls away as the movement continues (clasp-knife).
- *Akinesia.* There is difficulty in initiating movement (starting to walk, or rising from a chair). The face is expressionless and unblinking and may give the appearance of depression. Speech is slow and monotonous. The writing becomes small (micrographia) and tends to tail off at the end of a line.
- *Postural changes.* A stoop is characteristic and the gait is shuffling, festinant and with poor arm swinging. The posture is sometimes called 'simian', to describe the forward flexion, immobility of the arms and lack of facial expression. Balance is poor, with a tendency to fall.

Other features include dribbling of saliva, dysphagia, constipation, depression and dementia in the later stages.

There is gradual progression of the disease over 10–15 years, with death resulting most commonly from bronchopneumonia.

Investigations

The diagnosis is clinical. Investigations for other akinetic–rigid syndromes are only necessary in an atypical case, e.g. a young patient.

Management

Levodopa The treatment of choice is the dopamine precursor levodopa (L-dopa), in combination with a peripheral decarboxylase inhibitor, e.g. Madopar (L-dopa plus benserazide) or Sinemet (L-dopa plus carbidopa). This combined therapy reduces the peripheral side effects, principally nausea, of L-dopa and its metabolites. Over the years therapy may become less effective, even with increasing doses. Patients may also switch between periods of dopamine-induced dyskinesias (choreas and dystonic movements) and periods of immobility ('on–off' syndrome). This problem may be ameliorated by slow-release L-dopa; frequent small doses of L-dopa, or the addition of other antiparkinsonian drugs.

Other treatments

* Bromocriptine, a dopamine agonist
* Selegiline – a type B monoamine oxidase inhibitor – inhibits the catabolism of dopamine in the brain
* Amantadine increases the synthesis and release of dopamine and has a weak antiparkinsonian effect
* Anticholinergic drugs, e.g. benzhexol, have most effect on tremor and little effect on akinesia. They often cause mental confusion.

Surgical treatment Surgery to transplant dopamine-producing cells (fetal or autologous adrenal medulla) has not produced significant clinical improvement.

Other akinetic–rigid syndromes

Drug-induced parkinsonism

Reserpine, phenothiazines and butyrophenones block dopamine receptors and may induce a parkinsonian syndrome with slowness and rigidity, but usually with little tremor. These syndromes tend not to progress, they respond poorly to L-dopa, and the correct management is to stop the drug.

'Parkinsonism plus'

This describes rare disorders in which there is parkinsonism and evidence of a separate pathology. Progressive supranuclear palsy is the most common disorder and consists of axial rigidity, dementia and signs of parkinsonism, together with a striking inability to move the eyes vertically or laterally. There is a poor response to L-dopa.

Dyskinesias

Benign essential tremor

This is usually a familial (autosomal dominant) tremor of the arms and head (titubation) which occurs most frequently in elderly people. Unlike the tremor of Parkinson's disease it is not usually present at rest, but is most obvious when the hands adopt a posture such as holding a glass or a spoon. It is made worse by anxiety and improved by alcohol and propranolol.

Chorea

Chorea is a continuous flow of jerky, quasi-purposive movements, flitting from one part of the body to another. They may interfere with voluntary movements but cease during sleep. The causes of chorea are listed in Table 14.13. Treatment is with phenothiazines or tetrabenazine.

Huntington's disease

Huntington's disease is a rare autosomal dominant condition with full penetrance; the abnormal gene is on the short arm of chromosome 4. There is loss of neurons within the basal ganglia, leading to depletion of GABA (γ-aminobutyric acid) and acetylcholine but sparing dopamine. Symptoms begin in middle age and there is then a relentlessly progressive course, with chorea and personality change preceding dementia and death. There is no treatment that arrests the progression of the disease, and the management is symptomatic treatment of chorea and genetic counselling of family members.

Table 14.13 Causes of chorea

Huntington's disease

Sydenham's chorea (see Rheumatic fever)

Benign hereditary chorea in elderly people

Drug induced
  Phenytoin
  L-Dopa
  Alcohol

Systemic disease
  Thyrotoxicosis
  Systemic lupus erythematosus
  Pregnancy (chorea gravidarum)

Other CNS diseases
  Stroke
  Trauma
  Tumour

Hemiballismus

Hemiballismus (also called hemiballism) describes violent swinging movements of one side of the body, usually caused by infarction or haemorrhage in the contralateral subthalamic nucleus. Treatment is with tetrabenazine.

Myoclonus

Myoclonus is the sudden, involuntary jerking of a single muscle or group of muscles. The most common example is benign essential myoclonus, which is the sudden jerking of a limb or the body on falling asleep. Myoclonus may also occur with epilepsy and some encephalopathies.

Tics

Tics are brief, repeated stereotypical movements, usually involving the face and shoulders. Unlike other involuntary movements it is usually possible for the patient to control tics.

Dystonias

Dystonias are prolonged spasms of muscle contraction. They may occasionally occur as a symptom of neurological disease, e.g. Wilson's disease, but are usually of unknown cause and occur without other neurological problems, e.g. blepharospasm (spasms of forced blinking) or spasmodic torticollis (the head is turned and held to one side or drawn backwards or forwards). The treatment of choice for many dystonias is the injection of minute amounts of botulinum toxin (which inhibits the release of acetylcholine from nerve endings) into the muscle. Acute dystonic reactions are seen with phenothiazines, butyrophenones and metoclopramide, and can occur after a single dose of the drug. Spasmodic torticollis, trismus and oculogyric crises (i.e. episodes of sustained upward gaze) may occur. Acute dystonias respond promptly to an anticholinergic drug administered by intravenous or intramuscular injection, e.g. benztropine (1–2 mg) or procyclidine (5 mg).

Multiple sclerosis

Multiple sclerosis (MS) is a common disease of unknown cause in which there are multiple areas of demyelination within the brain and spinal cord. These are 'disseminated in time and place' (hence the old name 'disseminated sclerosis').

Epidemiology

The most common age of onset is between 20 and 35 years, the disease being more common in women. The prevalence varies widely (6 per 10 000 in England); it is rare in tropical countries.

Aetiology

The aetiology is unknown; viruses and autoimmune mechanisms have been implicated. The disease is more common in family members, although there is no clear-cut pattern of inheritance.

Pathology

The essential features are perivenular plaques of demyelination which have a predilection for the following sites within the brain:

- Optic nerves
- Brain stem and cerebellar connections
- Cervical cord
- Periventricular region.

The peripheral nerves are never affected.

Clinical features

Symptoms are variable and characteristically appear suddenly, before resolving either partially or completely. Inflammation of the optic nerve produces blurred vision and pain in and around the eye. A lesion in the optic nerve head produces disc swelling (optic neuritis) and pallor (optic atrophy) following the attack. When inflammation occurs in the optic nerve further away from the eye (retrobulbar neuritis) there are often no ophthalmoscopic features. Brain-stem demyelination produces diplopia, vertigo, dysphagia and nystagmus.

In some patients there will only be one or two attacks with little residual neurological deficit, and they remain very well for years. At the other extreme, in some patients an increasing neurological deficit accumulates and spastic tetraparesis, ataxia, brain-stem signs, blindness, incontinence and dementia characterize the final stages. Death follows from recurrent urinary tract infection, uraemia and bronchopneumonia.

Differential diagnosis

Initially individual plaques (e.g. in the optic nerve, brain stem or cord) may cause diagnostic difficulty and must be distinguished from compressive, inflammatory, mass or vascular lesions. In young patients with a relapsing and remitting course the diagnosis is straightforward, as few other diseases produce this clinical picture.

Investigations

The diagnosis is made on the basis of clinical findings taken in combination with the findings on investigation.

- Radiology. MRI is the first-line investigation and shows plaques, particularly in the periventricular area and brain stem. Lesions are rarely visible on CT scanning.
- Electrophysiological tests. Visual, auditory and somatosensory evoked potentials may be prolonged, even in the absence of any past or present visual symptoms.
- CSF is not usually obtained, as the diagnosis is made with MRI or evoked potentials. Protein concentration and white cell count are raised. The IgG portion of the

total protein is increased and electrophoresis reveals oligoclonal bands, which indicate the production of immunoglobulin (to unknown antigens) within the CNS.

Management

The treatment of MS is with interferon.

- Subcutaneous administration of β-interferon reduces the relapse rate by a third and may delay the time to severe debility. Treatment is prolonged, expensive and associated with side effects, such as 'flu-like symptoms'.
- Short courses of ACTH or corticosteroids (e.g. i.v. methylprednisolone 1000 mg/day for 3 days) may promote remission in relapse, but do not influence the outlook in the long term.
- Physiotherapy and occupational therapy maintain the mobility of joints and muscle relaxants (e.g. baclofen, dantrolene and benzodiazepines) reduce the discomfort and pain of spasticity. Urinary catheterization is eventually needed for those with bladder involvement.

INFECTIVE AND INFLAMMATORY DISEASE

Meningitis ND

Meningitis (inflammation of the meninges) can be caused by infection, drugs and contrast media, malignant cells and blood (following subarachnoid haemorrhage). The term is, however, usually reserved for inflammation caused by infective agents (Table 14.14).

Clinical features

There is usually a rapid onset of severe headache, photophobia (intolerance of light) and vomiting with malaise, fever and rigors. Neck stiffness and Kernig's sign are usually present. Consciousness is usually not impaired, although the patient may be delirious with a high fever. Papilloedema may occur. The presence of drowsiness, lateralizing signs and cranial nerve lesions indicates the existence of a complication, e.g. venous sinus thrombosis, severe cerebral oedema or cerebral abscess.

Table 14.14 Infective causes of meningitis in the UK

Bacteria	*Neisseria meningitidis* *****
	Steptococcus pneumoniae *****
	Haemophilus influenzae (rare)
	Staphylococcus aureus
	Listeria monocytogenes
	Gram-negative bacilli
	Mycobacterium tuberculosis
	Treponema pallidum
	Leptospira spp.
Viruses	Enteroviruses (echo, Coxsackie, polio)
	Mumps
	Herpes simplex virus
	HIV
	Epstein–Barr virus
Fungi	*Cryptococcus neoformans*
	Candida spp.

* These organisms account for most cases of pyogenic meningitis in otherwise healthy adults.

Acute bacterial meningitis Most cases in adults are caused by meningococci. The organism is carried asymptomatically in the nasopharynx and spread from person to person by respiratory droplets or direct spread. Meningitis occurs after the organism invades the bloodstream from the nasopharynx, to reach the meninges. Characteristically there is a sudden onset of the disease with high fever, and a petechial/purpuric skin rash is often present. In patients with fulminant meningococcal septicaemia there are often large ecchymoses and gangrenous skin lesions.

The pneumococcus is the most common cause of meningitis in elderly people, and may complicate pneumonia or other respiratory tract infections. Direct spread of the organism may occur from an infected middle ear or via a skull fracture. The features of meningitis appear rapidly and the mortality rate may be as high as 30%.

Viral meningitis is usually a benign self-limiting condition lasting for about 4–10 days. There are no serious sequelae.

Tuberculous meningitis is often a chronic illness with vague symptoms of headache, lassitude, anorexia and vomiting. Signs of meningism may be absent or appear late in the course of the disease.

Investigations

The diagnosis is confirmed by lumbar puncture (page 652) and urgent CSF microscopy and analysis for protein and glucose concentration. Typical changes are shown in Table 14.15. However, if there are focal neurological signs, papilloedema or loss of consciousness, a lumbar puncture should only be performed after an urgent CT scan has ruled out an intracranial mass lesion, e.g. an abscess. Additional investigations include blood cultures, blood glucose and viral serology.

Table 14.15 Typical changes in the CSF in meningitis

	Normal	Viral	Pyogenic	Tuberculous
Appearance	Clear	Clear/turbid	Turbid/purulent	Turbid/viscous
Mononuclear (cells/mm³)	<5	10–100	<50	100–300
Polymorph (cells/mm³)	Nil	Nil	200–3000	0–200
Protein (g/l)	0.2–0.4	0.4–0.8	0.5–2.0	0.5–3.0
Glucose (% blood glucose)	>50	>50	<50	<30

Management

Bacterial meningitis is an emergency with a high mortality rate (15%), even with treatment. If the diagnosis is suspected clinically antibiotics must be given immediately, with subsequent urgent investigations. As a result of the emergence of resistant organisms, cefotaxime is replacing penicillins and chloramphenicol for the initial treatment of bacterial meningitis. Subsequent treatment is given depending on the results of culture and the antibiotic sensitivities of the organism.

A scheme for the immediate treatment of acute bacterial meningitis is given in Table 14.16.

In children with haemophilus meningitis, dexamethasone reduces meningeal inflammation and limits sensorineural hearing loss in survivors. There are few data in adults and it is not recommended.

Table 14.16 Antibiotic and acute bacterial meningitis

Organism	Antibiotic	Alternative
Unknown pyogenic	Cefotaxime	Benzylpenicillin and chloramphenicol
Meningococcus	Benzylpenicillin	Cefotaxime
Pneumococcus	Cefotaxime	Penicillin
Haemophilus	Cefotaxime	Chloramphenicol

Tuberculous meningitis is treated for at least 9 months with triple antituberculous therapy (page 420).

Notification

All cases of meningitis must (by law) be notified to the local Public Health Authority; this allows contact tracing and provides data for epidemiological studies.

Meningococcal prophylaxis

Oral rifampicin is given to patients and close (usually household) contacts to eradicate nasopharyngeal carriage of the organism.

Encephalitis

Encephalitis is inflammation of the brain parenchyma. It is caused by a wide variety of viruses and may also occur in bacterial and other infections. In certain groups (e.g. homosexuals, intravenous drug abusers) HIV infection and opportunistic organisms (e.g. *Toxoplasma gondii* in patients with full-blown AIDS) are important causes.

Acute viral encephalitis

A viral aetiology is often presumed, although not confirmed serologically or by culture. In the UK the common organisms are Echo, Coxsackie, mumps and herpes simplex viruses.

Clinical features

Many of these infections cause a mild self-limiting illness with headache and drowsiness. Less commonly the illness is severe, with focal signs (e.g. hemiparesis, dysphasia), seizures and coma. Severe encephalitis, which has a mortality rate of about 20% even with treatment, is most commonly caused by herpes simplex virus (HSV1).

Investigations

- CSF analysis shows a moderate increase in mononuclear cells (5–500 cells/mm^3). Protein may also be increased.
- Viral serology of blood and CSF may identify the causative virus.
- HSV DNA detection by PCR has a sensitivity of 95% in early HSV encephalitis. It is recommended that a 0.5 ml sample of CSF be sent for HSV PCR in all suspected cases.
- CT may show areas of oedema.
- EEG often shows non-specific slow–wave activity.

Treatment

Suspected herpes simplex encephalitis is immediately treated with intravenous acyclovir (10 mg/kg every 8 hours). If the patient is in a coma the prognosis is poor, whether or not treatment is given.

Intracranial abscesses

An abscess may develop in the epidural, subdural or intracerebral sites. Epidural abscesses are uncommon; subdural abscess presents similarly to intracerebral abscess (see below).

Cerebral abscess

Cerebral abscess may follow the direct spread of organisms from a skull fracture or a focus of infection in the paranasal sinuses or middle ear. Alternatively, haematogenous spread of infection may occur from the lung (e.g. bronchiectasis), heart (e.g. endocarditis) or bone (e.g. osteomyelitis). Frequently no cause is found. The most common organisms are streptococci, *Bacteroides* spp., staphylococci and enterobacteria. Infection with tubercle bacilli may result in chronic caseating granulomata (tuberculomas) presenting as intracranial mass lesions.

Clinical features

Presenting features include fever, seizures, focal neurological signs, and symptoms and signs of raised intracranial pressure (page 604).

Investigations

CT or MRI will usually outline the abscess. Lumbar puncture is not performed if an abscess is suspected because of the danger of coning in the presence of raised intracranial pressure (page 605).

Management

Treatment involves a combination of intravenous antibiotics and surgical drainage.

Neurosyphilis

Syphilis is described on page 29. Neurosyphilis occurs late in the course of untreated infection. It is now rarely seen in the UK because most cases of syphilis are recognized in the early stages and treated with penicillin. The different clinical syndromes (summarized in Table 14.17) may occur alone or in combination.

Management

Treatment is with parenteral benzylpenicillin for 3 weeks, which may arrest (but not reverse) the neurological disease. High-dose steroid cover is usually given to reduce the severity of a Jarisch–Herxheimer reaction (page 30).

Creutzfeldt–Jakob disease (CJD)

This is a progressive dementia, usually developing after 50 years of age, characterized pathologically by spongiform changes in the brain. It is one example of a prion (a proteinaceous infectious particle) disease and the pathology is similar to bovine spongiform encephalopathy (BSE) of cattle. The transmissible agent is resistant to many of the usual processes that destroy proteins. CJD occurs as a sporadic form or an iatrogenic form as a result of contaminated material such as corneal grafts or human growth hormone. There is no known treatment and death is invariable, usually within 6 months of onset.

Table 14.17 The clinical syndromes of neurosyphillis

Asymptomatic neurosyphilis	Positive CSF serology without symptoms or signs
Meningovascular syphilis 3–4 years after primary Infection	Subacute meningitis with cranial nerve palsies and papilloedema Raised intracranial pressure and focal deficits caused by an expanding intracranial mass (gumma) Paraparesis caused by spinal meningovasculitis
General paralysis of the insane 10–15 years after primary infection	Progressive dementia Brisk reflexes Extensor plantar responses Tremor
Tabes dorsalis 10–35 years after primary infection (caused by demyelination in the dorsal roots)	Lightning pains: short, sharp stabbing pains in the legs Ataxia, loss of reflexes and sensory loss Neuropathic joints (Charcot's joints) Argyll–Robertson pupils (page 563) Ptosis and optic atrophy

A new variant of CJD has been recognized which presents with neuropsychiatric symptoms, followed by ataxia and dementia, and affecting a younger age group. The appearance of this new variant has led to the speculation that there has been transmission from the animal to the human food chain, with infection from BSE-infected cattle to humans.

INTRACRANIAL TUMOURS

Primary intracranial tumours account for 10% of all neoplasms, and about one-quarter of all intracranial tumours are metastatic. Primary intracranial tumours may be derived from the skull itself, from any of the structures lying within it, or from their tissue precursors. They may be malignant on histological investigation but rarely metastasize outside the brain. The most common intracranial tumours occurring in adults are listed in Table 14.18.

Table 14.18 Relative frequency of intracranial tumours in adults on the basis of clinical presentation

Tumour	Relative frequency (%)

Primary malignant
  Astrocytoma
  Oligodendroglioma
	40

Benign
  Meningioma
  Neurofibroma
	30

Metastases
  Bronchus
  Breast
  Stomach
  Prostate
  Thyroid
  Kidney
	25

Clinical features

The clinical features of a cerebral tumour are the result of the following:

- Progressive focal neurological deficit
- Raised intracranial pressure
- Focal or generalized epilepsy.

Neurological deficit is the result of a mass effect of the tumour and surrounding cerebral oedema. The deficit depends on the site of the tumour, e.g. a frontal lobe tumour will initially cause personality change, apathy and intellectual deterioration. Subsequent involvement of the frontal speech area and motor cortex produces expressive aphasia and hemiparesis. Rapidly growing tumours destroy cerebral tissue, and loss of function is an early feature.

Raised intracranial pressure produces headache, vomiting and papilloedema. The headache is typically most severe on waking and decreases as the patient stands up, thereby lowering intracranial pressure. It is made worse by coughing, straining and sneezing.

As the tumour grows there is downward displacement of the brain and pressure on the brain stem, causing drowsiness, which progresses eventually to respiratory depression, bradycardia, coma and death.

Distortion of normal structures at a distance from the growing tumour leads to focal neurological signs (false localizing signs). The most common are a third and sixth cranial nerve palsy (page 565) resulting from stretching of the nerves by downward displacement of the temporal lobes.

Epilepsy Fits may be generalized or partial in nature. The site of origin of a partial seizure is frequently of value in localization.

Differential diagnosis

The main differential is from other intracranial mass lesions (cerebral abscess, tuberculoma, subdural haematoma and intracranial haematoma) and a stroke, which may have an identical clinical presentation.

Investigations

- Radiology. CT with contrast enhancement is the investigation of choice when a tumour is suspected. MRI is of particular value in investigation of tumours of the posterior fossa and brain stem. Cerebral angiography is sometimes necessary to define the site or blood supply of a mass, particularly if surgery is planned. Plain skull radiographs are rarely of diagnostic value, with the exception of pituitary tumours.
- Other investigations. These include routine tests, e.g. chest radiograph if metastatic disease is suspected. Lumbar puncture and examination of the CSF is rarely helpful and is contraindicated in this situation. The danger is of immediate herniation of the cerebellar tonsils, impaction within the foramen magnum and compression of the brain stem ('coning').

Management

- Surgery. Surgical exploration, and either biopsy or removal of the mass, is usually carried out to ascertain its nature. Some benign tumours, e.g. meningiomas, can be removed in their entirety without unacceptable damage to surrounding structures.
- Radiotherapy is usually recommended for gliomas and radiosensitive metastases.

- Medical treatment. This is palliative to reduce the symptoms related to cerebral oedema and raised intracranial pressure. Dexamethasone (either orally or intravenously), a very potent corticosteroid, may produce a dramatic improvement in symptoms. The prognosis is very poor in patients with malignant tumours, with only 50% surviving 1 year.

HYDROCEPHALUS

Hydrocephalus is a condition marked by an excessive amount of CSF within the cranium. CSF is produced in the cerebral ventricles and normally flows downward into the central canal of the spinal cord and then out into the subarachnoid space, from where it is reabsorbed. Hydrocephalus occurs when there is obstruction to the outflow of CSF; rarely it is the result of increased production of CSF.

Aetiology

In children, hydrocephalus may be caused by a congenital malformation of the brain (e.g. Arnold–Chiari malformation), meningitis or haemorrhage causing obstruction to the flow of CSF. In adults hydrocephalus is caused by:

- A late presentation of a congenital malformation
- Cerebral tumours in the posterior fossa or brain stem which obstruct the aqueduct or fourth-ventricle outflow
- Subarachnoid haemorrhage, head injury and meningitis
- Normal-pressure hydrocephalus, in which there is dilatation of the cerebral ventricles without signs of raised intracranial pressure. It presents in elderly people with dementia, urinary incontinence and ataxia.

Clinical features

The features are of headache, vomiting and papilloedema caused by raised intracranial pressure. There may be ataxia and bilateral pyramidal signs.

Management

Treatment is by the surgical insertion of a shunt between the ventricles and the right atrium or peritoneum (ventriculoatrial or ventriculoperitoneal).

Migraine

Migraine is the term used for recurrent headache associated with both visual and gastrointestinal disturbance; in spite of the origin of the word, it does not invariably mean unilateral headache.

Epidemiology

The prevalence of migraine is approximately 10%; some patients have a strong family history. Onset is usually before the age of 30 years.

Pathogenesis

The cause of migraine remains controversial. The headache is believed by some to result from vasodilatation or oedema of blood vessels, with stimulation of the nerve endings near affected extracranial meningeal arteries. The prodromal symptoms are the result of vasospasm and cerebral ischaemia. There is some evidence that the neurotransmitter serotonin is important in pathogenesis.

Clinical features

The diagnosis of migraine is clinical. The classic symptoms are of transient prodromal symptoms followed after 15–60 minutes by a throbbing headache accompanied by nausea, vomiting and photophobia. Prodromal symptoms are usually visual: scotomata, unilateral blindness, hemianopic field loss, flashes and fortification spectra. Other prodromal symptoms include aphasia, tingling, numbness and weakness of one side of the body. Migraine may also occur without these prodromal symptoms. The most common way in which a migraine attack resolves is through sleep.

Differential diagnosis

The sudden onset of headache may be similar to meningitis or subarachnoid haemorrhage. The hemiplegic, visual and hemisensory symptoms must be distinguished from thromboembolic TIAs. In TIAs the maximum deficit is present immediately and headache is unusual (page 581).

Management

General measures Patients should avoid precipitating factors (chocolate, cheese, too much or too little sleep).

Women taking the oral contraceptive pill may be helped by stopping the drug or changing the brand.

Treatment of the acute attack

- Simple analgesia, e.g. paracetamol, and an antiemetic, e.g. metoclopramide, may be all that is necessary for many patients
- Sumatriptan, naratriptan and zolmitriptan are serotonin or 5-hydroxytryptamine (5-HT) agonists which constrict the cranial arteries. They are used in patients not responding to simple analgesia and may be given orally, by subcutaneous injection or intranasal spray. Occasionally patients have developed cardiac-like chest pain, and rarely myocardial infarction, after using sumatriptan. Its use is contraindicated in patients with ischaemic heart disease
- Ergotamine is less commonly used since the introduction of sumatriptan. It may be given orally, rectally, intravenously or by nasal inhalation. Its use is absolutely contraindicated in patients with ischaemic heart disease and peripheral vascular disease.

Prophylaxis Prophylaxis is indicated for frequent attacks (more than two per month) which do not respond rapidly to treatment. The options are:

- β-blockers, e.g. propranolol
- Serotonin antagonists: pizotifen and methysergide.

An occasional side effect of methysergide is retroperitoneal fibrosis, which precludes its use for more than 6 months

Giant cell arteritis (cranial arteritis, temporal arteritis)

This is a granulomatous arteritis of unknown aetiology occurring chiefly in those over the age of 60 and affecting in particular the extradural arteries. Giant cell arteritis is closely related to polymyalgia rheumatica (page 225), and these can occur in the same patient.

Clinical features

There is headache, scalp tenderness (e.g. on combing the hair) and occasionally pain in the jaw and mouth which is characteristically worse on eating (jaw claudication). The superficial temporal artery is tender to touch, pulsation is soon lost and the artery becomes hard, tortuous and thickened. The great danger is sudden and irreversible blindness, caused by inflammation and occlusion of the ciliary and/or central retinal artery, which occurs in 25% of untreated cases. Systemic features include weight loss, malaise and a low-grade fever.

Investigations

- ESR is almost always elevated >50 mm/h.
- Full blood count may show a normochromic/normocytic anaemia.
- Histology. A temporal artery biopsy, which can be performed under local anaesthetic, usually confirms the diagnosis. However, the granulomatous changes may be patchy and therefore missed.

Management

High doses of steroids (oral prednisolone, initially 60–100 mg daily) should be started immediately in a patient with typical features and a temporal artery biopsy obtained as soon as possible (the histological changes remain for up to a week after starting treatment). The steroid dose is gradually reduced, guided by symptoms and the ESR, and can usually be stopped after some months to several years.

Facial pain

The face is richly supplied with pain-sensitive structures – the teeth, gums, sinuses, temporomandibular joints, jaws and eyes – disease of which causes facial pain. Trigeminal nerve lesions (see Table 14.15) may also present with facial pain, and this is suggested by the presence of trigeminal sensory or motor loss on physical examination.

Trigeminal neuralgia

Trigeminal neuralgia (tic douloureux) is a condition of unknown cause, seen most commonly in old age.

Clinical features

Severe paroxysms of knife-like pain occur in one or more divisions of the trigeminal nerve (page 567), although rarely in the ophthalmic division. Each paroxysm is stereotyped, brought on by stimulation of a specific 'trigger zone' in the face. The stimuli may be minimal, and include washing, shaving and eating. There are no objective physical signs and the diagnosis is based on the history.

Management

The anticonvulsant carbamazepine suppresses attacks in most patients. If this fails, thermocoagulation of the trigeminal ganglion or section of the sensory division may be necessary.

Differential diagnosis

Similar pain may occur with structural lesions involving the trigeminal nerve. These lesions are often accompanied by physical signs, e.g. a depressed corneal reflex.

DISEASES OF THE SPINAL CORD

The spinal cord extends from C1 (its junction with the medulla) to the vertebral body of L1. The spinal canal below L1 is occupied by lumbar and sacral nerve roots, which group together to form the cauda equina and ultimately extend into the pelvis and thigh (Figure 14.11). Paraplegia (weakness of both legs) is almost always caused by a spinal cord lesion, as opposed to hemiplegia (weakness of one side of the body), which is usually the result of a lesion in the brain.

Spinal cord compression
Clinical features

Patients present with spastic paraparesis: there is upper motor neuron weakness in the legs (page 553), loss of sphincter control and sensory loss below the level of the lesion. The onset may be acute (hours to days) or chronic (weeks to months), depending on the cause.

Aetiology

The causes of spinal cord compression are listed in Table 14.19; the most common causes in developed countries are highlighted. Spinal tuberculosis is a frequent cause in areas where TB is common, e.g. India, Asia and Africa.

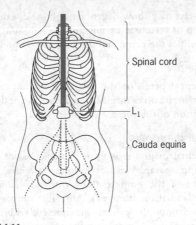

Figure 14.11
The spinal cord and cauda equina. (From Parsons, M. (1993) A Colour Atlas of Clinical Neurology. London, Mosby Wolfe.)

Table 14.19 Causes of spinal cord compression

Vertebral body neoplasms	Metastases, e.g. from lung, breast, prostate
	Myeloma
Disc and vertebral lesions	Trauma
	Chronic degenerative disease
Inflammatory	Epidural abcess
	Tuberculosis (Pott's paraplegia)
	Granuloma
Spinal cord neoplasms	Primary cord neoplasm, e.g. glioma, neurofibroma
	Metastases
Rarities	Paget's disease, bone cysts, osteoporosis
	Epidural haemorrhage

Investigations

Urgent investigation is essential in a patient with suspected cord compression, especially with acute or subacute onset, because irreversible paraplegia may follow if the cord is not decompressed.

- Spinal X-rays may show degenerative bone disease and destruction of vertebrae by infection or neoplasm.
- MRI identifies the cause and site of cord compression.

Management

The treatment depends on the cause, but in most cases the initial treatment involves surgical decompression of the cord and stabilization of the spine.

Differential diagnosis

The differential diagnosis is from intrinsic lesions of the cord causing paraparesis. Transverse myelitis (acute inflammation of the cord resulting from viral infection, syphilis or radiation therapy), anterior spinal artery occlusion and multiple sclerosis may present with a rapid onset of paraparesis. A more insidious onset occurs with motor neuron disease, subacute combined degeneration of the cord, and as a non-metastatic manifestation of malignancy.

Very rarely a parasagittal cortical lesion, e.g. meningioma, may cause paraplegia.

Syringomyelia and syringobulbia

Fluid-filled cavities within the spinal cord (myelia) and brain stem (bulbia) are the essential features of these conditions.

Aetiology

The most frequent cause is blockage of CSF flow from the fourth ventricle in association with an Arnold–Chiari malformation (congenital herniation of the cerebellar tonsils through the foramen magnum). The normal pulsatile CSF pressure waves are transmitted to the delicate tissues of the cervical cord and brain stem, with secondary cavity formation. Hydrocephalus may also occur as a result of disturbed CSF flow.

Clinical features

Patients usually present in the third or fourth decade with pain and sensory loss (pain and temperature) in the upper limbs. The clinical features are demonstrated in Figure 14.12.

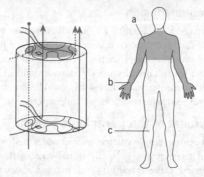

Figure 14.12
Production of physical signs in syringomyelia. Expanding cavities distend the cord. Pain and temperature (a) fibres crossing at that level are destroyed, but sensory fibres in the posterior columns (other sensory modalities) and those that enter the spinothalamic tract at a lower level are spared. Sensory loss is therefore 'dissociated' and confined to the upper trunk and limbs. Further extension damages the anterior horn cells (b), the pyramidal tracts (c) and the medulla, causing wasting in the hands, a spastic paraplegia, nystagmus and a bulbar palsy. (From Parsons, M. (1993) A Colour Atlas of Clinical Neurology. London, Mosby Wolfe.)

Investigation

MRI is the investigation of choice and demonstrates the intrinsic cavities.

Treatment

Surgical decompression of the foramen magnum sometimes reduces the rate of deterioration.

Friedreich's ataxia

This is the most common of the hereditary spinocerebellar degenerations. There is a progressive degeneration of the spinocerebellar tracts and cerebellum causing cerebellar ataxia, dysarthria and nystagmus. Degeneration of the corticospinal tracts causes weakness and an extensor plantar response. The tendon reflexes are absent as a result of peripheral nerve damage. Loss of the dorsal columns causes absent joint position and vibration sense. Other features are pes cavus, optic atrophy, cardiomyopathy, and death by middle age.

Cauda equina lesion

Spinal damage at or distal to L1 (a common cause is central prolapse of an intervertebral disc at the lumbosacral junction) injures the cauda equina, which is formed by the lumbar and sacral nerve roots. This produces various mixtures of flaccid paralysis (compare spastic paralysis of a cord lesion above L1), sacral numbness, urinary retention and impotence.

Management of the paraplegic patient

Regular turning, ripple mattresses and water beds will help to prevent pressure sores. In the initial stages patients may need urinary catheterization and manual evacuation of faeces. This may become unnecessary as reflex emptying of the bladder and rectum develops. Passive physiotherapy is helpful in preventing limb contractures. Severe spasticity may be helped by dantrolene sodium, baclofen or diazepam. Many patients graduate to a wheelchair and maintain some degree of independence.

....

DEGENERATIVE DISEASES

Motor neuron disease

The symptoms of motor neuron disease (MND) are caused by a relentless and unexplained destruction of upper motor neurons and anterior horn cells in the brain and spinal cord, which is usually fatal within 3 years. Most die from respiratory failure as a result of bulbar palsy and pneumonia.

It presents in middle age and is more common in men.

Clinical features

Three clinical patterns may be identified at diagnosis; however, as the disease progresses most patients develop a mixed picture.

- *Progressive muscular atrophy* is a predominantly lower motor neuron lesion of the cord causing weakness, wasting and fasciculation in the hands and arms.
- *Amyotrophic lateral sclerosis* is a combination of disease of the lateral corticospinal tracts and anterior horn cells producing a progressive spastic tetraparesis or paraparesis with added lower motor neuron signs (wasting and fasciculation).

- *Progressive bulbar palsy* results from destruction of upper (pseudobulbar palsy) and lower (bulbar palsy) motor neurons in the lower cranial nerves. There is dysarthria, dysphagia with wasting, and fasciculation of the tongue

There is no involvement of the sensory system or motor nerves to the eyes and sphincters.

Investigations

The diagnosis is clinical. An EMG shows muscle denervation, but this is not a specific finding.

Differential diagnosis

The most important differential is a cervical spine lesion, which may present with upper and lower motor neuron signs in the arms and legs. It is often distinguished by the presence of sensory signs.

Management

Excessive extracellular glutamate, the principle excitatory neurotransmitter, has been proposed as a mediator of neuronal injury and cell death in MND. This theory has led to the development of Riluzole, which decreases glutamate release from astrocytes and neurons, as a therapy for MND. Riluzole probably slows progression but does not arrest the disease process.

Spinal muscular atrophies

This is a group of rare disorders which destroy the anterior horn cell of the spinal cord. Two forms present in adult life, causing a slowly progressive wasting and weakness of the limbs.

DISEASES OF THE PERIPHERAL NERVES

Mononeuropathies

Mononeuropathy is a process affecting a single nerve, and multiple mononeuropathy (or mononeuritis multiplex) is a process affecting several or multiple nerves. Mononeuropathy may be the result of acute compression, particularly where the nerves are exposed anatomically (e.g. the common peroneal nerve at the head of the fibula), or entrapment, where the nerve passes through a relatively tight anatomical passage (e.g. the carpal tunnel). It may also be caused by direct damage, e.g. major trauma, surgery or penetrating injuries.

Carpal tunnel syndrome

Carpal tunnel syndrome is the most common entrapment neuropathy. It results from pressure on the median nerve as it passes through the carpal tunnel.

Aetiology

It is usually idiopathic but may be associated with hypothyroidism, diabetes mellitus, pregnancy, obesity, rheumatoid arthritis and acromegaly.

Clinical features

The history is of pain and paraesthesiae in the hand, typically worse at night, when it may wake the patient. On examination there may be no physical signs or weakness and wasting of the thenar muscles, and sensory loss of the palm and palmar aspects of the radial three and a half fingers. Tapping on the carpal tunnel may reproduce the pain (Tinnel's sign).

Management

Treatment with nocturnal splints or local steroid injections gives temporary relief. Surgical decompression is the definitive treatment unless the condition is likely to resolve (e.g. with pregnancy, obesity).

Compression neuropathies may also affect the ulnar nerve (at the elbow), the radial nerve (caused by pressure against the humerus) and the common peroneal nerve (resulting from pressure at the head of the fibula).

Mononeuritis multiplex

Mononeuritis multiplex often indicates a systemic disorder (Table 14.20); treatment is that of the underlying disease.

Polyneuropathy

Polyneuropathy describes a diffuse, usually symmetrical, disease process that may be acute or chronic and may involve motor, sensory and autonomic nerves, either alone or in combination. Sensory symptoms include numbness,

Table 14.20 Causes of mononeuritis multiplex

Diabetes mellitus

Leprosy (the most common cause worldwide)

Connective tissue disease
  Rheumatoid arthritis
  Systemic lupus erythematosus
  Polyarteritis nodosa
  Sarcoidosis
  Non-metastatic manifestation of malignancy
  Amyloidosis
  Neurofibromatosis
  AIDS

tingling, 'pins and needles', pain in the extremities and unsteadiness on the feet. Numbness typically affects the distal arms and legs in a 'glove and stocking' distribution. Motor symptoms are usually those of weakness. Autonomic neuropathy causes postural hypotension, urinary retention, impotence, diarrhoea (or occasionally constipation), diminished sweating, impaired pupillary responses and cardiac arrhythmias.

Many varieties of neuropathy affect autonomic function to some degree, but occasionally autonomic features predominate. This occurs in diabetes mellitus, amyloidosis and the Guillain–Barré syndrome. A classification of polyneuropathy is given in Table 14.21.

Peroneal muscular atrophy

Peroneal muscular atrophy (Charcot–Marie–Tooth disease) is a common clinical syndrome in which there is distal limb

Table 14.21 Classification of polyneuropathy

Idiopathic (the majority of cases)
Postinfective (Guillain–Barré syndrome)
Drugs: isoniazid, nitrofurantoin, metronidazole, vincristine
Toxins: excess alcohol, lead poisoning
Metabolic: diabetes mellitus, uraemia, liver disease, amyloidosis
Vitamin deficiency: B_1, B_6, B_{12}
Non-metastatic manifestation of malignancy
Autonomic neuropathies
Neuropathies in connective tissue disease
Hereditary sensorimotor neuropathy

wasting and weakness that progresses over many years, mostly in the legs, with variable loss of sensation and reflexes. In advanced cases the distal wasting below the knees is so marked that the legs resemble 'inverted champagne bottles'. The most common form is inherited in an autosomal dominant fashion.

Postinfective polyneuropathy (Guillain–Barré syndrome)

This is the single most common acute neuropathy. *Campylobacter jejuni*, which causes a diarrhoeal illness, is the chief precipitant of Guillain–Barré syndrome (26% of cases). Most other cases are precipitated by a viral infection.

Clinical features

There is weakness and numbness in the distal limbs which ascends over days or weeks. Disability ranges from mild to very severe, with involvement of the respiratory and facial muscles. Autonomic features, such as postural hypotension, ileus and bladder atony, are sometimes seen.

Pathogenesis

It is thought to be caused by a cell-mediated immune response directed at normal peripheral myelin, and this may be provoked in some cases by preceding infection.

Investigations

The diagnosis is usually based on clinical grounds.

- CSF protein is typically elevated, with a normal sugar and cell count.
- Nerve conduction studies show a slowing of motor conduction consistent with segmental demyelination.

Management

- Intravenous and plasmapheresis IgG both accelerate recovery and are probably of equal efficacy.
- Treatment is also supportive and ventilation may be required if the respiratory muscles are involved. Involvement of the respiratory muscles should be monitored with regular measurement of vital capacity.

- Corticosteroids are *not* of proven benefit.
- Visiting and counselling services are offered by past patients through the Guillain–Barré support group

Prognosis

Gradual recovery over months is the norm. The mortality rate as a result of respiratory, cardiac and autonomic complications is about 5–10%.

Vitamin deficiency neuropathies

Thiamine (vitamin B₁)

Alcohol abuse is the most common cause of thiamine deficiency in the west. Presentation is with the Wernicke–Korsakoff syndrome (page 468). Severe deficiency causes the clinical syndrome of beri-beri (polyneuropathy, Wernicke's encephalopathy and cardiac failure), rarely seen in western countries.

Pyridoxine (vitamin B₆)

Deficiency causes mainly a sensory neuropathy. It may be precipitated during isoniazid therapy (which complexes with pyridoxal phosphate) for tuberculosis in those who acetylate the drug slowly.

Vitamin B₁₂

Deficiency causes the syndrome of subacute combined degeneration of the cord. This comprises distal sensory loss (particularly the posterior column), absent ankle jerks (as a result of the neuropathy) and evidence of cord disease (exaggerated knee jerk reflexes, extensor plantar responses). Treatment is with intramuscular vitamin B₁₂, which reverses the peripheral nerve damage but has little effect on the CNS (cord and brain signs).

DISEASES OF VOLUNTARY MUSCLE

Myopathies

Weakness is the predominant feature of a myopathy. The myopathies are divided into those that are inherited (muscular dystrophies), inflammatory lesions (the most common is polymyositis, page 223) and those associated with drugs, toxins and endocrine disease (Table 14.22). The

Table 14.22 Causes of a proximal myopathy

Prolonged high-dose steroid therapy
Cushing's syndrome
Thyrotoxicosis
Hypothyroidism (occasionally)
Osteomalacia
Hypokalaemia
Prolonged alcohol abuse
Other drugs, e.g. diamorphine, lithium, quinine, chloroquine

second group usually produces weakness of the limb girdles (proximal myopathy); however, severe hypokalaemia may produce a generalized flaccid weakness.

Muscular dystrophies

Muscular dystrophies are progressive genetically determined disorders of skeletal and sometimes cardiac muscle. The most common is Duchenne muscular dystrophy, which presents in early childhood and progresses to severe disability with death in the late teens. The milder dystrophies present later in life and are summarized in Table 14.23.

Table 14.23 Limb girdle and facioscapulohumeral dystrophies

	Limb girdle	Facioscapulohumeral
Inheritance	Autosomal recessive	Autosomal dominant
Onset	10–20 years	10–40 years
Muscle affected	Shoulder and pelvic girdle	Face, shoulder and pelvic girdle
Progress	Severe disability in 20–25 years	Normal life expectancy
Pseudohypertrophy	Rare	Very rare
Serum CPK levels	Slightly raised	Slightly raised or normal

CPK, creatinine phosphate kinase.

Myasthenia gravis

Myasthenia gravis is an acquired condition characterized by weakness and fatiguability of proximal limb, ocular and bulbar muscles. The heart is not affected. It occurs most commonly in the third decade and is twice as common in women as in men.

Aetiology

The cause is unknown. Serum IgG antibodies to acetylcholine receptors, in the postsynaptic membrane of the neuromuscular junction, cause receptor loss. Myasthenia gravis is associated with thymic hyperplasia in about 70% of patients under 40 years of age, and in about 10% a thymic tumour is found.

Clinical features

Fatiguability is the most important feature, with the proximal limb muscles, extraocular muscles and muscles of mastication, speech and facial expression being most commonly involved. The ocular muscles are the first to be involved in about 65% of patients, resulting in ptosis and complex ocular palsies.

Investigations

- Acetylcholine receptor antibodies are specific for myasthenia gravis and are found in the serum in 90% of cases of generalized myasthenia gravis.
- The Tensilon test is positive. (Injection of 10 mg edrophonium, an anticholinesterase, results in rapid temporary improvement in weakness).
- Nerve stimulation tests show a characteristic decrement in evoked potential following stimulation of the motor nerve.

Management

Anticholinesterases (pyridostigmine, neostigmine) form the mainstay of treatment and the dose is determined by the patient's response.

In patients without thymoma Anticholinesterase medication alone is given in mild disease. In patients under 45 with more severe disease thymectomy is usually indicated. This results in improvement in about 65% of cases. Immunosuppressive treatment with steroids and/or azathioprine should be considered in those who fail to respond to thymectomy.

In patients with thymoma Thymectomy is indicated in these patients because of the ability of the tumour to invade locally. It is unusual for myasthenia to improve following surgery, and immunosuppressive treatment is usually required.

MYOTONIAS

These conditions are characterized by myotonia, i.e. continued muscle contraction after the cessation of voluntary effort. They are important because the patient tolerates general anaesthetics poorly. The two most common forms are dystrophia myotonica and myotonia congenita, described below.

Dystrophia myotonica

Dystrophia myotonica is an autosomal dominant condition characterized by progressive distal muscle weakness with myotonia, ptosis, facial muscle weakness and thinning. Other features commonly present are cataracts, frontal baldness, cardiomyopathy, mild mental handicap, glucose intolerance and hypogonadism.

Myotonia congenita

Myotonia congenita is also an autosomal dominant disorder characterized by mild isolated myotonia occurring in childhood and persisting throughout life. The myotonia is often accentuated by rest and cold.

DEMENTIA AND DELIRIUM

Delirium (toxic confusional state)

Delirium is an acute or subacute condition in which impairment of consciousness is accompanied by abnormalities of perception and mood. Impairment of consciousness can vary in severity and often fluctuates (compare with dementia). Confusion is usually worse at night and may be accompanied by hallucinations, delusions, restlessness and aggression. Many diseases (Table 14.24) can be accompanied by delirium, particularly in the elderly.

Management

Investigation and treatment of the underlying disease should be undertaken. General measures include

Table 14.24 Some causes of delirium

Systemic infection	
Drug/alcohol withdrawal	
Metabolic disturbance	Hepatic failure
	Renal failure
	Disorders of electrolyte balance
	Hypoxia
	Hypoglycaemia
Vitamin deficiency	Vitamin B_{12}
	Vitamin B_1 (Wernicke–Korsakoff syndrome)
Brain damage	Trauma
	Tumour
	Abscess
	Subarachnoid haemorrhage
Drug intoxication	Anticonvulsants
	Anticholinergics
	Anxiolytics/hypnotics
	Opiates

withdrawing all drugs where possible, rehydration, and adequate pain relief and sedation. Benzodiazepines are usually the drugs of choice, although in severe delirium intramuscular haloperidol may be preferred.

Dementia

Dementia is characterized by a disturbance of multiple higher cortical functions, including memory, thinking, orientation, comprehension, calculation, learning capacity, language and judgement. Consciousness is not, however, clouded. Dementia affects about 10% of those aged 65 and over, and 20% of those over 80. There are numerous causes of dementia (Table 14.25), although by far the most common is Alzheimer's disease which accounts for 70%.

Alzheimer's disease
Alzheimer's disease is a primary degenerative cerebral disease of unknown aetiology. A relationship with the ingestion or accumulation of aluminium has been suggested, though not proven.

Table 14.25 Some common causes of dementia

Alzheimer's disease
Multiple cerebral infarction
Alcohol (Wernicke–Korsakoff syndrome)
Hypothyroidism
Intracranial mass, subdural haematoma, hydrocephalus
Chronic traumatic encephalopathy
Vitamin B_{12} deficiency
Syphilis
CJD
Huntington's chorea
HIV
Late Parkinson's

Clinical features

There is an insidious onset with steady progression over years. Short-term memory loss is usually the most prominent early symptom, but subsequently there is slow disintegration of the personality and intellect, eventually affecting all aspects of cortical function. There are characteristic pathological features, which include neuronal reduction in several areas of the brain, neurofibrillary tangles, argentophile plaques, consisting largely of amyloid protein, and granulovacuolar bodies.

Investigations

The presence of dementia is usually diagnosed clinically by a simple assessment of the mental state (Table 14.26).

Management

In most cases there is no specific therapy although the associated anxiety and depression often need treatment. Patients should be managed in the community as much as possible, with appropriate support and help for carers.

Acetylcholinesterase inhibitors, e.g. donepezil, have a modest benefit and slow intellectual deterioration in patients with mild to moderate Alzheimer's disease.

Prognosis

The typical course is one of progressive decline. The average survival is 8–10 years.

Table 14.26 Simple clinical assessment of the mental state

Function	Question
Orientation	What is the time/day/month/year? Where are you? What is the place? Whom do you recognize?
Concentration	Repeat months of the year backwards Take 7 serially from 100 (serial 7s) Repeat a span of digits (e.g. 5-figure: 43701; 6-figure 732156)
Memory *Short-term* *Medium/long-term*	 Recall test name and address after 2 and 5 min Current affairs (e.g. name of prime minister, occupant of the throne, dates of World War II)
Intelligence	Simple arithmetic sums Meaning of words Meaning of proverbs Ability to read and write
Higher cortical function	Spatial awareness – drawing 3D objects Naming of objects Right–left discrimination (touch your left ear with your right hand)

Vascular (multi-infarct) dementia

This is the second most common cause of dementia and can be distinguished by its history of onset, clinical features and subsequent course. There is usually a history of transient ischaemic attacks, although the dementia may follow a succession of acute cerebrovascular accidents or, less commonly, a single major stroke.

Dermatology

....

INTRODUCTION

Skin diseases are extremely common, although their exact
prevalence is unknown. There are over 1000 different
entities described, but two-thirds of all cases are the result of
fewer than 10 conditions. The most common include acne,
eczema, psoriasis, warts and infections caused by bacteria,
fungi and viruses. Some conditions may be part of normal
development, e.g. acne; others may be inherited, e.g.
Ehlers–Danlos syndrome; still others are part of a systemic
disease, e.g. the rash of systemic lupus erythematosus.

Only the most common skin conditions will be described
in the following sections.

Acne vulgaris

Acne vulgaris is a common condition affecting almost 90%
of adolescents. It is thought to result from hyperactivity of
the sebaceous glands leading to increased production of
sebum with blockage of the follicular openings and the
formation of comedones (blackheads), inflammatory
papules, nodules and cysts. Normal skin bacteria, principally
Propionibacterium acnes, within the blocked follicle are capable
of producing proinflammatory mediators and lipolytic
enzymes, which may be responsible for producing the
clinical lesions.

Clinical features

Non-inflammatory lesions include open and closed
comedones. Closed comedones (whiteheads) are flesh-
coloured papules with an apparently closed overlying
surface. Open comedones (blackheads) appear as black plugs
which distend the follicular orifice, the pigmentation being
provided by oxidation of melanin pigment. These are often

the forerunners of the more severe inflammatory lesions, such as papules, pustules, nodules and cysts. Other features that may be present include hypertophic or keloidal scarring, and hyperpigmentation, which occurs predominantly in patients with darker complexions.

Management

Acne should be actively treated to avoid unnecessary scarring and psychological distress. There are a variety of approaches to treatment, the choice of which depends on the severity of the disease.

Topical treatments

- Local applications such as abrasives, astringents or exfoliatives are useful in mild disease.
- Tretinoin applied topically is useful in reversing abnormal follicular keratinization and reducing microcomedo formation. Clinical efficacy may take 3–4 months to become apparent.
- Antibiotics such as clindamycin and erythromycin applied topically are useful in mild to moderate inflammatory disease.
- Other agents, such as salicylic acid, benzoyl peroxide and, more recently, topical isotretinoin, are occasionally used.

Systemic treatments

- Oral antibiotics, e.g. tetracycline or erythromycin, are indicated in those with moderate to severe disease, where topical treatment has failed, and those with involvement of the shoulders and back. Treatment over several months is often necessary.
- Isotretinoin (a vitamin A analogue given orally) is used in severe cystic disease that is unresponsive to other treatments. Although highly effective it is associated with several adverse effects. Most importantly this drug is highly teratogenic and is absolutely contraindicated during pregnancy. All women of child bearing age should be given the oral contraceptive pill during treatment with isotretinoin.
- Hormonal treatment with the oral contraceptive pill or an antiandrogen such as cyproterone acetate may be useful in women.

Psoriasis

Psoriasis is a chronic hyperproliferative disorder characterized by the presence of well demarcated silvery-scaled plaques over extensor surfaces such as the elbows and knees, and in the scalp. It can affect any group with equal sex incidence, and occurs in about 2% of people in temperate zones.

Aetiology

The cause of the condition is unknown, although genetic factors are felt to be important. It is associated with several HLA-specific antigens, particularly HLA-CW6. Trigger factors in genetically susceptible individuals include infections (particularly streptococcal), local trauma, drugs such as lithium carbonate and β-blockers, and probably also stress.

Clinical features

Several clinical patterns are recognized:

- Plaque psoriasis is the most common, occurring as well demarcated, salmon–pink silvery scaling lesions on the extensor surfaces of the limbs, particularly the elbows and knees. Scalp involvement is common and is most often seen at the hair margin or over the occiput. Nail involvement, which can occur alone or in association with psoriasis elsewhere, is manifest as pitting and onycholysis (separation of the nail from the underlying vascular bed). The arthropathy associated with psoriasis is described on page 214.
- Flexural psoriasis presents as pinkish glazed lesions that are well demarcated and non-scaly. The groin, perianal and genital skin are most commonly involved.
- Pustular psoriasis most commonly affects the palms or soles. There are areas of well demarcated scaling and erythema associated with white, yellow or green pustule formation. Identical features are seen as one of the cutaneous features of Reiter's syndrome (keratoderma blenorrhagica, page 213).
- Erythrodermic psoriasis is a severe and potentially life-threatening condition. The trunk and limbs may be involved by an almost universal scaling, sometimes

associated with generalized pustule formation. This disease occurs classically following corticosteroid therapy.

Management

The approach depends on the severity of the disease. As no treatment is universally effective, simple local treatment is used for mild disease, with systemic therapy reserved for severe or pustular psoriasis.

Local therapy Topical steroids, dithranol (inhibits DNA synthesis), calcipotriol (topical vitamin D_3) and occasionally coal tar may all be useful for relatively mild disease, and are suitable for use on an outpatient basis.

Systemic therapy

- Oral retinoic acid derivatives, e.g. acitretin or etretinate, are useful in severe erythrodermic or pustular psoriasis. Although effective, these agents are potentially toxic and also teratogenic. They should not therefore be used in women of childbearing ages.
- Low-dose oral methotrexate (7.5–20 mg once a week) can be highly effective, particularly in psoriatic arthritis. Other immunosuppressive agents, such as cyclosporin and tacrolimus, are sometimes useful in severe intractable disease, although toxicity often limits their long-term use.

PUVA Psoralens (photosensitizing agents taken by mouth) and high-intensity ultraviolet A light (UVA) are usually highly effective for treating extensive psoriasis. Repeated treatments, however, carry the risk of UV-induced skin cancer.

Eczema

Eczema is characterized by superficial skin inflammation with vesicles (when acute), redness, oedema, oozing, scaling and usually pruritus. The terms 'dermatitis' and 'eczema' are usually used interchangeably, as both conditions show similar inflammatory changes in the skin.

Eczema may arise from several different stimuli, but most commonly it is classified as:

- Endogenous (atopic)
- Exogenous due to allergy or chemical irritation.

Atopic eczema

Aetiology

The cause of this condition is unknown, although there is a capacity to hyperreact to many environmental factors. There are high levels of serum IgE antibodies, although their significance in contributing to the pathogenesis is unclear. There is also a significant hereditary predisposition.

Clinical features

The disease may start in the first few weeks of life with erythema, weeping, itching and scaling. In adults the flexures at the neck, elbow, wrist and knee are commonly involved.

Management

The offending agents should be removed if possible. Regular use of emollients, such as aqueous cream or emulsifying ointments, is useful in hydrating the skin. Corticosteroid creams, e.g. 1% hydrocortisone, form the mainstay of treatment.

Exogenous eczema (contact dermatitis)

In this condition there is acute or chronic skin inflammation, often sharply demarcated, produced by substances in contact with the skin. It may be caused by a primary chemical irritant, or may be the result of a type IV hypersensitivity reaction. Common chemical irritants are industrial solvents used in the workplace, or cleaning and detergent solutions used in the home. With allergic dermatitis there is sensitization of T lymphocytes over a period of time, which results in itching and dermatitis upon re-exposure to the antigen.

Clinical features

An unusual pattern of rash with clear-cut demarcation or odd-shaped areas of erythema and scaling should arouse suspicion and, in combination with a careful history, should indicate a cause. Patch testing, where the suspected allergen is placed in contact with the skin, is often useful in identifying a suspected allergen.

Management

Causative agents should be removed where possible. Steroid creams are useful for short periods in severe disease. Antipruritic agents are used for symptomatic relief of itching.

Erythema nodosum

Erythema nodosum is an acute and sometimes recurrent paniculitis which produces painful nodules or plaques on the shins, with occasional spread to the thighs or arms. Adult females are most commonly affected. Histological features suggest that this is an immunological reaction with immune complex deposition within dermal vessels. In 50% of cases no obvious cause is found. Other causes are listed in Table 15.1

Table 15.1 Some causes of erythema nodosum

Drugs	Sulphonamides
	Oral contraceptive pill
	Penicillin
Systemic diseases	Sarcoidosis*
	Inflammatory bowel disease*
Infection	Bacteria and viruses*
	Streptococcal*
	Tuberculosis
	Leprosy
	Cat scratch disease
	Tularaemia
	Chlamydia spp.
	Psittacosis
	Lymphogranuloma venereum
	Fungal
	Histoplasmosis
	Coccidioidomycosis
	Blastomycosis
Pregnancy	

* The most common causes.

Clinical features

Painful nodules or plaques up to 5 cm in diameter appear in crops over 2 weeks, and slowly fade to leave bruising and staining of the skin. Systemic upset is common, with malaise, fever and arthralgia.

Management

NSAIDs such as indomethacin should be given to lessen the pain associated with cutaneous and joint symptoms. Recovery may take weeks, and recurrent attacks can occur.

Erythema multiforme.

This is an acute self-limiting condition affecting the skin and mucosal surfaces which is probably related to the deposition of immune complexes. Children and young adults are most commonly affected. The disease is commonly associated with:

- Herpes simplex infection
- *Mycoplasma pneumoniae*
- Drugs, e.g. sulphonamides, sulphonylureas and barbiturates
- Connective tissue diseases.

Clinical features

Symmetrically distributed erythematous papules occur most commonly on the back of the hands, the palms and the forearms. The lesions may show central pallor associated with oedema, bulla formation and peripheral erythema. Severe mucosal disease may predominate in, for example, infection with *Mycoplasma pneumoniae*. Eye changes include conjunctivitis, corneal ulceration and uveitis.

The Stevens–Johnson syndrome is a severe erythema multiforme with oral and genital ulceration and marked constitutional symptoms.

Management

The disease is usually self-limiting although the Stevens–Johnson syndrome can be fatal. Offending drugs should be withdrawn and the underlying disease treated. In severe cases intravenous fluids and feeding may be required.

....

OTHER DISEASES AFFECTING THE SKIN

Marfan's syndrome

Marfan's syndrome is an autosomal dominant disorder of collagen synthesis. Fragility of the skin may lead to bruising. The most obvious abnormalities are skeletal: tall stature, arm span greater than height, arachnodactyly (long spidery fingers), sternal depression, lax joints and a high arched palate. There is often upward dislocation of the lens as a result of weakness of the suspensory ligament. Cardiovascular complications (ascending aortic aneurysm formation, aortic dissection and aortic valve incompetence) are responsible for a greatly reduced lifespan.

Ehlers–Danlos syndrome

Inherited defects of collagen lead to fragility and hyperelasticity of the skin, with easy bruising, 'paper-thin' scars and hypermobility of the joints. The walls of the aorta and gut are weak and may rarely rupture with catastrophic results.

Neurofibromatosis

Neurofibromatosis is an autosomal dominant disease with distinctive clinical features.

- Type 1 (von Recklinghausen's disease), with the abnormal gene on chromosome 17. Clinical features include multiple cutaneous neurofibromas, multiple 'café-au-lait' spots (light-brown macules of varying size), axillary freckling, scoliosis, and an increased incidence of a variety of neural tumours, e.g. meningioma, eighth-nerve tumours and gliomas.
- Type 2, with the abnormal gene on chromosome 22. Typically bilateral acoustic neuromas and other neural tumours occur.

Practical procedures 16

The purpose of this chapter is to describe some of the common practical procedures you may have to undertake as a house officer or, for a few of them, as a medical student. Before attempting them alone you should first perform them with a more experienced colleague. Because of space restrictions only a limited number of procedures have been listed and they are the ones that are carried out on a daily basis or which may have to be performed as an emergency. Elective procedures and those usually performed by more senior colleagues are not discussed.

GENERAL PRINCIPLES FOR ALL PROCEDURES

A simple and concise explanation of the procedure must be given to the patient. In some cases, e.g. liver biopsy, it is usual to obtain written informed consent, which includes an explanation to the patient of the risks associated with the procedure. At the end of a procedure all needles, syringes and trocars should be disposed of in a sharps bin.

Sterile procedures

Some procedures are performed under strict aseptic conditions to minimize the risks to the patient of introducing infection. The equipment and methods are similar in each case. The operator washes his or her hands thoroughly with a disinfecting agent such as povidone–iodine (Betadine) or chlorhexidine (Hibiscrub), and wears sterile gloves for the procedure. An assistant, who maintains a no-touch technique, helps to open dressing packs and gives needles and syringes to the operator. The operative field is cleaned with aqueous Betadine or 0.5% chlorhexidine in alcohol and the skin of the selected entry site is isolated with sterile towels.

Local anaesthesia

A preparation of 1% lignocaine is usually used for local anaesthesia. The maximum amount used in an adult should be less than 20 ml, although usually much less is necessary. After cleaning the skin a 25 gauge (orange) needle is inserted intradermally and a small bleb raised before infiltrating the deeper tissues with a 23 gauge (blue) needle. Before each injection the plunger of the syringe should be pulled back to ensure that a blood vessel has not been entered.

Venepuncture

Equipment

- Syringe
- 21 gauge (green) needle
- Tourniquet
- Labelled tubes for the blood.

Many hospitals now employ a vacutainer system where the tubes contain a vacuum and are attached to the needle while it is in the vein. This reduces the chances of a needle-stick injury to the operator.

Methods

The antecubital vein in the forearm is an ideal site and, if unsuccessful, more distal sites may be attempted. The tourniquet is applied proximally and the skin over the venepuncture site cleaned with a swab. The skin is rendered tense with the operator's left hand, thus immobilizing the vein. The syringe with the needle attached is held in the right hand and the needle, with the bevel upwards, is passed obliquely to the skin and pointed in the direction of blood flow. Loss of resistance is felt when the vein is entered. The required amount of blood is drawn slowly (to prevent haemolysis) up into the syringe. At the end of the procedure the tourniquet is removed, a dry swab is applied to the venepuncture site and the needle removed from the vein while applying pressure on the swab. The needle is removed from the syringe before expelling the blood into the tubes. A butterfly cannula which can be left in situ is used for repeated sampling over a short time period, e.g. a glucose tolerance test.

If you fail...

It is often easier to palpate a suitable vein than to see it. Vasodilatation may be achieved by exercising the arm or placing it in warm water. Try other sites, e.g. a vein in the foot.

Setting up an intravenous (i.v.) cannula

Indications

- Fluid replacement
- Administration of intravenous drugs (e.g. antibiotics)
- To ensure i.v. access in case of emergency (e.g. coronary care)
- Short-term feeding via a peripheral vein.

Equipment

- Cannula
- Alcohol swab
- Adhesive tape
- Tourniquet
- Infusion fluid already run through a giving set.

Procedure

Place the tourniquet around the upper arm and search carefully for a vein. Aim for a palpable vein, preferably away from joints and in the non-dominant arm. Clean the skin with an alcohol swab and, if a large-bore cannula is being inserted (e.g. 14–16 gauge), anaesthetize the entry site with 2–3 ml of lignocaine injected intradermally with a 25 gauge needle. Once the cannula enters the vein, blood will flash back into the cannula. It can then be advanced along the vein while gently withdrawing but not completely removing the trocar. Remove the tourniquet, occlude the tip of the cannula by pressing on the vein at the tip of the cannula with your finger. Remove the trocar and attach the plastic cap or giving set. Ensure that the fluid is running adequately, or alternatively flush with 5–10 ml of 0.9% saline. Secure the cannula carefully with tape and dispose of sharps in sharps bin.

Complications

- 'Tissuing' of drip
- Thrombophlebitis.

If you fail...

- Come back and try later.
- Place the arm in some warm water to dilate the veins.
- Ask a colleague for help.
- Consider subcutaneous fluids: glucose and 0.9% saline, but not drugs, can be administered subcutaneously via a butterfly needle.

Arterial sampling

Indications

- Blood gas and acid–base analysis
- Very occasionally if blood cannot be obtained from a vein.

Equipment

- Dedicated blood gas syringe or standard syringe with 2–3 ml of heparin
- 23 gauge needle
- Cotton-wool balls
- Alcohol swab
- Disposable gloves.

Procedure

Note the concentration of any inspired oxygen the patient may be receiving. Decide on the site for arterial puncture: brachial, radial or femoral artery. The brachial or radial artery in the non-dominant arm is the preferred choice in most cases. The femoral artery is more likely to be involved with atheroma, especially in the elderly. Clean the area with the alcohol swab and expel excess heparin from the blood gas syringe. Clean and anaesthetize the skin using local anaesthetic (page 636). Palpate with three fingers over the course of the artery to determine the area of maximum pulsation. Insert the needle, bevel up, at about 45° to the skin. Once the artery is entered, blood will pulsate into the syringe. If no blood is obtained after the needle has been advanced an appropriate distance, withdraw the needle, exerting gentle traction on the plunger, as blood often enters on removal. If this is not successful the needle must be redirected. Once 1.5–2 ml of blood have been obtained, remove the needle and ask an assistant to apply firm pressure with the cotton wool to the puncture site for 5 minutes. Remove the needle from the syringe and expel any air bubbles. The syringe should be capped and sent for immediate analysis.

Complications

- Arterial spasm and ischaemia
- Dislodgment of atheroma from femoral artery.

If you fail...

Do not persist with several attempts but ask a colleague for help.

Central venous cannulation
Indications

- Measurement of central venous pressure (CVP)
- Infusion of substances irritant to small veins and tissues, e.g. dopamine
- Difficulty in obtaining peripheral venous access
- Administration of drugs during a cardiac arrest
- Modified central venous lines are used for administration of intravenous feeding, insertion of a Swan–Ganz catheter and temporary transvenous cardiac pacing.

Contraindications

There are no absolute contraindications, but the cannula is placed away from an area of skin sepsis if possible.

Equipment

- Materials for a sterile procedure performed under local anaesthetic (page 635)
- Scalpel and blade
- Central line pack (e.g. Leader-Cath)
- Infusion fluid already run through a giving set, and a three-way tap
- CVP monitoring set if required.

Method

The aim of central venous cannulation is to place the tip of the cannula in the right atrium or superior vena cava. This is usually achieved by percutaneous puncture of the right internal jugular or subclavian vein. The internal jugular vein is preferred in patients with respiratory disease (the risk of pneumothorax is less than with subclavian vein cannulation) or a bleeding tendency (bleeding can be more easily controlled by direct pressure in the neck if there is inadvertent arterial puncture).

This is a sterile procedure performed under local anaesthesia (page 635). The patient is placed in a slightly head-down position and a small skin incision (see site, later) made with a scalpel blade in the anaesthetized skin. A needle, used to locate the vein, is attached to a saline-filled syringe and gentle aspiration is maintained as the needle is advanced through the skin and subcutaneous tissues towards the vein. Once in the vein the syringe is removed and the needle occluded with a finger to prevent air embolism. The flexible end of the guidewire is passed down the needle into the vein and the needle removed leaving the guidewire in place. The cannula is loaded on to the guidewire and slid into the vein, before the wire is removed leaving the cannula in position. The giving set is attached to the cannula, which is secured in position by a stitch and transparent adhesive dressing. A chest X-ray is taken as soon as possible after insertion to demonstrate the correct position of the cannula tip and exclude complications such as a pneumothorax.

When removing a central line, remember to place the patient in the head-down position.

Internal jugular vein puncture The internal jugular vein runs behind the sternomastoid lateral to the carotid artery. The line of the carotid artery is located with the fingers of the left hand and the site of cannula insertion is chosen as a point at or just above an imaginary line drawn across the cricoid membrane; this avoids damage to structures in the root of the neck. With the right hand the needle is advanced just lateral to the fingers of the left hand and passed parallel to the midline at an angle of 45° to the skin.

Subclavian vein puncture The needle is inserted just below the midpoint of the clavicle and advanced along its posterior surface towards the suprasternal notch. The needle and syringe are kept parallel to the coronal plane at all times to avoid puncturing the pleura or subclavian artery.

Complications

- Puncture of major arteries, pleura and thoracic duct
- Air and catheter embolism
- Catheter-related sepsis
- Venous thrombosis.

If you fail...

Do not persist with several attempts but ask a senior colleague or anaesthetist for help.

Measurement of central venous pressure

The CVP is the pressure in the right atrium and may be measured continuously using a pressure transducer, or intermittently using a manometer. A constant zero-reference level is essential for accurate measurement; either the midaxillary line or the sternal angle is usually used. The normal value is between 0–4 and 3–7 cm H_2O, measured from the sternal angle and midaxillary line, respectively, as the zero-reference points (Figure 16.1)

1. The manometer is filled with fluid by opening the three-way tap to the infusion fluid.
2. The manometer tube is connected to the patient by closing off the three-way tap to the infusion fluid.

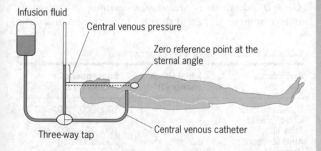

Infusion fluid

Central venous pressure

Zero reference point at the sternal angle

Three-way tap

Central venous catheter

Figure 16.1
Measurement of central venous pressure using the sternal angle as zero-reference point.

3. The meniscus in the manometer will drop steadily until it moves with respiration above and below a mean pressure. The pressure at the end of respiration is the CVP.
4. The infusion is reconnected to the patient via the three-way tap, thus isolating the manometer.

Electrical cardioversion

Indications

- Elective cardioversion
  Atrial tachyarrhythmias
- Emergency cardioversion
  Atrial tachyarrhythmias causing haemodynamic compromise, e.g. hypotension,
  pulmonary oedema
  Ventricular tachycardia
  Ventricular fibrillation (VF).

Contraindications

Digitalis toxicity (relative contraindication).

Equipment

- Defibrillator
- Self-adhesive monitor–defibrillator pad electrodes
- Intravenous cannula in situ.

Method

General anaesthesia is necessary in a conscious patient to induce amnesia and avoid the pain of the tetanic muscular

Table 16.1 Energy requirements for arrhythmias

Arrhythmia	Initial shock energy (J)	Subsequent shocks (J)
Supraventricular tachycardia	50	100, 200, 300, 360
Atrial flutter	50	100, 200, 300, 360
Atrial fibrillation	100	200, 300, 360
Ventricular arrhythmias	200	200, 360

contraction induced by the electric current through the thorax. The two electrodes are placed in a position that will maximize transmyocardial current flow, and this is usually achieved by placing one at the apex of the heart and the other over the right second intercostal space. For all arrhythmias except VF the defibrillator should be enabled to deliver a synchronized shock, i.e. the shock is delivered on the R wave of the QRS complex. Failure to deliver a synchronized shock may induce VF. Energy selection in cardioversion is arrhythmia dependent (Table 16.1). Before delivering the shock the operator must make sure that no-one, including him or herself, has any contact with the patient either directly or indirectly, e.g. by touching the bed on which the patient is lying. The operator usually calls 'stand back' before delivering the shock.

Complications

- Superficial burns to the skin
- Induction of arrhythmias
- Systemic embolization after cardioversion of AF (page 334)
- Myocardial damage from excessive energy.

If it fails...

Ensure the electrodes have been correctly placed. Consider a change of electrode position, e.g. anterior and posterior chest walls. Stop the procedure after a maximum of seven shocks in elective cardioversion. Consider chemical cardioversion with antiarrhythmic drugs.

A difficult decision is when to stop resuscitation and defibrillation efforts in a patient who is not responding. This depends on the patient, the circumstances of the arrest and how long the patient has had a non-perfusing cardiac rhythm. In general, if a patient arrests in hospital and resuscitation has not resulted in a perfusing cardiac rhythm after 30 minutes then further attempts are unlikely to be successful. The prognosis is poorer in patients who arrest outside hospital. There are exceptions: resuscitation is continued for longer in a hypothermic patient.

Pleural aspiration

Indications

- Diagnostic
  - To investigate the cause of a pleural effusion. A pleural biopsy is sometimes performed at the same time, as this increases the diagnostic yield
- Therapeutic
  - To drain large effusions for symptom relief
  - To instil therapeutic agents such as sclerosants.

Equipment

- Materials for a sterile procedure performed under local anaesthesia (page 635)
- Specimen containers
- For diagnostic tap: 20 ml syringe with 21 gauge needle
- For therapeutic tap
  - 50 ml syringe with Luer-Lock fitting
  - Three-way tap
  - 14 guage cannula
  - Receiver for fluid.

Method

This is a sterile procedure performed with a local anaesthetic (page 635). The patient should be sitting up and leaning over a suitably placed bed table with the arms folded in front of the body. The upper limit of the effusion posteriorly is determined from the chest X-ray and by percussion. The skin and subcutaneous tissues overlying the intercostal space at the chosen level are infiltrated with lignocaine and the area anaesthetized down to the pleura. The needle is passed over the upper border of the rib to avoid damaging the subcostal neurovascular bundle. For a diagnostic tap 20 ml of fluid is aspirated, placed into appropriate containers and sent for microscopy and culture, cytology and protein concentration.

If it fails ...

If you cannot obtain any fluid try a different space, usually higher up. If fluid cannot be aspirated or only a small amount is obtained (e.g. with a loculated effusion) an ultrasound examination will identify whether fluid is actually present and, if so, the most promising site for aspiration can be marked.

Complications

- Pneumothorax
- Pulmonary oedema; the risk is greatest with the rapid removal of large quantities of fluid (>1 litre)
- Damage to the neurovascular bundle which lies in the subcostal groove.
- Infection
- Seeding of malignant cells along the tract with a malignant effusion.

Chest drain insertion

Indications

- Aspiration of air (pneumothorax)
- Aspiration of fluid (blood, effusions, pus).

Equipment

- Materials for a sterile procedure performed under local anaesthetic (page 635)
- Scalpel blade
- Chest drain
- Underwater-seal bottle and connecting tubing
- '0' or '1' silk or nylon suture
- Artery forceps
- Dressings.

Procedure

This is a sterile procedure performed under local anaesthetic. The 4th–5th intercostal space in the midaxillary line is preferred, although the second interspace in the midclavicular line can be used in an emergency. For the former approach the patient should be sitting up and leaning over a suitably placed bed table, with the arms folded in front of the body. A 28 French gauge or larger drain should be used for blood to minimize blockage. A 24 French gauge is adequate for air or low-viscosity effusions.

The skin, underlying muscle and pleura should be infiltrated with 8–10 ml of 1% lignocaine, advancing over the upper border of the rib below to avoid the subcostal neurovascular bundle. Aspiration should be applied intermittently until the pleural cavity is entered and the presence of air or fluid confirmed. A 1 cm incision is made with the scalpel and a purse string suture inserted loosely around the incision. Access to the pleural cavity through the intercostal muscles is obtained by blunt dissection using a pair of artery forceps, and the track widened to allow the passage of a finger. The length of tube required is measured and inserted, *without the use of the central trocar*, into the pleural cavity. The drain is connected to the underwater drainage system and secured with the purse string suture and taped to the chest wall. The tube is then connected to the underwater drainage system and unclamped. If correctly placed, bubbling, drainage of fluid if present, and respiratory swing should be evident. The position of the tube and expansion of the lung are then checked with a chest X-ray. To remove the chest drain, ask the patient to exhale, remove the drain, and tighten the purse string suture to close the incision.

Complications

- Injury to the neurovascular bundle
- Re-expansion pulmonary oedema
- Infection.

Nasogastric tube insertion

Indications

- To drain gastric secretions, e.g. prior to surgery, acute pancreatitis or for bowel obstruction
- For enteral feeding (using a fine-bore tube).

Equipment

- Nasogastric tube
- Lignocaine lubricating jelly
- Large-bore syringe
- Litmus paper
- Drainage bag
- Adhesive tape.

Procedure

Lubricate the distal end of the tube with jelly and place into the nostril, advancing slowly towards the occiput. As the tube enters the pharynx, ask the patient to take a sip of water and to swallow as you advance the tube into the oesophagus. Once the tube is in the stomach, aspirate fluid with the syringe and test for acid with litmus paper (blue to pink). It is not possible to aspirate through fine-bore feeding tubes, and therefore the correct position must be confirmed with a chest X-ray prior to commencing feeding. Remember to secure the tube to the nose with adhesive tape.

Complications

- Aspiration
- Gastro-oesophageal reflux
- Local trauma to nose.

If you fail...

- Try the other nostril
- Put tube in the refrigerator, which usually causes it to stiffen.

Digital examination of the rectum

Place the patient in the left lateral position with the buttocks at the edge of the couch and ask them to curl up with their knees towards the chest. Wear a disposable glove on the right hand and separate the patient's buttocks with both hands. Examine the perineum and anus for inflammation, skin tags, external piles, fissures, fistulae and sinuses. If a prolapse is suspected ask the patient to bear down and look for the rectal mucosa or bowel appearing through the anus.

Put some lubricant on the index finger of the right hand and place the pulp of the finger flat on the anus. Introduce the finger into the anal canal by pushing gently in a slightly backwards direction. Extreme pain and spasm of the anal sphincter at this stage suggests an anal fissure, which may make further examination impossible. The lower end of the fissure, which is usually situated posteriorly, may be visible if the buttocks are gently separated. To examine the rectum the finger is advanced and rotated through 180°C so that the pulp of the finger lies anteriorly. The walls of the rectum are normally smooth and soft, and any deviation, e.g. polyps, carcinoma, should be noted. Posteriorly the coccyx and sacrum can be felt through the rectal wall, and anteriorly the prostate gland in men and the cervix in women. The normal prostate gland is smooth and firm with a shallow midline groove separating two lateral lobes. A hard, irregular gland with loss of the median groove is characteristic of carcinoma.

After withdrawal the examining finger should be inspected for blood and the colour of the faeces noted.

Abdominal paracentesis
Indications

- To investigate the cause of ascites
- Rapid relief of large-volume ascites.

Equipment

- Materials for a sterile procedure performed under local anaesthetic (page 635)
- For diagnostic tap: 20 ml syringe with 21 gauge needle
- For therapeutic tap
  - Large-bore (14 gauge) cannula with three-way tap
  - Collecting system and specimen containers
  - Intravenous giving set and plasma expander.

Procedure

This is a sterile procedure performed under local anaesthesia (page 635). Lie the patient in a semirecumbent position and confirm the presence of ascites clinically.

Clean and anaesthetize the skin over the right flank. For a diagnostic tap, a standard 21 gauge (green) needle attached to a 20 ml syringe is introduced along the anaesthetized track to the peritoneal cavity and fluid aspirated and sent for white cell count, microscopy and culture, and measurement of protein and amylase. For therapeutic paracentesis a large-bore cannula is introduced in a similar fashion until fluid is aspirated. The stylet is then removed and a 50 ml syringe and collecting system is attached to the cannula via a three-way tap. Aspiration is continued until the desired volume of fluid is removed. If large-volume paracentesis is planned an intravenous drip should be set up and (>3–4 litres) albumin infused at a concentration of 8 g per litre of fluid removed. Following the procedure a simple dry dressing is applied.

Complications

- Infection
- Ascitic fluid leak
- Puncture of intra-abdominal viscus
- Renal impairment and encephalopathy after large-volume paracentesis in patients with cirrhosis.

If it fails...

Ask the radiologist to perform the procedure under ultrasound control.

Sengstaken tube insertion

Indications

Variceal bleeding not controlled pharmacologically or by injection sclerotherapy

Equipment

- Sengstaken tube
- 50 ml syringe
- Radio-opaque contrast material (e.g. Omnipaque)
- Length of string
- 0.5 litre bag of saline or glucose
- Large collection bowl.

Procedure

Familiarize yourself with the construction of the tube and identify the four ports: two for aspiration of the oesophagus and stomach, and two for inflation of the oesophageal and gastric balloons (Figure 16.2). Check the capacity of both the gastric and the oesophageal balloon. With the patient on the left lateral side, insert the tube into the mouth and guide into the pharynx with the fingers. The tube should pass easily down the oesophagus. On entry into the stomach, blood is usually readily aspirated through the gastric aspiration port. Insert the tube as far as possible and inflate the gastric balloon with the appropriate volume of fluid (150–250 ml). Using a mixture of water and contrast

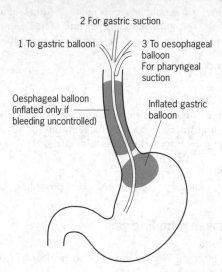

1 To gastric balloon

2 For gastric suction

3 To oesophageal balloon
For pharyngeal suction

Oesophageal balloon (inflated only if bleeding uncontrolled)

Inflated gastric balloon

Figure 16.2
Diagram of a Sengstaken tube in situ.

material aids radiological confirmation of correct placement. The tube is then withdrawn until resistance at the gastro-oesophageal junction is felt. At this stage the 0.5 litre bag of fluid is attached with string to the end of the tube and allowed to hang over the side of the bed, so that constant traction is applied to the balloon. It is not normally necessary to inflate the oesophageal balloon. The balloon should be left in place inflated for no longer than 24 hours to minimize the risk of pressure necrosis of the oesophagus.

Complications

- Oesophageal rupture
- Pressure necrosis leading to oesophageal ulceration and stricture
- Aspiration leading to pneumonia.

Urine collection and testing

Urine passed into a clean dry vessel is suitable for chemical tests. A midstream specimen of urine (MSU) is necessary for microscopy and culture. The urine should be analysed immediately or stored in a refrigerator to reduce the growth of contaminants.

Urine testing

Commercially prepared paper strips are available to test for urine specific gravity, pH, protein, glucose, ketones, bilirubin, urobilinogen and blood. Usually one strip is impregnated with dyes specific for each test. It is important that the strips are kept in sealed, dry containers and the test areas not handled. The manufacturers' instructions must be followed exactly. The strip is dipped briefly into the urine and its edge then run against the rim of the container to remove excess fluid. The strip is held horizontally (to prevent urine running down the strip and mixing the dyes) and the colour changes read at exactly the times specified by the manufacturer. The colour changes are compared with the colour charts supplied on the outside of the strip containers.

Bladder catheterization (urethral)
Indications

- Relief of urinary retention
- To monitor urinary output in the critically ill
- Urinary incontinence
- Collection of an uncontaminated urine specimen for bacteriological analysis.

Equipment

- Catheter pack (usually prepacked)
- Sterile lignocaine gel with nozzle
- 16–18 gauge catheter (usually Foley type)
- Sterile gloves
- 20 ml syringe with sterile water
- Catheter bag.

Procedure

Place the patient in a supine, slightly reclining position. Women should have their knees flexed and the thighs apart. In the female use one gloved hand to cleanse the urethral meatus while holding the labia apart with the other. In the male the foreskin, if present, should be retracted in order to cleanse the meatus with sterile saline. Apply sterile lignocaine gel to the tip of a 16–18 gauge catheter and into the urethra. Place a kidney dish between the legs in readiness. Insert the catheter into the urethra, holding the penis perpendicular to the body. Gentle pressure is required to advance the catheter into the bladder, at which point urine should flow into the kidney dish. Any resistance should prompt withdrawal and reinsertion. The catheter should be inserted almost to the side arm before inflating the balloon with the volume of sterile water indicated on the catheter. The catheter is then withdrawn to lie at the bladder neck. Reposition the foreskin in uncircumcised men, and record the volume of urine drained.

Complications

- Infection
- Urethral trauma.

If you fail...

Do not make repeated attempts in the male, as damage to the longer urethra can occur. Ask advice of surgeons/urologists for consideration of a suprapubic approach.

Lumbar puncture
Indications

- To obtain a sample of CSF for detection of infection, blood, malignant cells or abnormal proteins
- To introduce contrast material, e.g. myelography
- Administration of chemotherapeutic drugs.

Equipment

- Materials for a sterile procedure performed under local anaesthetic (page 635)
- 23–24 gauge spinal needle
- Manometer
- Three separate numbered sterile collection bottles.

Procedure

This is a sterile procedure performed under local anaesthetic. Position the patient on their left side on the edge of the bed with the knees curled up to the chest.

Identify the L3–L4 interspace by palpating the anterior superior iliac spine and marking the interspace perpendicularly below it. Having cleansed and anaesthetized the skin, insert the spinal needle in the interspace with the stylet in place aiming for the umbilicus. Resistance is usually felt at the spinal ligaments and again at the dura. The stylet can then be removed, at which stage clear colourless fluid should emerge. The manometer is then attached to measure pressure (normally 80–180 mmH$_2$O). Fluid is collected into the three separate numbered bottles. A decreasing concentration of red blood cells from bottles 1 to 3 indicates a traumatic tap, rather than blood in the CSF. Fluid should be sent for microscopy and culture, protein, and glucose concentration with a simultaneous plasma glucose sample. Additional investigations may be appropriate depending on the suspected diagnosis. The patient should lie flat for 12 hours after the procedure to avoid a headache that may develop.

Complications

- Post–procedure headache
- Infection
- Herniation of the brain stem through the foramen magnum ('coning').

If you fail...

Try with the patient sitting upright on the edge of the bed (CSF pressure cannot be measured in this position)

Diagnosis of death

When asked to confirm a patient's death it is important to see the body and to confirm the identity of the patient with the nursing staff.

Confirmation of death involves the demonstration of:

- Fixed and dilated pupils
- Absent carotid pulse
- No breath sounds over 1 minute
- No heart sounds over 1 minute
- No response to painful stimuli, e.g. pressing firmly on the sternum.

Record these details in the notes, giving the time and date of confirmation of death, and sign your name clearly.

Death certification and referral to the Coroner

A death certificate is usually completed on the day following death. It is signed by a doctor who attended the deceased in his or her last illness, and that doctor must have seen the patient both within 14 days before death and after death. Although there is no legal requirement for a doctor to inform the Coroner of a death (this is the legal responsibility of the Registrar of Deaths), it is usual to inform the Coroner of a death under particular circumstances. These include:

- Uncertain cause of death
- The patient has not been seen by the doctor within 14 days before death
- The death was suspicious
- Death occurred within 24 hours of admission to hospital without a firm diagnosis being made
- Deaths due to accidents, injuries, suicide, neglect, poisoning or drug or alcohol overdose
- Death of persons in legal custody
- Death related to medical treatment or within 24 hours of an anaesthetic.

Cremation forms

If the patient is to be cremated you will be asked to complete form B, the Certificate of Medical Attendance of the cremation form. You must have attended the patient within 14 days prior to death and you must see the patient after death (ensuring that there are no pacemaker implants in the body); make certain that the cause of death on the cremation form is identical to that on the death certificate.

Final medicine examination: Questions

....

INFECTIOUS DISEASES AND TROPICAL MEDICINE

1. Discuss the management of an otherwise healthy 32-year-old man who has just been found to be HIV positive.

2. What are the early symptoms and signs of rubella? Write short notes on its prevention.

3. How would you investigate and treat a young male patient presenting with urethral discharge?

4. Write short notes on diarrhoea 1 week after return from the Far East.

5. Describe briefly the intestinal infections produced by:
   (a) *Campylobacter* sp.
   (b) *Yersinia* sp.
   (c) *Clostridium difficile*

6. A 1-year-old boy has been unwell for 6 hours, temperature 40.5°C with eight petechial spots on the trunk and legs. He is drowsy, with systolic blood pressure of 45 mmHg.
   (a) What is the probable diagnosis?
   (b) What immediate treatment would you give?
   (c) What treatment would you give the rest of the family?
   (d) Can the disease be prevented in this age group?
   (e) What complications would you examine for at an outpatient visit 6 weeks later?

Answers

1. Most patients are found to be positive on antibody testing. Before any patient is tested for evidence of HIV infection they must be counselled by a trained person

(often a nurse), and a full explanation is given of what a positive test means. Some patients will require this information to be discussed again when they are subsequently found to have a positive test. They must be told that the result is confidential and will only be known by those staff involved with the care. A risk history must be established (e.g. intravenous drug abuse, sexual history) and advice given about avoiding transmission to others (i.e. non-penetrative sex, no sharing of needles). This patient is said to be healthy, but a full physical examination must be carried out to look for evidence of AIDS. A full list of those diseases that indicate AIDS in an HIV-positive patient is given in Table 1.9.

The natural history of the disease must be discussed (see page 32). Baseline investigations include FBC, CD4 count and HIV RNA to assess viral load. The mainstay of treatment is antiretroviral therapy, Examples of these drugs and indications for their use are given on page 38.

2. The clinical features of rubella are discussed on page 5. Prevention is active (live attenuated rubella vaccine given with mumps and measles as a single dose at 1–2 years of age) or passive (human immunoglobulin reduces symptoms but does not reduce teratogenic effects).

3. This is discussed on pages 28–29.

4. This is traveller's diarrhoea and the causes are listed in Table 1.5. This question does not say whether this is bloody diarrhoea, but the presence of blood narrows the differential diagnosis. Most cases are self-limiting but antibiotics may be necessary for severe infections. Ciprofloxacillin covers most of these organisms. Metronidazole is given for amoebiasis or giardiasis.

5. (a) The only campylobacter producing intestinal infection is *Campylobacter jejuni*, which belongs to the genus *Vibrio* (other members are *Vibrio cholerae* and *Vibrio parahaemolyticus*). *Campylobacter* and *Salmonella* species account for most cases of food poisoning (poultry is the main source of infection in both). Campylobacter infection produces a prodromal febrile infection lasting 1–4 days, followed by a diarrhoeal phase which may last 1–2 weeks. Severe abdominal pains often accompany the

diarrhoea, which may be bloodstained. Septicaemia may occur, but rarely death. Sigmoidoscopy may show an acute colitis resembling ulcerative colitis. Diagnosis is made by microscopy (seen as motile rods) and culture of faeces. Infection is usually self-limiting antibiotic treatment with erythromycin is given to those with systemic symptoms. Complications include cholecystitis, pancreatitis and reactive arthritis.

(b) There are three main *Yersinia* species in humans, all of which are uncommon in Britain. *Y. pseudotuberculosis* and *Y. enterocolitica* cause diarrhoea, terminal ileitis and mesenteric adenitis (may be confused with appendicitis). Diagnosis is usually by serology, demonstrating a rise in antibody titre on paired samples. The illness is usually self-limiting, but tetracycline may be helpful for treating a severe infection. The third species, *Y. pestis*, causes plague.

(c) *Clostridium difficile* produces pseudomembranous colitis, which is an uncommon complication of antibiotic therapy. *Cl. difficile* is present in the colon of some healthy individuals, and colitis has been attributed to the selection of drug-resistant *Cl. difficile* that proliferates in the colon and produces a necrotizing toxin. Diagnosis is by demonstration of the toxin in stool and by typical sigmoidoscopic appearances (pseudomembranous on an erythematous background). Treatment is with oral metronidazole or vancomycin.

6. The temperature and hypotension indicate septicaemic shock. The petechial spots suggest this is caused by infection with *Neisseria meningitidis* (not all of these infections produce meningitis).

(a) Fulminant meningococcaemia is a severe life-threatening illness with a rapidly progressive downhill course.

(b) The initial treatment is intravenous benzylpenicillin, which must be started immediately the diagnosis is clinically suspected. In addition, shock should be treated urgently (page 442).

(c) Family contacts should receive prophylaxis with rifampicin 600 mg twice daily for 2 days.

(d) A vaccine is available but offers only short-term protection and is generally only given when travelling to high-risk places, e.g. Africa, Asia, South America and the Middle East, or during institutional outbreaks.

(e) A small number of patients develop chronic complications, e.g. arthritis, vasculitis and pericarditis, which may be due to immune complex disease.

....

GASTROENTEROLOGY

1. State the causes of bloody diarrhoea. What are the most common infectious causes and what specific antibacterial therapy is available to treat them?

2. Write short notes on the management of massive haematemesis.

3. A 30-year-old man presents with a 10-week history of discomfort in the right iliac fossa. He has also noticed some weight loss. The ESR is raised (50 mm/h). What are the likely causes? What imaging tests might be appropriate?

4. A 23-year-old beautician, who is otherwise well, gives a 5-year history of alternating morning diarrhoea, constipation, flatulence and left lower quadrant abdominal pain. What is the most likely diagnosis and how would you manage the problem?

5. A man of 30 presents with a 3-month history of difficulty in swallowing. What features of the history and clinical examination would help in making a diagnosis?

6. How would you investigate and manage a 44-year-old patient found to have a lesser curve gastric ulcer on a barium meal examination?

7. A 45-year-old man presents with a 6-month history of loose, pale, bulky offensive stools associated with mild abdominal discomfort. Discuss the differential diagnosis and your approach to investigation and treatment.

Answers

1. Bloody diarrhoea strongly suggests colonic disease. The common causes are inflammatory bowel disease and

infections, although colon cancer (usually blood mixed in with the stools, not frank diarrhoea) and acute intestinal ischaemia should be borne in mind. The infectious causes of bloody diarrhoea are *Compylobacter jejuni*, *Shigella* sp. (bacillary dysentery), *Entamoeba histolytica* (amoebic dysentery, occurring in the tropics), some types of *Escherichia coli* and, rarely, *Salmonella* sp. and *Clostridium difficile*. Ciprofloxacillin will cover the common organisms except *Entamoeba histolytica*, which is treated with metronidazole.

2. Massive haematemesis is usually the result of bleeding from varices or large peptic ulcers. Patients are usually shocked on presentation and must be aggressively resuscitated, initially with plasma expanders (page 442) and subsequently with whole blood. After adequate resuscitation the source of bleeding is localized at gastroscopy; further management depends on the cause (page 59).

3. In a young person right iliac fossa discomfort associated with weight loss and a raised ESR strongly suggests Crohn's disease (page 70). An appendix mass must be considered, although the history is long. In immigrants, ileocaecal tuberculosis should be considered (page 66). Amoebiasis may sometimes cause right iliac fossa pain, usually with the formation of an 'amoeboma', and this should be considered in travellers from the tropics. Imaging is with abdominal ultrasonography and small-bowel follow-through.

4. These features, particularly in a young, otherwise healthy female, are very suggestive of irritable bowel syndrome. The approach to management is outlined on page 84.

5. The causes of dysphagia are listed on page 45. Progressive dysphagia associated with weight loss is suggestive of malignancy, although this would be unusual in a young man. A preceding history of heartburn suggests reflux with a complicating peptic stricture. Chest pain, regurgitation and dysphagia for liquids points to a motility disorder such as achalasia. Oesophageal candidiasis or cytomegalovirus infection may cause dysphagia in patients with AIDS.

6. The investigation and management of gastric ulceration is described on pages 54–55. Benign gastric ulcers may appear radiologically similar to gastric cancer, and therefore endoscopy with multiple biopsies is usually recommended. Ulcers associated with *Helicobacter pylori* infection are treated by eradicating *H. pylori*. Ulcers that are *H. pylori* negative, e.g. those associated with NSAID ingestion, are treated with acid-suppressing drugs such as ranitidine or omeprazole. Gastric ulcers must be followed up (by endoscopy) to ensure healing. An ulcer that is resistant to treatment raises the question of malignancy (initial biopsies may be negative because of sampling error), and repeat biopsies must be taken. Remember that NSAIDs are an important cause of gastric ulceration, so these should be withdrawn if possible.

7. These features are strongly suggestive of malabsorption, which may result from either chronic pancreatic insufficiency (page 137) or disease of the small intestine. A careful history may elucidate the cause (? family history, travel abroad?, heavy alcohol consumption?) Initial screening tests would include the measurement of stool fat and stool weight, and an FBC including B_{12} and red cell folate. Small intestinal causes of malabsorption are discussed on pages 62–66. Assessment of pancreatic structure and function is dealt with on page 138.

LIVER, BILIARY TRACT AND PANCREATIC DISEASES

The most common types of questions all relate to the differential diagnosis and appropriate investigations in a jaundiced patient.

1. A 50-year-old woman complains of itching, passing dark urine and pale stools, and is deeply jaundiced. What causes should be considered in the first instance and how would you investigate these?

2. A 36-year-old woman presents with a 4-day history of painless jaundice. There is no previous history of medical illness and, apart from marked jaundice, there are no abnormal physical signs. Initial investigations show:

Hb 11.5 g/dl, WCC 36 × 10^9/l, MCV 106 fl,
platelets 41 × 10^9/l
Serum sodium 129 mmol/l, potassium 2 mmol/l,
urea 1.4 mmol/l Serum bilirubin 190 mmol/l,
alkaline phosphatase 350 U/l, ALT 108 U/l,
gGT 250 U/l.

Hepatitis B and A antibody titres are not elevated.
Serum vitamin B$_{12}$ and folate are normal.
What is the probable diagnosis and what further tests
would be useful? What is the initial management?

Other questions relate to the management of complications
that may develop in chronic liver disease.

3. Discuss the immediate and subsequent management of a
   patient with haematemesis caused by oesophageal varices.

4. Describe the factors underlying the formation of ascites.
   Describe the principles of management when the ascites
   results from chronic liver disease.

Answers

1. The jaundice is associated with pruritus, dark urine and
pale stools, and is therefore cholestatic. The next step is to
establish whether this is intrahepatic or extrahepatic. The
causes are listed in Table 3.1. Information obtained from a
detailed clinical history and physical examination may well
point to one of these as the probable cause; ultrasonography
is the initial key investigation (Figure 3.2).

2. The most probable diagnosis is alcoholic hepatitis
superimposed on a background of chronic alcoholic liver
disease (even in the absence of physical signs). The raised
MCV (with a normal vitamin B$_{12}$ and folate), very high
γGT and thrombocytopenia all suggest alcohol abuse. The
very high WCC is typical of alcoholic hepatitis. The
sodium is probably low because of inability to excrete a
free water load and dilutional hyponatraemia (page 259).
Further investigations and initial management are discussed
on page 125. In addition, thiamine must be given to
prevent Wernicke's encephalopathy (page 468).

3. The answers to these are discussed on pages 59 and 114,
respectively.

DISEASES OF THE BLOOD AND HAEMATOLOGICAL MALIGNANCIES

The most common questions relate to the investigation and differential diagnosis of patients presenting with anaemia, usually microcytic or macrocytic. The anaemia of chronic disease frequently appears, but the emphasis in these questions is usually on the investigation of the underlying pathology (Q4).

1. Discuss the causes of hypochromic/microcytic anaemia.

2. You are asked to assess a 25-year-old woman who is found to have a low haemoglobin at her first antenatal booking clinic. There are no physical abnormalities. The values are as follows: Hb 10.7 g/dl, MCV 64 fl, WBC 7.2×10^9/l, platelets 202×10^9/l. What diagnoses do you consider and what simple investigations would you request in the first instance? Why are they important?

3. A 36-year-old woman complains of being easily tired over 6 months, and her stools have become more frequent. An FBC shows a Hb of 8 g/dl, MCV 110 fl. Describe your investigations and treatment.

4. A 65-year-old woman comes to see you complaining of severe headaches for several weeks, and of now having lost vision in one eye. Initial investigations show: Hb 10.5 g/dl, WBC 8.0×10^9/l, ESR 90 mm.
   (a) What features would you pay attention to in the physical examination?
   (b) What is the probable diagnosis?
   (c) What further diagnostic investigation would you arrange?
   (d) What treatment would you give?
   (e) What possible complications of this treatment would concern you in a patient of this age?

Other common questions are listed below.

5. Discuss the diagnostic considerations in investigating an adult presenting with non-accidental bruising.

6. Discuss the investigation and management of a 50-year-old man found to have a raised haematocrit (packed cell volume or PCV) on routine blood count.

7. Discuss the causes and investigation of persistent enlargement of the cervical lymph nodes in a man aged 25 years.

8. A 60-year-old woman with repeated sore throats has a blood count carried out by her general practitioner who seeks your advice. Investigations reveal: Hb 9.1 g/dl, WBC 2.0×10^9/l, platelets 80×10^9/l. What does it show and what causes should you consider?

Answers

1. The causes of hypochromic/microcytic anaemia are discussed on pages 142–145. Iron deficiency is the most common cause.

2. This woman has a mild microcytic anaemia. The most probable causes are thalassaemia trait (particularly with the very low MCV) and iron-deficiency anaemia. Iron requirements increase during pregnancy (2 mg/day) as a result of transfer of iron to the fetus and an increased red cell mass. These processes occur largely in the second trimester, and therefore it is likely that she was iron deficient before pregnancy (if this is the cause of the anaemia). In a young woman the most probable cause of iron deficiency is heavy menstrual blood loss (suggested by frequent periods, the passage of clots and frequent changes of pads/tampons). Investigations are Hb electrophoresis and iron studies (page 144).

3. Anaemia with an MCV >100 fl is most probably the result of vitamin B_{12} or folate deficiency. The frequent stools suggest gastrointestinal disease. Taking these two together, the most likely diagnosis is small bowel disease, either Crohn's or coeliac disease (pages 70 and 62). Initial investigations are the measurement of serum vitamin B_{12}, red cell folate, serum antiendomysial antibodies, small-bowel follow-through and jejunal biopsy. There may also be malabsorption of iron, and iron deficiency must be excluded (page 144). Treatment is that of the underlying disease and the replacement of haematinics (pages 72, 64, 148 and 149).

4. The most probable diagnosis is giant cell arteritis (page 608) causing central retinal artery occlusion and anaemia of chronic disease. Examine the temporal arteries, the eyes (milky-white fundus as a result of oedema) and generally (fever, weight loss). The diagnosis and treatment are discussed on page 609. Complications of steroid treatment are: osteoporosis and fractures, diabetes mellitus, hypertension, depression, psychosis and risk of peptic ulceration, particularly when taken together with NSAIDs.

5. The causes and investigation of a bleeding disorder are discussed on pages 177–178. Bruising suggests a platelet or vascular problem. Inherited clotting factor deficiency usually presents with mucosal bleeding, bleeding after surgery and haemarthroses. The probable cause may be suggested after thorough history and examination (e.g. female or male patient, age, family history, concomitant disease, drugs, alcohol).

6. This is polycythaemia and is discussed on page 166.

7. Persistent enlargement of a group of nodes makes most infections unlikely. In a young man this is most probably the result of Hodgkin's disease, leukaemia, or possibly TB. Non-Hodgkin's lymphoma is uncommon in a young person. If there are risk factors, HIV infection (usually generalized lymphadenopathy) must be considered. Initial investigations: FBC and blood film, ESR, lymph node biopsy for histological examination. Further investigation, which includes chest radiograph, CT, bone marrow and HIV test, would depend partly on initial results.

8. This elderly woman has pancytopenia, the causes of which are listed in Table 4.7. The probable cause may be suggested by a detailed history (particularly drugs) and physical examination. A bone marrow trephine biopsy is the key investigation.

....

RHEUMATOLOGY

1. Describe a typical attack of gout. How would you confirm the diagnosis and treat the patient?

2. Write short notes on the investigation and treatment of an acute arthritis of one ankle in a man aged 50 years.

3. A 45-year-old woman with a long-standing history of rheumatoid arthritis presents with a 6-month history of increasing dyspnoea. She does not experience orthopnoea. The venous pressure is not elevated and her heart sounds are normal. Her electrocardiogram is normal. Blood gases on air show an arterial P_{O_2} 7.7 kPa, venous P_{CO_2} 4.9 kPa, pH 7.45.
   (a) What is the probable diagnosis?
   (b) What other physical signs would you look for?
   (c) What other investigations would be helpful and what would you expect the results to show?

4. A 72-year-old woman with known breast cancer presents with dehydration, confusion and vomiting. Her corrected serum calcium is 3.8 mmol/l. Discuss your approach to management.

5. Write short notes on the causes of tetany in a 23-year-old woman.

6. A woman of 55 presents with backache which proves to be osteoporotic in origin. What features would lead to this diagnosis, what are the predisposing factors and how would you treat her?

7. A 60-year-old woman with a long history of alcohol abuse presents because she can no longer climb stairs or rise from chairs. She has recently begun treatment with NSAIDs given by her general practitioner for presumed osteoarthritis of both hips. Biochemical investigations reveal the following data: serum sodium 142 mmol/l, potassium 4.2 mmol/l, chloride 102 mmol/l, urea 8 mmol/l, creatinine 60 mmol/l, corrected calcium 2.2 mmol/l, phosphate 0.5 mmol/l, alkaline phosphatase 1000 U/l. Discuss these results. What do you consider to be the most probable diagnosis? Describe appropriate investigations to support your diagnosis and discuss what might be the best treatment.

Answers

1. A typical attack of gout is described on page 228. The diagnosis is confirmed by joint aspiration (page 230). The

serum uric acid is measured, but may be normal in an acute attack. Radiographs are rarely helpful; they are normal in the early stages, but in chronic disease there may be periarticular erosions. Treatment is (a) of the acute attack, (b) general advice, and (c) consideration for long-term therapy if there have been many previous attacks or evidence of chronic gouty tophi on physical examination (page 230).

2. The causes and immediate investigation of a large joint monoarthritis are discussed on page 201. Subsequent tests would depend on the findings on joint aspiration, and may include radiography of the joint and the measurement of serum uric acid concentration.

3. The probable diagnosis is fibrosing alveolitis, a rare complication of rheumatoid arthritis. Less probably it is drug induced (rare side effects of gold and methotrexate). She has type I respiratory failure (page 449). Physical signs to look for are central cyanosis, clubbing, reduced chest expansion and end-expiratory crackles at the lung bases. Investigations to confirm the diagnosis are listed on page 426.

4. Severe hypercalcaemia such as this is a medical emergency and almost certainly related to malignancy. Management is discussed in Emergency Box 5.1. Other causes of hypercalcaemia are listed in Table 5.13.

5. In a 23-year-old, presumably otherwise healthy, woman the most probable cause is respiratory alkalosis secondary to hyperventilation. Alkalosis causes tetany by reducing ionization of calcium salts (ionized calcium is physiologically active). Other causes of tetany – hypocalcaemia (page 244), hypokalaemia (page 262) and hypomagnesaemia (page 265) – are much less likely, but must be considered.

6. Backache occurs in osteoporosis as a result of vertebral collapse or a crush fracture (not osteoporosis per se), which is seen on plain radiograph. Bone densitometry is used to confirm the diagnosis of osteoporosis and measure the response to treatment. The predisposing factors are listed on page 240; of these, the most important is early

menopause. The treatment is analgesia in the short term and, in the long term, hormone replacement therapy, maintenance of calcium intake, and bisphosphonates (page 241).

7. There is a borderline low serum calcium, a very low serum phosphate and markedly raised alkaline phosphatase. The diagnosis is probably osteomalacia (resulting from vitamin D deficiency), causing a proximal myopathy. Against this is the very high alkaline phosphatase, which is usually only moderately raised in osteomalacia. The myopathy may be the result of alcohol, but this does not explain the very high alkaline phosphatase. The serum urea is raised and the creatinine is at the lower end of the normal range. This picture is seen with dehydration or a gastrointestinal bleed (possibly related to ingestion of NSAIDs).

....

WATER AND ELECTROLYTES

1. A 39-year-old woman is admitted to a hospital with a 3-week history of nausea, vomiting and weakness following a chest infection. She has a past history of depression and hypothyroidism, for which she was taking thyroxine. On examination she is dehydrated, drowsy and pigmented with a blood pressure of 70/40 mmHg. She is oliguric and investigation shows: haemoglobin 14.9 g/dl, white blood cells 7.4×10^9/l, urea 22.8 mmol/l, creatinine 290 mmol/l, sodium 118 mmol/l, potassium 5.7 mmol/l, bicarbonate 23 mmol/l, thyroxine 29.6 mmol/l, free T_4 4.5 pmol/l, TSH >50 mU/l.
   (a) What are the probable diagnoses and their cause?
   (b) What further investigations are indicated?
   (c) What is the initial treatment?

2. Write short notes on potassium deficiency.

3. What are the possible causes of a low plasma sodium concentration and how may they be distinguished? What clinical effects may be attributable to this abnormality?

Answers

1 (a) This presentation is typical of an Addisonian crisis precipitated by the chest infection. The patient is markedly hypotensive and dehydrated on clinical examination. The raised urea and creatinine are compatible with dehydration and prerenal acute renal failure (page 299). The serum sodium is very low and, in combination with the clinical findings, suggests that the cause is salt and water loss (page 257), from either the kidney or the gastrointestinal tract. The combination of pigmented skin, a history of probable autoimmune disease (the most common cause of hypothyroidism is autoimmune) and hyperkalaemia suggests Addison's disease (page 499) resulting from autoimmune adrenal destruction. The thyroid function tests show evidence of hypothyroidism (low thyroxine, low T_4 and raised TSH).

(b) Blood glucose (to look for hypoglycaemia), random plasma cortisol and ACTH, chest radiograph, blood cultures, serum adrenal autoantibodies.

(c) The immediate and subsequent management of an Addisonian crisis is given in Emergency box 12.3.

2. Potassium deficiency (which implies total body depletion) is not the same as hypokalaemia (which means a low serum concentration and may be caused by deficiency or redistribution into cells). Depletion occurs with excess losses or inadequate intake (rare) and the causes are listed in Table 6.7.

3. The causes, investigation and symptoms of hyponatraemia are discussed on pages 257–260. Management of hyponatraemia resulting from water excess is given in Emergency box 6.1.

RENAL DISEASE

Three topics occur commonly and with almost equal frequency. These are chronic renal failure, the causes and management of acute renal failure, and the causes of proteinuria and the nephrotic syndrome.

1. What are the clinical features of 'end-stage' renal failure, and how may it be treated?

2. What clinical and other evidence would lead you to suspect the diagnosis of chronic renal failure in a 50-year-old man? How would you determine the cause of renal failure?

3. In a patient presenting with a plasma creatinine of 500 µmol/l which of the following features would suggest that the renal failure is chronic, rather than acute?
   (a) Reduced renal size detected by ultrasonography.
   (b) A urine sodium concentration of less than 10 mmol/l.
   (c) Elevated serum alkaline phosphatase and subperiosteal erosions on radiograph of the hands.
   (d) A haemoglobin of 14 g/l.
   (e) The presence of ureteric obstruction on renal ultrasonography.
   (f) Evidence of polyneuropathy.

4. List the causes of renal failure resulting from poor perfusion of the kidneys. What are the clinical and laboratory features?

5. What factors contribute to the development of acute renal failure in a patient with multiple injuries following a road traffic accident? Outline your management during the first 24–48 hours.

6. You have been asked to see a 45-year-old man with a creatinine of 530 µmol/l whose urinary output has fallen to 150 ml over 24 hours. Discuss the differential diagnosis and your approach to investigation.

7. A 50-year-old man presents with bilateral ankle swelling and is found to have a serum albumin of 28 g/l. Discuss the differential diagnosis in terms of history, possible physical findings and further helpful investigations.

Other questions are:

8. Describe how patients with glomerulonephritis may present.

9. Discuss the presentation and management of recurrent urinary tract infection in women.

Answers

1. The clinical features and treatment of end-stage renal failure are discussed on pages 305–309.

2. A patient presenting with any of the complications discussed on page 305 would lead you to suspect chronic renal failure (CRF), but the usual ways in which patients present are with hypertension, nocturia and polyuria, or with symptoms of anaemia. The investigations for renal failure are discussed on page 305. A renal biopsy is performed in patients with normal-sized kidneys. Small kidneys are technically difficult to biopsy, histological investigations are hard to interpret, and at this late stage the prognosis would not be influenced by treatment of the underlying condition.

3. (a), (c) and (f) suggest chronic renal failure. The urine sodium concentration is very low, and this may occur with prerenal acute renal failure (when the kidney is conserving sodium) and with chronic renal failure when the concentrating ability of the kidney is lost and large amounts of dilute urine are produced. The normal Hb is in favour of acute renal failure.

4. This is discussed on page 299. Poor perfusion of the kidneys is usually caused by hypovolaemia; other causes include pump failure (cardiogenic shock) or shock resulting from a pulmonary embolism. The clinical and laboratory features are described on pages 299 and 300.

5. The most probable cause is poor renal perfusion secondary to hypovolaemia from blood loss. Other causes include rhabdomyolysis (extensive crush injury to muscle leads to the release of myoglobin, which is directly toxic to renal tubular cells), ruptured urethra (suspect with severe pelvic fractures and anuria) and later septicaemia and drugs (e.g. gentamicin). Initial management is to correct hypovolaemia with whole blood (measurement of central venous pressure will guide replacement) followed by a bolus of frusemide (page 300) if the patient remains oliguric. If urine output does not increase and urethral rupture is excluded as the cause of oliguria, then treatment is as far established acute tubular necrosis (page 304). The

investigations must include measurement of the muscle enzyme creatinine phosphokinase.

6. The short history of oliguria and decline of renal function suggests acute renal failure. The aetiology and investigations are discussed on pages 293–303.

7. Hypoalbuminaemia is caused by decreased synthesis (liver disease) or increased loss from the kidneys or, rarely, the gut (protein-losing enteropathy). The main differential is between liver disease and nephrotic syndrome. Important points in the history are risk factors for chronic liver disease (e.g. alcohol, intravenous drug abuse) and diseases that may be associated with nephrotic syndrome (e.g. diabetes, chronic infections and amyloidosis, drugs). Signs of chronic liver disease must be looked for on physical examination. Initial investigations are liver biochemistry and measurement of urinary protein excretion.

8. This is discussed on page 278.

9. This is discussed on pages 285–286.

....

CARDIOVASCULAR DISEASE

1. What simple screening tests are justified in a 45-year-old man presenting with hypertension? What are the causes of secondary hypertension, and how could your investigations demonstrate them?

2. A 55-year-old man presents with retrosternal chest pain radiating to the left arm and jaw. The character of the pain is suggestive of myocardial ischaemia.
   (a) What additional features in the clinical history would suggest that the pain is angina rather than myocardial infarction?
   (b) What features in the history would suggest that this is unstable angina?
   (c) Describe the management of a patient with unstable angina.

3. A 28-year-old married man with a family history of ischaemic heart disease presents with exertional chest pain. Discuss the investigation and management.

4. (a) How would you try to differentiate acute
       pericarditis from acute myocardial infarction
       clinically?
   (b) Pericarditis may be a complication of myocardial
       infarction. When after the infarction does it
       typically occur?
   (c) What are the most common causes of acute
       pericarditis in the UK?

5. A 60-year-old woman presents with breathlessness and
   clinical features of mild heart failure. She is found to
   have atrial fibrillation with an uncontrolled ventricular
   response (130 beats/min).
   (a) Give four possible causes for the atrial fibrillation.
   (b) Name three drugs that may be used to control the
       ventricular response.
   (c) What investigations would you order?

6. A 44-year-old woman is admitted to hospital with
   malaise and fever. She has felt unwell for 6 months.
   Examination shows pallor, an apical pansystolic
   murmur and splenomegaly. A blood count sent by the
   general practitioner shows a haemoglobin of 8.4 g/dl,
   WBC 7.2×10^9/l and platelets 394×10^9/l.
   (a) What investigations are required?
   (b) How might treatment be monitored?

7. (a) Discuss the clinical features of an acute attack of
       left ventricular failure.
   (b) Name three physical findings that would be of
       most value in distinguishing it from other causes
       of severe shortness of breath.

8. What are the key points to the management of acute
   pulmonary oedema?

9. A 50-year-old man complains of a painful red swollen
   calf.
   (a) What factors may be responsible?
   (b) How would you discriminate between the causes?

10. A 61-year-old man is admitted following a year's
    history of dizziness on exertion, culminating in a
    black-out while cutting the lawn. On admission he
    has a slow rising pulse and a systolic ejection murmur.
    There is no history of angina.

(a) What is the likely diagnosis?
(b) How would you estimate its clinical severity?
(c) What is the most probable pathology?
(d) What is the treatment?

Answers

1. If the history or physical examination does not suggest a secondary cause for hypertension the screening tests in a middle-aged man are a chest radiograph, serum urea, creatinine and electrolytes, and stix testing of the urine to look for protein and blood. The secondary causes of hypertension are listed on page 385 and the relevance of these investigations discussed on page 511. An ECG is also performed to look for end-organ damage (left ventricular hypertrophy), which is an indication for early treatment rather than observation in a patient with mild hypertension.

2. (a) The pain of angina is usually less severe than that of myocardial infarction. Classic angina comes on with exercise and is relieved by rest, and the pain is usually not accompanied by other symptoms such as sweating, nausea or vomiting. The pain of myocardial infarction may come on at rest, is persistent and may last several hours, and is often accompanied by sweating, nausea and vomiting.

(b) Unstable angina is angina of recent onset (less than 1 month), worsening angina or angina at rest.

(c) This is discussed on page 353.

3. The nature of the chest pain and the positive family history suggest a diagnosis of angina resulting from ischaemic heart disease. He is very young and every effort should be made to confirm the diagnosis, identify risk factors and determine the extent and site of coronary artery stenosis. A resting ECG, and usually an exercise ECG, is performed (page 351). Risk factors (page 349) are identified from the history, physical examination and measurement of serum cholesterol and blood glucose; every effort must be made to correct abnormalities. In younger people (<50 years) coronary angiography is often performed to document the site and extent of coronary artery stenosis, which will guide future management. In patients with left main stem or multivessel disease, coronary artery bypass grafting is of

clear prognostic benefit compared to medical therapy. Treatment is medical (page 351) in the first instance in the absence of these lesions. His siblings and children should also be screened for risk factors, e.g. familial hypercholesterolaemia.

4. (a) Acute pericarditis and myocardial infarction are discussed on pages 382 and 353. They can usually be differentiated on the basis of the nature, the site and radiation of the pain, and the presence of associated symptoms and signs (e.g. nausea, vomiting, breathlessness, pericardial rub on auscultation).

   (b) Pericarditis is common in the first few days, particularly in anterior wall infarction. Postmyocardial infarction syndrome (Dressler's syndrome) is much less common. It occurs weeks or months after an acute myocardial infarction and consists of pericarditis, fever and a pericardial effusion. It is caused by an autoimmune response to damaged cardiac tissue.

   (c) Coxsackie viral infection and myocardial infarction.

5. The causes of atrial fibrillation are listed on page 331. In an elderly woman the probable causes are ischaemic heart disease, mitral valve disease, thyrotoxicosis and cardiomyopathy. The drugs usually used to control the ventricular rate are those that slow conduction through the AV node: digoxin, β-blockers and verapamil. Digoxin is the only one not to have a negative inotropic action, and can thus be used in heart failure. Investigations are an ECG (which will show fibrillation and may show evidence of ischaemia or mitral valve disease, Figure 8.7), a chest radiograph (which will confirm the clinical diagnosis of heart failure and may show evidence of mitral valve disease, Figure 8.14), an echocardiogram, and thyroid function tests.

6. This combination of clinical signs suggests infective endocarditis affecting the mitral valve. Investigations are discussed on page 374. Treatment is monitored clinically (patient well being, temperature charts, evidence of heart failure) and by regular blood counts, ESR and echocardiography. Antibiotic doses are adjusted according

to bacteriological studies (minimum bactericidal concentration) and gentamicin levels (to ensure therapeutic levels are obtained but without toxic levels likely to cause side effects).

7. (a) Clinical features of acute left ventricular failure are listed on page 347.

(b) A gallop rhythm, widespread crackles and pulsus alternans differentiate pulmonary oedema from other causes of acute shortness of breath (listed in Table 9.1). In pulsus alternans the arterial pressure alternates between high and low systolic peaks. Its presence indicates severe left ventricular failure.

8. The key points to the management of pulmonary oedema are listed in Emergency Box 8.2.

9. (a) The differential diagnosis of a swollen calf includes deep venous thrombosis (DVT), cellulitis or a ruptured Baker's cyst. Oedema in heart failure or hypoalbuminaemia also causes a swollen calf, but this is usually bilateral. A Baker's cyst (popliteal cyst) is a synovial cyst in the popliteal fossa which sometimes occurs in patients with a knee effusion. Rupture of the cyst produces sudden and severe pain, swelling and tenderness of the upper calf.

(b) The diagnosis of a ruptured Baker's cyst is often missed and treated inappropriately with anticoagulants. An ultrasound will distinguish a ruptured cyst from a DVT.

10. (a) The history and examination are typical of aortic stenosis (page 368). As in this case, presentation is usually in the sixth decade.

(b) The presence of symptoms indicates at least moderately severe aortic stenosis. A longer ejection systolic murmur, clinical and ECG evidence of left ventricular hypertrophy all indicate more severe stenosis. The severity may be more accurately assessed by Doppler echocardiography.

(c) The most likely pathology is a calcified bicuspid aortic valve.

(d) Treatment in a symptomatic patient is valve replacement.

RESPIRATORY DISEASE

1. A 17-year-old girl presents to Accident and Emergency with an acute exacerbation of asthma.
   (a) What features on clinical examination would suggest a severe attack of asthma?
   (b) How would your findings influence the management of this patient?

2. A 45-year-old woman develops breathlessness and wheezing following a cold. What features would you seek to support a diagnosis of asthma?

3. Describe your approach to the investigation and management of pneumonia in a 50-year-old ventilation engineer.

4. (a) What are the main causes of haemoptysis?
   (b) How would you investigate a patient with this complaint?

5. (a) List the four conditions which you consider most likely to account for acute shortness of breath in a 50-year-old man.
   (b) What are the most important physical signs for each condition?
   (c) Which initial investigation is likely to be most helpful, together with the clinical history and examination, in distinguishing between these causes?

6. Discuss your management of a 25-year-old man presenting with acute right pleural pain, in whom the radiograph shows air in the pleural cavity and a completely collapsed right lung.

7. A 28-year-old previously healthy Caucasian female presents with a persistent dry cough for 4 weeks. She has also recently developed a nodular rash on her legs. She does not smoke and works in an office. Physical examination reveals coarse crackles at both lung bases and a rash on her legs. A chest X-ray shows prominent bilateral hilar lymphadenopathy and reticulonodular infiltrates in both lung fields.

(a) What is the most likely diagnosis?

(b) What is the most likely cause of the rash on the legs?

(c) If a lung biopsy was obtained, what would you expect it to show?

8. A 35-year-old woman is admitted as an emergency with acute onset of shortness of breath and central chest pain. She was recently discharged from hospital after a cholecystectomy. On examination she is obese, pale, sweating, pulse 120/min and BP 80/50. The JVP is raised by 4 cm and there is a left parasternal heave. She smokes 30 cigarettes per day and takes the combined oral contraceptive pill.

(a) What is the most likely diagnosis?

(b) In this patient, what are the risk factors for the presumed diagnosis?

(c) What is the immediate treatment of this condition?

Answers

1. (a) Features of a severe attack of asthma are:
- Inability to complete a sentence in one breath
- Pulse >110 beats/min
- Respirations ≥25 breaths/min
- PEFR 33–50% of predicted value or 33–50% of patient's best.

There are additional clinical features which suggest that the attack is life-threatening, and these are listed on page 402.

(b) Acute severe asthma is a medical emergency and an indication for urgent hospital admission. The management is discussed in Emergency Box 9.1.

2. A positive family history, previous wheezing on exposure to allergens and other clinical features discussed on page 399 support a diagnosis of asthma.

3. The causes of pneumonia in a healthy adult are listed on page 413. Pneumonia in a ventilation engineer may be the result of any of the causes of community-acquired pneumonia, but he is particularly at risk of infection with *Legionella* sp. The initial treatment must cover this organism, and investigations performed must look

particularly for evidence of this infection (page 416). Additional treatment includes oxygen therapy to correct hypoxaemia and treatment of complications, e.g. acute renal failure, hyponatraemia.

4. The causes of haemoptysis and investigation are listed on page 393.

5. (a) Acute means onset over hours or days. The most probable causes are pulmonary oedema, pneumothorax and pneumonia (although cough is often the predominant symptom). Pulmonary embolism may occur, particularly in a patient with risk factors (page 185).

(b) A patient with pulmonary oedema is acutely breathless, wheezy (cardiac asthma) and may cough up frothy blood-tinged sputum. They may be sweating profusely, and on auscultation there is a gallop rhythm and wheezes and crackles are heard throughout the chest. Pneumonia and pulmonary embolism may produce pleuritic chest pain and a pleuritic rub may be present. The patient with pneumonia will probably have a temperature. The clinical features of pneumothorax and pulmonary embolism are described on pages 437 and 376, and vary according to the size of the pneumothorax or embolism.

(c) The most useful investigation in the first instance is a chest X-ray.

6. The chest X-ray appearances describe a pneumothorax. The initial treatment in a patient with complete collapse is aspiration (page 437) with insertion of a chest drain (page 645) if this is unsuccessful.

7. (a) There are many causes of hilar lymphadenopathy. However, the clinical history together with the bilateral hilar enlargement suggest sarcoidosis.

(b) Erythema nodosum.

(c) Lymphocytes, macrophages and sometimes fibrosis. Non-caseating granulomas are the key histopathologic feature of sarcoidosis and are found in lymph nodes and in a lymphatic distribution in the lung.

8. (a) The history and examination findings are suggestive of a massive pulmonary embolism with acute right heart

strain. A similar clinical picture may also be seen with a right ventricular infarct, but she has a number of risk factors which are more in favour of pulmonary embolism.

(b) Recent surgery, smoking, obesity and the combined oral contraceptive pill.

(c) 100% oxygen and pain relief with diamorphine. This patient has a massive embolism with hypotension and right heart strain (raised JVP and right ventricular heave) and you should consider giving thrombolysis. She may also require intravenous fluids to try and raise the filling pressure of the right ventricle, thereby increasing cardiac output. Treatment with heparin and subsequently warfarin should also be given to reduce the chance of further emboli.

INTENSIVE CARE MEDICINE

1. A man aged 55 years who underwent right hemicolectomy for carcinoma of the caecum 4 days ago has developed acute circulatory failure ('shock'), with an arterial pressure of 65/40 mmHg and heart rate of 120/min.
   (a) List the probable causes of this occurrence.
   (b) Indicate the clinical features that would aid you in distinguishing between them, and outline your initial management of the situation.

2. Write short notes on the management of cardiogenic shock.

3. Compare the clinical manifestations of acute haemorrhagic, acute cardiogenic and acute bacterial (septicaemic) shock.

Answers

1. The two most likely causes are sepsis or a massive pulmonary embolism. Less likely are gastrointestinal haemorrhage and a perioperative myocardial infarction complicated by cardiogenic shock. The clinical features of each of these conditions are discussed on pages 442, 377, and 441, respectively. Management involves:
- Emergency resuscitation with 60% oxygen, large-bore intravenous cannulae and administration of colloid

- Make a diagnosis: temperature charts and physical examination will often reveal the cause. Consider: ECG, blood gases, chest radiograph
- Further treatment depends on the response to fluids and the likely cause.

2. Cardiogenic shock is an extreme form of cardiac failure ('pump failure'), often secondary to a myocardial infarction in which there has been extensive damage to the left ventricular muscle. The mortality rate is 90%. Management therefore involves admission to the ICU, oxygen therapy, relief of pain and intensive monitoring (Emergency Box 10.1), including a Swan–Ganz catheter. Dobutamine and dopamine are given for their inotropic action and to promote renal perfusion (Table 10.2). If PCWP is below 18 mmHg fluid is cautiously infused so as to optimize the filling pressures of the heart. Vasodilators are sometimes given (page 444).

3. This is discussed on pages 441–442.

....

POISONING, DRUG AND ALCOHOL ABUSE

1. After a disagreement with her boyfriend, a 20-year-old woman was seen to ingest 50 tablets of aspirin (i.e. 15 g total) and was brought to hospital 4 hours later. You find her alert and complaining of mild tinnitus only. The salicylate concentration in a blood sample taken in the Accident and Emergency department is within the therapeutic range. She wishes to return home and regrets the whole incident; in particular, she assures you that she has no suicidal intent. Briefly outline the major points of management.

2. A girl aged 17 is admitted after a suicide attempt with a single drug. Initial blood gases were: P_aO_2 13.7 kPa, P_aCO_2 3.7 kPa, pH 7.49.
   (a) What is the metabolic abnormality?
   (b) What drug has this woman taken?
   (c) What acid–base changes may occur later?
   (d) When she has recovered, what features would alert you to the risk of a further life-threatening suicide attempt?

3. Outline the effects and management of paracetamol poisoning.

4. (a) Outline the various physical disorders that may occur as a result of excessive alcohol consumption.
   (b) What features in a routine haematological screen would lead you to suspect alcohol abuse?

Answers

1. Ingestion of 10–20 g of aspirin may produce severe toxicity. This case represents a very serious overdose and serum levels are within the normal range because intestinal absorption is still taking place (see page 458). Initial management is with gastric lavage and then administration of repeated doses of activated charcoal. Intravenous fluids should be started immediately to initiate a diuresis; further management depends on the salicylate concentration in a repeat blood sample taken 6 hours after drug ingestion (page 461). More than one drug is often taken in overdose cases, and this should be sought from the history and measurement of plasma paracetamol levels. Several points suggest that the overdose is not a serious suicide attempt (page 460) and psychiatric referral is probably not necessary.

2. (a) The patient has a respiratory alkalosis.
   (b) Aspirin.
   (c) Respiratory alkalosis is due to direct stimulation of the respiratory centre by salicylates. Initially renal excretion of bicarbonate will bring the pH towards normal, producing some compensation of the alkalosis. Subsequently a combined respiratory and metabolic acidosis develops because:

- Hypotension and dehydration impair renal function with retention of organic acids,
- Salicylates interfere with carbohydrate, fat and protein metabolism, as well as with oxidative phosphorylation. This gives rise to increased lactate, pyruvate and ketone bodies, all of which contribute to the acidosis.
- Salicylate and its metabolites are acidic and further enhance the metabolic acidosis.
- Severe overdose produces depression of the respiratory centre and a respiratory acidosis.
   (d) Risk factors for suicide are listed in Table 11.2.

3. This is discussed on pages 461–463.

4. (a) The physical complications of alcohol abuse are discussed on page 468.

(b) Macrocytosis and, less commonly, thrombocytopenia are seen with alcohol abuse.

....

ENDOCRINOLOGY

1. An otherwise healthy 36-year-old woman presents with 8 months of feeling anxious and tremulous. On examination her pulse is 115 per minute, BP 155/90 and there is a moderately enlarged, non-tender, non-nodular thyroid and hyperreflexia.
   (a) What is your clinical diagnosis?
   (b) What tests would you order? What would you expect the results to be?
   (c) What are the main treatment options for this patient?

2. A 29-year-old man presents with 5 days of pain and tenderness over the thyroid gland. He feels jittery but otherwise well. On examination, he is afebrile, pulse 120 per minute, BP 140/90. His thyroid is enlarged and diffusely tender, with no evidence of nodules.
   (a) What is your clinical diagnosis and how would you confirm it?
   (b) How would you treat this patient?
   (c) What is his prognosis?

3. (a) What are the clinical features of myxoedema?
   (b) How would you confirm or refute the diagnosis?

4. An 85-year-old woman is found lying on the floor of her unheated flat; hypothermia is suspected.
   (a) How would you confirm the diagnosis?
   (b) What abnormality might there be on ECG?
   (c) What would be your management? What measures would you avoid?

5. A 64-year-old smoker presents with haemoptysis and a 4-week history of proximal muscle weakness. On examination he is noted to have a plethoric complexion, hypertension, abdominal striae and skin

bruising. The chest X-ray shows a mass in the right lower zone. The plasma potassium is 2.9 mmol/l and blood glucose 16 mmol/l.

(a) What diagnosis do you suspect?

(b) How would you confirm the endocrine abnormality?

Answers

1. (a) Hyperthyroidism which, clinically and epidemiologically, is likely to be Graves' disease.

(b) Serum TSH will be low, often undetectable. Serum T_4 and T_3 will be high. Anti-TSH receptor antibodies will be present in the serum in most cases of Graves' disease.

(c) Antithyroid drugs given for about 2 years in the hope that the disease remits on its own. These include:

Carbimazole, most often used in the UK

Methimazole, the active metabolite of carbimazole, used in the USA

Propylthiouracil, occasionally used.

β-blockers for symptomatic relief, but they do not alter the course of the disease.

Radioiodine: preferred therapy for definitive treatment of Graves' disease. Surgery: reserved for those who cannot or will not take the above treatment.

2. (a) The presence of diffuse swelling and tenderness of the thyroid gland, together with the history of pain, suggests de Quervain's thyroiditis. Inflammation of the gland leads to the release of preformed hormone. The serum TSH would be low. A radioactive iodine uptake scan would show reduced uptake by the thyroid because the gland is not actively synthesizing thyroid hormone. This test is not routinely performed, but in other cases of hyperthyroidism there would be increased uptake.

(b) The disease is generally mild and limited to a few weeks, so definitive therapy is rarely needed. β-blockers are used for symptomatic relief. Patients may become transiently hypothyroid during recovery.

(c) Spontaneous remission in a few weeks.

3. (a) The symptoms and signs of myxoedema are listed on page 491.

(b) Almost all cases of hypothyroidism are the result of disease of the thyroid gland; much less commonly it is caused by hypothalamic–pituitary disease. In primary hypothyroidism measurement of serum TSH (which will be high because of loss of feedback inhibition of secretion by T_4) and free T_4 (which will be low) will confirm the diagnosis.

4. (a) The diagnosis and management of hypothermia are discussed on page 516. Hypothermia is diagnosed when the core (rectal) temperature is <35°C measured with a low-reading rectal thermometer.

(b) The ECG abnormalities are 'J' waves (pathognomic of hypothermia), a tachycardia with a bradycardia developing at temperatures <32°C. At very low temperatures there may be ventricular arrhythmias.

(c) The treatment is described on page 517. Alcohol must be avoided because it may cause confusion, lead to vasodilatation (and heat loss) and precipitate hypoglycaemia.

5. The history of haemoptysis in a smoker with an abnormal chest X-ray is highly suggestive of bronchial carcinoma. The proximal muscle weakness, hypertension, striae, bruising, hypokalaemia and high blood sugar suggest Cushing's syndrome, which is most likely due to ectopic ACTH production by a small cell lung cancer. A low-dose dexamethasone suppression test and measurement of serum ACTH will confirm the diagnosis.

....

DIABETES MELLITUS AND OTHER DISORDERS OF METABOLISM

1. A 45-year-old West Indian woman weighing 95 kg and 160 cm (5 feet 4 inches) tall is found, on routine examination, to have glycosuria without ketonuria, and a random blood glucose of 17 mmol/l.
   (a) What is the diagnosis?
   (b) What type do you suspect?
   (c) What is the initial management?

2. A man of 56 has been diabetic since the age of 20. He now complains of bilateral ankle swelling.

(a) What is the differential diagnosis?

(b) How would you investigate and manage this patient?

3. A 18-year-old man who is a known diabetic is admitted as an emergency. His parents say that he has become unwell over the last 3 days, with vomiting and confusion. Laboratory investigations reveal a blood glucose 36 mmol/l, serum sodium 147 mmol/l. urea 12 mmol/l, potassium 5.0 mmol/l and arterial blood pH 7.1.

(a) What is the diagnosis?

(b) Considering the serum potassium concentration, is his total body potassium high, low or normal?

(c) Outline your initial treatment of this patient.

4. A 20-year-old woman complains of being very thirsty and passing large quantities of urine.

(a) What are the likely causes?

(b) How would you establish the diagnosis?

5. (a) What are the features of an attack of hypoglycaemia? Suggest the mechanism of each manifestation

(b) What causes of a series of proven attacks ought to be considered?

6. A 37-year-old man presents for an evaluation because his brother recently died of coronary disease in his early 40s. The patient's father also has a history of elevated cholesterol and early coronary disease. The patient denies smoking cigarettes and has eliminated high-fat dairy products, most red meat and alcohol from his diet. There is no history of hypertension and physical examination is unremarkable. Measurement of plasma lipids shows a triglyceride of 1.5 mmol, total cholesterol 9.0 mmol/l, LDL-cholesterol 6.8 mmol/l, HDL-cholesterol 1.5 mmol/l.

(a) What lipid abnormality do you suspect?

(b) What other tests would you perform?

(c) A dietitian considers the changes to his diet have been adequate and there is little more dietary advice that can be offered. What drug therapy would you prescribe in order to lower the cholesterol?

7. Describe the changes on serum cholesterol of changes in:
   (a) dietary saturated fat
   (b) dietary unsaturated fat
   (c) dietary cholesterol
   (d) sugar.

Answers

1. (a) The random blood sugar confirms the presence of diabetes mellitus.

(b) Her age, obesity (body mass index >30) and absence of symptoms or ketosis suggest that this is type 2 diabetes mellitus.

(c) Initial management involves patient education and weight reduction, achieved with a 1000–1600 kcal diet planned in conjunction with a dietitian. Diabetic complications must be sought by physical examination, blood tests and urinalysis (page 531). Oral hypoglycaemics (page 523) are necessary if blood glucose remains high in spite of weight loss having been achieved.

2. (a) The most probable causes of leg oedema in this patient are complications resulting from long-standing diabetes, i.e. nephrotic syndrome (page 533) or heart failure (secondary to ischaemic heart disease).

(b) These will be distinguished by physical examination, chest radiograph, urinalysis and measurement of the serum albumin. Further management depends on the cause and is described on page 283 and 343.

3. (a) This is diabetic ketoacidosis, as shown by the high blood glucose and acidosis. This is the typical hyperglycaemic emergency of the young diabetic.

(b) The serum potassium concentration is a poor indicator of total body potassium because most potassium is intracellular. Total body potassium is low with diabetic ketoacidosis because of increased potassium excretion in the urine and loss in the vomit.

(c) The initial treatment is with intravenous saline, soluble insulin and potassium supplements (page 526).

4. (a) Frequency of micturition must not be confused with polyuria (usually >3 l/day); a 24-hour urine output chart is helpful if there is doubt.

(b) The first and most simple test to perform is a random blood sugar, which will be high if polyuria is secondary to diabetes mellitus. Other causes are primary or hysterical polydipsia (a relatively common cause of polyuria and polydipsia in young women), cranial diabetes insipidus (CDI), nephrogenic DI (page 509) and chronic renal failure. A full history and examination must include a drug history (e.g. lithium causes nephrogenic DI). Investigations, other than a blood glucose, include serum osmolality, urine osmolality, serum urea, electrolytes and calcium. A water deprivation test may be necessary (page 510).

5. (a) Symptoms are the result of secretion of counterregulatory hormones (catecholamines cause hunger, sweating, pallor and tachycardia) and neuroglycopenia (e.g. confusion, drowsiness, fits and eventually coma).

(b) The causes of hypoglycaemia are listed on page 538. In an otherwise healthy person (e.g. in the absence of cancer, severe liver or renal failure), the most likely causes of recurrent hypoglycaemia are drugs, factitious hypoglycaemia, alcoholic binges and insulinoma. Often the cause will be apparent from the history, physical examination and measurement of blood glucose and plasma insulin during a hypoglycaemic episode. A supervised fast with measurement of glucose and insulin may be needed (page 537).

6. (a) The patient may have monogenic familial hypercholesterolaemia caused by a defect in the LDL receptor gene (page 541), or he may have a polygenic predisposition to elevated LDL-cholesterol. The distinction is not clinically important.

(b) It is important to identify causes of secondary hyperlipidaemia. Screening for diabetes mellitus (with a fasting blood glucose) and hypothyroidism (with a serum TSH) should be performed.

(c) Drugs of choice are the HMG Co-A reductase inhibitors and bile acid-binding resins.

7. Serum cholesterol is mainly derived from endogenous synthesis (page 539) and thus any dietary modification will

have only a moderate effect. Hypercholesterolaemia is reduced by restricting the intake of cholesterol and saturated fat (both found in animal fat) and replacing with vegetable fat (containing unsaturated fats). Carbohydrate restriction reduces serum triglyceride levels.

NEUROLOGY

1. A lady of 70 wakes one morning with weakness in the right arm and some difficulty in speaking. The symptoms are present the following day and her family bring her to the Accident and Emergency department.
   (a) What are the likely causes?
   (b) How would you manage this patient?
   (c) What information would you give to the patient and relatives?

2. A man of 65 suddenly develops weakness and numbness of the left arm, which gradually passes off after 15 minutes.
   (a) What are the likely causes?
   (b) How might they be investigated?

3. A 16-year-old girl presents with a 1-day history of severe headache with fever, nausea, vomiting, muscle and joint pains. Over the last 6 hours she had become disorientated and developed a rash. Findings on examination were pulse 125/minute, BP 95/55, temperature 39.5°C. Petechiae and purpura were present on the hands and legs.
   (a) What is your clinical diagnosis?
   (b) What is your immediate management?
   (c) Despite treatment she deteriorated rapidly and developed a widespread haemorrhagic rash, BP 70/40, disseminated intravascular coagulation (DIC) and anuria. What is this condition called?

4. A 40-year-old known alcoholic is brought into Accident and Emergency unconscious and smelling of alcohol.
   (a) What are the most likely causes of coma in this patient?

(b) Describe your management?

5. (a) List the potentially treatable or reversible causes of apparent dementia.
   (b) What features of the history and clinical findings might arouse your suspicions?

6. A 34-year-old homosexual man with a previous episode of *P. carinii* pneumonia first noted 1 week previous to admission poor control of his left hand, and would walk to his left. He also noticed difficulty in remembering events, understanding what was read, and dressing apraxia. He had also had early morning headaches. On examination he was afebrile, he had oral thrush, and fundal examination showed white exudates. He had a left-sided weakness, left homonymous hemianopia and left-sided neglect.
   (a) Do you think this patient has AIDS?
   (b) The history and examination is suggestive of a space-occupying lesion. Where is it situated?
   (c) A brain CT scan shows a ring enhancing lesion with surrounding oedema and some compression of the adjacent ventricle. What is your differential diagnosis in this patient?

7. A 23-year-old woman was admitted through Accident and Emergency with a 2-day history of symmetrical leg weakness and paraesthesiae. Later she was unable to sit up in bed and reported difficulty in coughing and stiffness of the face.
   (a) What is the most likely diagnosis?
   (b) What confirmatory tests would you obtain?
   (c) What is the most common antecedent infection to this condition?
   (d) What is the management of this condition?

8. Give three common causes of ptosis and mention the associated features in each case.

9. What are the features of Horner's syndrome? Briefly describe the anatomical pathways involved. What underlying causes may be responsible?

10. A 30-year-old Asian is admitted with headache and neck stiffness. CSF findings: pressure 23 mmH$_2$O, red

blood cells 0, white cells 290×10^6/l (lymphocytes 82%, monocytes 10%, neutrophils 8%), protein 2 g/l, glucose 1.8 mmol/l, blood glucose 6 mmol/l.

(a) What are the abnormalities?

(b) What is the diagnosis?

Answers

1. (a) The history is of sudden onset of right-sided weakness and dysphasia, which is almost certainly due to a vascular lesion (i.e. stroke). The causes of stroke are discussed on page 576; in a woman of this age it is most likely to be due to thrombosis at the site of atheromatous degeneration in the middle cerebral artery (page 578).

(b) The investigations and treatment of stroke are discussed on pages 579–580. A brain CT scan will differentiate between infarction and haemorrhage. Aspirin is given to patients with infarction to reduce the risk of further attacks.

(c) The family must be told that some recovery of function is expected. Any recovery of speech is likely to be within the first few days.

2. (a) This is a transient ischaemic attack (TIA), probably in the territory of the right middle cerebral artery.

(b) The causes and investigation of a TIA are listed on page 581.

3. (a) Meningitis. The petechial skin rash suggests meningococcal meningitis.

(b) Immediate intravenous benzylpenicillin should be given. In the presence of a typical skin rash lumbar puncture is not usually necessary and the organism is found on blood cultures. A CT scan should be performed if there is any suspicion of an intracranial mass lesion.

(c) The rapid downhill course is suggestive of fulminant meningococcaemia (Waterhouse–Friderichsen syndrome). Haemorrhage into the adrenal glands may or may not be present.

4. (a) Coma must never be ascribed to excess alcohol until a thorough history (from relatives, ambulance staff), physical examination and investigation have ruled out other causes. The most likely causes (Table 14.8) in this

case are alcohol, drug overdose (with alcohol as a second agent), hypoglycaemia, intracerebral haemorrhage, infarction and Wernicke–Korsakoff syndrome (page 468).

(b) The initial management consists of emergency resuscitation to stabilize the patient (page 572). Intravenous glucose and thiamine (see later) are given. Further assessment (page 572) and investigations (page 574) are performed to find the cause of coma. Further management consists of treatment of the underlying cause and care of the unconscious patient (page 575).

5. The causes of dementia are listed in Table 14.25. Treatable causes include hypothyroidism, vitamin B_{12} deficiency, uraemia, hepatic failure, operable cerebral tumour, subdural haematoma and normal pressure hydrocephalus (page 606). Depression may produce a clinical picture that is indistinguishable from dementia (pseudodementia) and resolves with treatment. Neurosyphilis (page 603) and Wernicke–Korsakoff syndrome (page 468) may cause dementia; treatment should always be given, as the disease process may be arrested but rarely reversed. Young age, focal neurological signs, a history of head injury and evidence of anaemia or hypothyroidism should arouse suspicion that this is not Alzheimer's disease (the usual cause of dementia).

6. (a) The history of *P. carinii* pneumonia and oral thrush occurring in a gay man suggests AIDS.
(b) Right parietal lobe.
(c) Ring enhancing lesions in HIV infected patients may be caused by *T. gondii*, bacteria or lymphoma. Ring enhancement is non-specific and indicates increased vascularity. This patient in fact had a brain abscess caused by infection with *Toxoplasma gondii* due to reactivation of a previous infection.

7. (a) The distal weakness progressing proximally is the typical picture of Guillain–Barré syndrome (GBS, acute inflammatory polyneuropathy) (page 618), the commonest cause of acute generalized muscle weakness.
(b) The diagnosis is made clinically, by nerve conduction studies and examination of the CSF obtained at lumbar puncture (page 618).

(c) Recent studies have identifed *Campylobacter jejuni* as a major cause of antecedent infection in GBS patients, and may be associated with a more severe form that tends to be exclusively motor.

(d) The management is:

- *General*: frequent monitoring of vital capacity to monitor respiratory muscle function in case ventilation is needed, cardiac monitoring to detect arrhythmias, chest and general physiotherapy, prompt treatment of infections, anticoagulation with heparin when bedbound and usual good nursing care. In this particular case the difficulty in coughing suggests involvement of the respiratory muscles, and ventilation may well be necessary.

- *Specific*: All patients with any but the mildest deficit should have either plasma exchange or intravenous immune globulin, started as early as possible. Which one is given will often depend on local preference and circumstances.

8. The causes of ptosis are third-nerve lesions (usually complete unilateral ptosis with other eye signs, page 564), sympathetic paralysis (partial unilateral ptosis with other features of Horner's syndrome, page 563), myopathy (partial bilateral), congenital (present since birth, usually partial, no other neurological signs) and syphilis (tabes dorsalis, page 603).

9. The features and causes of Horner's syndrome are described on page 563.

10. (a) There is a CSF lymphocytosis, reduced glucose (in the absence of hypoglycaemia), markedly raised protein and raised CSF pressure. A raised CSF protein occurs with any inflammatory lesion of the CNS. A reduced CSF glucose occurs with bacterial or tuberculous meningitis, and rarely with viral and fungal infections and malignancy. The CSF lymphocytosis is against bacterial meninigitis unless it has been partially treated.

(b) The findings are most likely to be due to tuberculous meningitis, which is particularly common in Asians.

DERMATOLOGY

1. What are the features and common causes of erythema nodosum? How would you investigate a patient with this condition?

2. Write short notes on the management of psoriasis.

Answers

1. The causes and clinical features of erythema nodosum are listed on page 632. Sarcoidosis and inflammatory bowel disease are the most common causes in the UK. A history of recent antibiotic ingestion, oral contraceptives or alteration in bowel habit should be sought. Basic investigations should include a full blood count, ESR and chest radiograph. Further investigations will depend on the history and associated clinical findings. For instance, in a patient who also has diarrhoea it would be reasonable to perform a small bowel barium follow-through examination to look for Crohn's disease. In a patient who is otherwise well and with a single attack, further investigation may be unnecessary.

2. The management of psoriasis is outlined on page 630.

Dictionary of terms

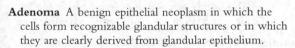

Adenoma A benign epithelial neoplasm in which the cells form recognizable glandular structures or in which they are clearly derived from glandular epithelium.

Adjuvant Term applied to chemotherapy or hormone therapy given after local treatment, in tumours where dissemination is undetectable but can be assumed to have occurred. If effective, it should lead to an increase in cure rate or overall disease-free survival.

Afterload The load against which the cardiac muscle exerts its contractile force, i.e. the peripheral vascular tree.

Allogeneic transplantation When another individual acts as the donor.

Annular lesions Lesions occurring in rings.

Antegrade pyelography A catheter is passed percutaneously into a renal calyx. This allows the injection of contrast medium to demonstrate upper urinary tract obstruction and drainage of an obstructed system.

Antibody An immunoglobulin molecule that has a specific amino acid sequence by virtue of which it interacts only with the antigen that induced its synthesis in cells of the lymphoid series (especially plasma cells), or with antigen closely related to it.

Antigen Any substance, organism or foreign material recognized by the immune system as being 'non-self', which will provoke the production of a specific antibody.

Antineutrophil cytoplasmic antibodies (ANCAs) These are detected on fixed human neutrophils. There are two types:

- Antibodies directed against proteinase 3 (PR3-ANCA), formerly called cytoplasmic or cANCA. Present in 90% of patients with Wegener's granulomatosis.
- Antibodies directed against myeloperoxidase, formerly called perinuclear or pANCA. Present in 60% of some other vasculitides, such as microscopic polyangiitis and Churg–Strauss syndrome. Also found in inflammatory bowel disease and rheumatological disease which is not associated with a vasculitis.

Antinuclear antigens (ANA) Represent a wide spectrum of autoantibodies. They are non-specific and may occur at low titre (e.g. 1:10) in healthy individuals.

Anuria A condition in which no urine is voided. It suggests complete urinary tract obstruction.

Apoptosis Programmed cell death, as signalled by the nuclei in normally functioning cells when age or state of cell health dictates.

Aphasia (dysphasia) A disturbance of the ability to use language, whether in speaking, writing or comprehending. It is caused by left frontoparietal lesions, often a stroke.
- Broca's aphasia (expressive aphasia) is due to a lesion in the left frontal lobe. There is reduced fluency of speech, with comprehension relatively preserved. The patient knows what he/she wants to say but cannot get the words out.
- Wernicke's aphasia (receptive aphasia) is due to a left temperoparietal lesion. The patient speaks fluently but words are put together in the wrong order, and in the most severe forms the patient speaks complete rubbish with the insertion of non-existent words. Comprehension is severely impaired.
- Global aphasia is due to widespread damage to the areas concerned with speech. The patient shows combined expressive and receptive dysphasia.

Apraxia Loss of the ability to carry out familiar purposeful movements in the absence of paralysis or other motor or sensory impairment.

Ataxia is due to failure of coordination of complex muscular movements despite intact individual movements and sensation.

Atrophy Thinning (e.g. of the skin).

Autoantibody An antibody that reacts with an antigen which is a normal component of the body.

Autologous When the patient acts as his or her own source of cells.

Behçets disease A rare multisystem chronic recurrent disease characterized by ulceration in the mouth and genitalia, iritis, uveitis, arthritis and thrombophlebitis. Often treated with immunosuppressive therapy (corticosteroids, chlorambucil).

Bone marrow is obtained for examination by aspiration from the anterior iliac crest or sternum. In many cases a trephine biopsy (removal of a core of bone marrow tissue) is also necessary.

Bronchoalveolar lavage At bronchoscopy a lung segment is washed with saline and the fluid retrieved for cell analysis.

Bulla A large vesicle.

Carcinoma A malignant neoplasm arising from epithelium.

Cardiac catheterization The passage of a small catheter through a peripheral vein (for study of right-sided heart structures) or artery (for study of left heart structures) into the heart, permitting the securing of blood samples, measurement of intracardiac pressures and determination of cardiac anomalies.

Cardiac nuclear imaging uses radiotracers (injected intravenously) which diffuse freely into myocardial tissue or attach to red blood cells.
- Thallium-201 is taken up by cardiac myocytes. Ischaemic areas (produced by exercising the patient) with reduced tracer uptake are seen as 'cold spots' when imaged with a γ camera.

- Technetium-99 m is used to label red blood cells and produce images of the left ventricle during systole and diastole.

Caseating Developing a necrotic centre.

CD (cluster differentiation) antigens Antigens on the cell surface that can be detected by immune reagents and which are associated with the differentiation of a particular cell type or types. Many cells can be identified by their possession of a unique set of differentiation antigens, e.g. CD4, CD8.

Chronotropic Positively chronotropic means to increase the *rate* of contraction of the heart; negatively chronotropic is the opposite.

Constructional apraxia Inability to copy simple drawings: often seen in hepatic encephalopathy, when the patient is unable to copy a five-pointed star.

C-reactive protein (CRP) is synthesized in the liver and produced during the acute-phase response. It is quick and easy to measure and is replacing measurement of the ESR in some centres.

Crust Dried exudate on the skin.

Cryoglobulins Immunoglobulins that precipitate when cold or during exercise. They may be monoclonal or polyclonal, e.g. mixed essential cryoglobulinaemia, and result in a cutaneous vasculitis or occasionally a multisystem disorder.

Cytokines Soluble messenger molecules which enables the immune system to communicate through its different compartments. Cytokines are made by many cells, such as lymphocytes (lymphokines) and other white cells (interleukins). Examples of cytokines, other than interleukins, include tumour necrosis factor (TNF), interferons and granulocyte–colony-stimulating factor (G-CSF).

Dysarthria Disordered articulation. Any lesion that produces paralysis, slowing or incoordination of the muscles of articulation, or local discomfort, will cause dysarthria. Examples are upper and lower motor lesions of the lower cranial nerves, cerebellar lesions, Parkinson's disease and local lesions in the mouth, larynx, pharynx and tongue.

Dysplasia Abnormal cell growth or maturation of cells.

Ecchymoses Bruises >3 mm in diameter.

Echocardiography A non-invasive method of recording the position and motion of the structures of the heart by echo obtained from beams of ultrasonic waves directed through the chest wall.

- Transoesophageal echo uses miniaturized transducers incorporated into special endoscopes. It allows better visualization of some structures and pathology, e.g. aortic dissection, prosthetic valve endocarditis.
- Doppler echocardiography uses the Doppler principle (in this case, the frequency of ultrasonic waves reflected from blood cells is related to their velocity and direction of flow) to identify and assess the severity of valve lesions.

Ejection fraction The fraction of the ventricular end-diastolic volume that is ejected during systole. It is usually equal to about 60%.

Ehlers–Danlos syndrome A group of inherited connective tissue disorders. Clinical features include hyperextensile skin, hypermobile joints, fragility of blood vessels with easy bleeding and, rarely, aortic rupture.

Electroencephalogram (EEG) Electrodes applied to the patient's scalp pick up small changes in electrical potential which, after amplification, are recorded on paper or displayed on a video monitor. It is used in the investigation of epilepsy and diffuse brain disorders.

Electromyography (EMG) A needle electrode is inserted percutaneously into voluntary muscle. Amplified action potentials are recorded on an oscilloscope. Normal resting muscle shows no activity, and during increasing muscle contractions progressively larger numbers of motor units are recruited. EMG is useful in the diagnosis of primary muscle disease (myopathies and dystrophies, individual motor unit potentials are small) and of lower motor neuron lesions (denervation, spontaneous activity appears at rest).

End-diastolic volume The volume of blood in the ventricle at the end of diastole.

Enzyme-linked immunosorbent (ELISA) assay A serologic test used for the detection of particular antibodies or antigens in the blood. ELISA technology links a measurable enzyme to either an antigen or antibody. In this way it can then measure the presence of an antibody or an antigen in the bloodstream.

Eosinophilia (normal range $0.04–0.44 \times 10^9$/l, 1–6% of total white cells) occurs in asthma and allergic disorders, parasitic infections (e.g. *Ascaris*), skin disorders (urticaria, pemphigus and eczema), malignancy and the hypereosinophilic syndrome (restrictive cardiomyopathy, hepatosplenomegaly and very high eosinophil count).

Epidemiology The study of the distribution and determinants of health-related states and events in populations.

Epitope That part of an antigenic molecule to which an antibody or T-cell receptor responds.

ERCP Endoscopic retrograde cholangiopancreatography. The ampulla of Vater is cannulated, and after injection of radio-opaque contrast medium the pancreatic and common bile ducts (CBD) can be visualized. The sphincter of Oddi may be cut (*sphincterotomy*) to facilitate the removal of stones and insertion of stents.

Erythema Redness.

Erythrocyte sedimentation rate (ESR) The rate of fall of red cells in a column of blood; a measure of the acute-phase response. The speed is mainly determined by the concentration of large proteins, e.g. fibrinogen. The ESR is higher in women and rises with age. It is used in a wide variety of systemic inflammatory and neoplastic diseases. The highest values (>100 mm/h) are found in chronic infections (e.g. TB), myeloma, connective tissue disorders and cancer.

Erythroderma Widespread redness of the skin, with scaling.

Euthanasia The illegal act of killing someone painlessly especially to relieve suffering from an incurable disease.

Excoriation Linear marks caused by scratching.

Excretion urography (intravenous urography (IVU) or intravenous pyelography (IVP). Serial radiographs are taken of the kidney and the full length of the abdomen, following intravenous injection of contrast, usually an organic iodine-containing medium.

Extractable nuclear antigens (ENA) Nuclear components that are soluble in saline. Examples are Sm, Ro, La and ribonucleoprotein (RNP) antigen. The presence of serum anti-Sm antibodies is highly specific for SLE. Anti-Ro (SS-A) and anti-La (SS-B) occur in patients with Sjögren's syndrome and in some patients with SLE.

Generic drugs Non-proprietary drugs. They should usually be used when prescribing in preference to proprietary titles.

Glomerular filtration rate (GFR) This is the most widely used test of renal function. In routine clinical practice the most reliable index of GFR is measurement of endogenous creatinine clearance, which is calculated from a 24-hour urine collection and measurement of a single serum creatinine value during the 24 hours.

Histocompatibility antigens Genetically determined isoantigens present on the membranes of nucleated cells. They incite an immune response when grafted on to genetically disparate individuals, and thus determine the compatibility of cells in transplantation.

Howell Jolly bodies DNA remnants in peripheral RBCs seen postsplenectomy, in leukaemia and megaloblastic anaemia.

Human leucocyte antigens (HLA) Human histocompatibility antigens determined by a region on chromosome 6. There are several genetic loci, each having multiple alleles, designated HLA-A, HLA-B, HLA-C, HLA-DP, -DQ and -DR. The susceptibility to some diseases is associated with certain HLA alleles (e.g. HLA-B27 in 95% of patients with ankylosing spondylitis), although their exact role in aetiology is unclear.

Hyperplasia The abnormal multiplication or increase in the *number* of normal cells in normal arrangement in a tissue.

Hypertrophy The enlargement or overgrowth of an organ or part due to an increase in *size* of its constituent cells.

Idiopathic Of unknown cause.

Incidence An expression of the rate at which a certain event occurs as the number of new cases of a specific disease occurring during a certain period.

Inotropic Positively inotropic means increasing the *force* of cardiac muscle contraction.

Left shift Immature white cells appear in the peripheral blood, e.g. with infection.

Leucocytosis An increase in the total circulating white cells ($>11 \times 10^9$/l).

Leucoerythroblastic reaction Immature red and white cells appearing in the peripheral blood. It occurs in marrow infiltration (e.g. malignancy), myeloid leukaemia and severe anaemia.

Leucopenia A decrease in the total circulating white cells ($<4.0 \times 10^9$/l).

Leukaemoid reaction A reactive but excessive leucocytosis characterized by the presence of immature cells in the peripheral blood.

Kawasaki disease An acute febrile illness (lasting more than 5 days) of unknown aetiology that occurs mainly in children. Features include damage to the coronary arteries which is reduced by treatment with aspirin and intravenous γ-globulin.

Macule A flat circumscribed area of discoloration.

Maculopapule A raised and discoloured circumscribed lesion.

Marfan's syndrome Autosomal dominant connective tissue disorder associated with mutations in the fibrillin I gene on chromosome 15. Up to one-third are new mutations. Clinical features include tall stature, long thin digits (arachnodactly), high arched palate, hypermobile joints, lens subluxation, incompetence of aortic and mitral valve, aortic dissection and spontaneous pneumothorax.

Metaplasia A change in the type of cells in a tissue to a form which is not normal for that tissue.

Micturating cystocopy Used mainly for the evaluation of vesicoureteric reflux in children. Contrast medium is instilled into the bladder via a catheter, and the ureters and kidneys are then screened during micturition.

Monocytosis (normal range 0.04–0.44×10^9/l, 1–6% of total white cells) occurs in chronic bacterial infections (e.g. TB), myelodysplasia and malignancy, particularly chronic myelomonocytic leukaemia.

Necrosis Morphological changes indicative of cell death and caused by the progressive degradative action of enzymes; it may affect groups of cells or part of a structure or an organ.

Neutropenia (normal range 2–7.5×10^9/l, 40–75% of total white cells). Causes include racial (in black Africans), viral infection, severe bacterial infection, megaloblastic anaemia, pancytopenia and drugs (marrow aplasia or immune destruction).

Neutrophil leucocytosis Occurs in bacterial infection, tissue necrosis, inflammation, corticosteroid therapy, myeloproliferative disease, leukaemoid reaction, leucoerythroblastic anaemia, acute haemorrhage and haemolysis.

Normoblasts Immature nucleated red blood cells (RBCs) seen in the peripheral blood with a leucoerthyroblastic reaction and severe anaemia.

Nodule A circumscribed large palpable mass >1 cm in diameter.

Oligoarticular Affecting a limited number of joints.

Oliguria The excretion of less than 300 ml of urine per day. Causes are extreme dehydration, hypotension, obstruction and acute renal failure.

Oncogene Gene coding for proteins which are either growth factors, growth factor receptors, secondary messengers or DNA-binding proteins. Mutation of the gene promotes abnormal cell growth.

Osmolarity The concentration of osmotically active particles expressed in terms of osmoles of solute per litre of solution.

Osmolality The concentration of osmotically active particles in solution expressed in terms of osmoles of solute per kilogram of solvent.

Pancytopenia Deficiency of all cell elements of the blood.

Papule A circumscribed raised palpable area.

Persistent vegetative state A condition of life without consciousness or will as a result of brain damage.

Petechiae Bruises <3 mm in diameter.

Plaque A disc-shaped lesion; can result from coalescence of papules.

Plasma The cell-free portion of blood in which particulate components are suspended. Plasma is the supernatant obtained after high-speed centrifugation of whole blood collected in a tube containing anticoagulant, e.g. heparin.

Polychromasia Blue tinge to red blood cells in the blood film caused by the presence of young red cells.

Polymerase chain reaction (PCR) Technique for rapid detection and analysis of DNA and, by a modification of the method, RNA. Using oligonucleotide primers and DNA polymerase minute amounts of genomic DNA can be amplified over a million times into measurable quantities.

Polyuria A persistent large increase in urine output, usually associated with nocturia. The causes are polydipsia, solute diuresis (e.g. hyperglycaemia with glycosuria), diabetes insipidus and chronic renal failure.

Preload The extent to which the heart muscle is stretched before contraction: this is in effect the end-diastolic volume.

Prevalence Total number of cases of a disease in existence at a certain time in a designated area.

Promyelocytes, myelocytes and metamyelocytes Immature white cells seen in the peripheral blood in leucoerythroblastic anaemia.

Purpura Extravasation of blood into the skin; does not blanch on pressure.

Pustule A pus-filled blister.

Radioimmunoassay Any system for testing antigen–antibody reactions in which use is made of radioactive labelling of antigen or antibody to detect the extent of the reaction.

Renal scintigraphy
- Static scanning is performed after an intravenous injection of technetium-99m-labelled dimercaptosuccinic acid (^{99m}Tc-DMSA), which is taken up by the kidneys. It allows an assessment of the function of each kidney
- Dynamic scanning is performed after an intravenous injection of technetium-99m-labelled diethylenetriamine pentaacetate (^{99m}Tc-DTPA), which is taken up by the kidneys and excreted into the collecting systems, ureter and bladder. It allows assessment of renal blood flow, estimation of GFR and assessment of obstructive uropathy.

Reticulocytes (normal range 0.2–2% of RBCs) Young red cells, recently released from the bone marrow, which still contain RNA. The reticulocyte count gives a guide to the erythroid activity in the bone marrow and is increased with haemorrhage, haemolysis and after the response to treatment with a specific haematinic.

Retrograde pyelography Following cystoscopy a catheter is placed in the ureteral orifice and contrast injected. It is used to investigate lesions of the lower ureter and to define the lower level of ureteral obstruction shown on ultrasound or antegrade studies.

Rheumatoid factors (RhF) Autoantibodies found in the serum, usually of the IgM class, which are directed against the *Fc* portion of human IgG. They are found in high titre in 70% of patients with rheumatoid arthritis. They may also be detected in other autoimmune rheumatic diseases, autoimmune hepatitis, chronic infections, and in elderly people at low titres.

Scales dried flakes of dead skin.

Serum The cell-free portion of blood from which fibrinogen has been separated in the process of clotting. Serum is the Supernatant obtained by high-speed centrifugation of whole blood collected in a plain tube.

Target cells ('Mexican hat cells') Red blood cells with central staining surrounded by a ring of pallor and an outer ring of staining. They occur in thalassaemia, sickle-cell disease and liver disease.

Telangiectasia A visible, small, dilated vessel on the skin.

TNM classification (tumour, node, metastasis) Staging system for many cancers. T is the extent of primary tumour, N is the involvement of lymph nodes and M indicates the presence or absence of metastases. For instance T0–T4 indicates increasing local tumour spread.

Tumour suppressor genes Genes whose protein products induce the repair or self-destruction (apoptosis) of cells containing damaged DNA. Unlike oncogenes, they restrict undue cell proliferation.

Vesicle A small, visible, fluid-filled blister.

Weal A transiently raised reddened area associated with scratching.

Index

W